Health Care:

An International Perspective

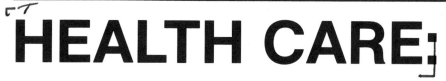

HEALTH CARE:

An International Perspective

Edited by
JOHN M. VIRGO

Atlantic Economic Society
Southern Illinois University at Edwardsville

Foreword by
MARGARET M. HECKLER
Secretary, Department of Health and Human Services

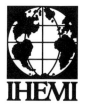

International Health Economics and Management Institute
Box 101, Southern Illinois University at Edwardsville
Edwardsville, Illinois 62026

© International Health Economics and Management Institute, 1984

Published by the International Health Economics and Management Institute, which assumes no responsibility for statements expressed by authors.

ISBN 0-914943-00-6
Library of Congress Catalog Card Number: 83-82337

Printed in the United States of America

Contents

Foreword

MARGARET M. HECKLER
Secretary, Department of Health and Human Services

Despite their rich historical and cultural diversity, the industrialized nations of the world have more social and economic features in common than one might think at first glance. That is why the papers assembled here on the international economics of health care are so valuable: they give us a common, helpful perspective and illume the possibilities for analyses, understanding, and taking action on the health care problems our societies face. These critiques not only help us understand each others problems, they help us in the search for solutions to our own and they stretch the canvas on which the delivery and financing issues of the coming century will be painted.

The problem of how to pay for increasing complex and expensive health care arises only because the economies of our countries have had such thrust and dynamism. We have discovered and shaped the advanced medical technologies and forged the innovations by which people are realizing longer and healthier lives. Our governments have used their expanding wealth to open the doors to equal access of quality health care to a greater and greater percentage of their citizenry and to improve their quality of life. As these papers so dramatically limn, industrialized nations have made dramatic progress toward these goals. The price of that progress is only just now coming into focus: *costs and the ability to pay*. This is true of both private and public expenditures for health care. Now, in both sectors, structural mechanisms for financing and social institutions for delivering health care are undergoing rapid almost cataclysmic change.

What was *need* has become *necessity* in that we must seek out ways our nations can set publicly-supported health care on footing that is more financially secure. The shared events of the last decade that include increased utilization of health care services, aging populations, soaring costs, and burgeoning medical care technologies now put that burden squarely on all of us.

In the last decade most of us have slowly absorbed a simple but significant lesson. Our health care resources are limited. We in the United States have had a particularly rude awakening to this notion of limitations. Our 15-year old Medicare program, which helps pay the medical care costs for virtually all (millions) of our elderly citizens, is threatened with insolvency. And the clock is ticking. Fortunately, there are many informed, thoughtful and visionary women and men who have dedicated themselves to the task of finding long-term solutions to the looming crisis so that Medicare for future generations will not be jeopardized.

We are entering a period of thriving change and challenge on all fronts, especially for the physicians who diagnose and order patient care, for hospitals where much of that care is provided, for the private and public insurers who pay for patient care. Tomorrow's health care answers are being framed by the questions of today, that is, questions about the quality of care, questions about access to care, and, above all, questions about the cost of care. Experiments are being made with new health care delivery models, as well as reimbursement and payment systems. Physicians are entering into innovative group practices even as hospitals embark on diversification strategies to better serve the people in their communities.

The key to more rational and cost-effective use of our limited resources is planning. As the restructuring of our nations' health care delivery and financing institutions begins, we must take care to assure our citizens that their basic health care needs will continue to be met. We also must deliver a clear message to physicians and hospitals upon whom we are so dependent for quality health care: that with careful, thoughtful planning it is possible to be accountable for the financial effects of patient care decisions without sacrificing the quality of that care.

The papers that follow plow important ground, raise the bedrock questions that will demand answers tomorrow, and provide a valuable forum for discussion and debate.

Introduction

JOHN M. VIRGO, Editor

The future of the health care sector will be one of dramatic change. Spiraling costs, esoteric technology, demographics, inflation, and rising consumer expectations will lead to economic, social, and political challenges in all industrialized countries. It is imperative that leaders in these countries initiate policies and programs to meet this changing health care environment.

A 25-nation conference was held in March 1983 where respected economists, health care professionals, government officials, and business leaders met to analyze, discuss and evaluate the future viability of health care in the industrialized world. Recommendations were made about future government policies and programs needed to alleviate the growing attitude that health care is becoming unmanageable, too costly, and inefficient. Basic social issues were raised: Who should receive health care? How much care is too much? Is health care a right or a privilege? Can a country afford unilateral care for the elderly and poor?

The conference was sponsored by the Atlantic Economic Society to increase awareness of the need to assess fundamental health care issues from an interdisciplinary, comparative point of view. Specialists in economics, management, finance, data processing, and marketing joined forces to discuss the future of health care around the world. The result was a realization that many countries, although having different political, social, and cultural values, share some of the same underlying problems. Much can be learned by discussing these fundamental difficulties and analyzing how other societies are responding to the challenge.

The success and interest stimulated by these meetings has led the Atlantic Economic Society to formalize the structure of a new health care management institute. At the end of the Paris conference, participants formed an International Steering Committee to stimulate similar worldwide meetings on the subject. Carolyne K. Davis, Administrator of the U.S. Health Care Financing

Administration and John M. Virgo, founder and Executive Vice-President of the Atlantic Economic Society, became the Chairpersons. Membership in the International Steering Committee is made up of representatives from six countries. Through the work of the committee, the new International Health Economics and Management Institute was formed in the latter part of 1983.

Objectives of the International Health Economics and Management Institute are: First, to provide a mechanism for hospital executives, educators, government officials, and business leaders to gain a better understanding of economic and health care problems around the world. Second, to increase the opportunity for the exchange of new ideas at both the theoretical and applied levels.

One international conference will be held each year in order to improve and expand knowledge in health economics and management systems. Every odd-numbered year the conference will be held in Europe and even-numbered year the conference will be held in the Caribbean in conjunction with the International Atlantic Economic Conference.

Contributors to this book exchanged a wealth of ideas at the Paris Conference. These new ideas were then incorporated into the authors' original manuscripts. It is hoped that the reader will also be able to profit from these new ideas. This book should be an indispensable aid to policy makers in their quest to overcome future challenges in the health care sector.

The editor would like to thank Jane A. Masters, Coordinating Editor of the *Atlantic Economic Journal,* who performed the substantial task of keeping him on schedule among the vast array of deadlines involved in a work of this magnitude. She tirelessly and good-naturedly gave of her time in typing and organizing the original manuscript in an efficient manner.

Kathy S. Virgo, Executive Administrator of the Atlantic Economic Society, must be commended for her genius in conceptualizing the project and as a kind and gentle critic of the editor. Beyond that she has shared with him from the early embryonic stages, the concept of a need for an international forum to bring policy makers together to openly discuss important health care issues. She has willingly given up vacations, holidays, and weekends to work on developing the new International Health Economics and Management Institute.

A special note of thanks to the editor's daughter, Deby, who generously gave her support and understanding throughout her summer vacation and whose light-hearted personality was a constant source of inspiration.

Finally, the quality of the book depends on the excellence of the authors, a willingness to meet deadlines, and an incorporation of the latest developments in the field into the authors' works. The extraordinary support of these individuals, and especially Harry Neer, has made this book possible.

Part One
The Issues

Chapter One

The Changing Health Care Sector

JOHN M. VIRGO

International Evolvement of Health Care

Many industrialized countries have followed a similar pattern of evolution in their health care systems. Initially, demand and supply factors, with price discrimination and charity, were in a competitive, private setting. Government activity increased through the introduction of public insurance and support within the private sector. Finally, substantial government involvement took place on both the demand and supply sides.

Cost containment measures are of increasing concern in the United States and Europe. Rising health care expenditures, coupled with growing taxpayer dissatisfaction, are causing all industrialized countries to reevaluate current health care systems. Planning, demand and control, and financial functions must be evaluated and changed. In most European countries, there is a renewed interest in private financing within public medicine.

Overall, there is now a movement, both in Europe and the United States, to sharply decrease the scope and methods of governmental involvement in health care. Scholars differ in their opinion of the extent of such a withdrawal. However, one can conclude that some increased competition and private financing will take place in all industrialized countries within a basic model of public supply.

France, England, Italy, and the United States provide good examples of the changing health care sector. Comparisons between countries are in many ways difficult to make. Differences in culture, political systems, and philosophies are important aspects to consider when making such comparisons. For example, the French health care system combines economic liberalism with governmental intervention. Economic liberalism exists because the physician has the freedom to choose where to practice, what to prescribe, and how much to charge. Governmental intervention exists through public hospitals and comprehensive health insurance.

There are a number of common factors among industrialized countries that have increased the cost of health care. Demand and supply factors are the most obvious. On the demand side, the aging of the population, prolonged

3

treatment of diseases which formerly resulted in quick death, increased problems from modern living and working conditions, a lowering of the pain and discomfort threshold, and a tendency to "medicalize" many social or psychological problems have caused increased costs.

Supply factors impacting on health care costs also have several commonalities among countries. Increased use of hospitals, fewer religious or charitable hospitals, higher salaries, professional upgrading, technological advancements, and the modernization of hospital plant and equipment have caused higher prices throughout all industrialized countries.

Claude E. Ameline (Chapter 2) states that there are also a number of factors in the French health care system that increase costs which are not usually found in other countries. For example, the number of French physicians has increased 66 percent in the last 10 years. They demand more hospital services and strongly contribute to increased expenses. Health insurance coverage has also grown because of a changing social environment that guarantees health care to the general population. Methods of payment for health care have caused a structural inflationary cycle to take place in France. Unions have caused an upward pressure on salaries, adding to the inflationary spiral.

The present French system, according to Ameline, has inefficient methods to control these rising costs. He feels that since health care is financed socially and based on mandatory contributions, costs must be controlled to avoid unacceptable levels of social sacrifice. Ameline suggests several ways through which the French health care system can be improved. He compares certain practices in the United States, Great Britain, and Sweden to see if they can be applied to the French system.

Ameline points out that in some ways the French system provides superior care over the U.S. system. For example, life expectancy in France is longer than in the U.S. and prenatal or infantile mortality rates are lower. The French system has its problems, however. The share of the national wealth given to health care has almost tripled, with an average rate of increase of 7.5 percent per year between 1950 and 1975. Its health insurance system is now in a deficit position creating dissatisfaction and demand for reform.

The National Health Service (NHS) of Britain has undergone change in recent years. A reorganization of NHS took place in 1974 when health authorities became responsible for all health services. This led to a new approach in planning, whereby "delegation downwards" was matched by "accountability upwards." The system established a comprehensive planning of health care services which was different from construction planning, manpower planning, or strategic issues planning. A five-step planning process looked at demand and supply, realism, consultation, compatibility, and flexibility. Yearly plans are prepared, reviewed, and adopted.

Robert J. Maxwell (Chapter 3) points out, however, that this new planning process fits a period of predictable growth of resources rather than a period of declining growth and retrenchment. He recommends some new approaches to facilitate planning under this type of economic environment: A mixed-scanning approach can synthesize the incremental view of problem solving. Planning for uncertainty using a Delphi technique might also be used. Structured public discussion can aid the planning process. Cost-benefit analysis can be used as a means of deciding which services should be reduced. Finally, the author suggests planning as a means of developing and debating key strategic concepts. Health care planning, he concludes, must be improved in the British system.

Italy's health care sector has undergone substantial revision since 1979 when a national health scheme was introduced, modelled after the British system. The long term stability of the Italian system is analyzed by Gilberto Muraro in Chapter 4. He considers the theoretical reasoning behind public health care, how it has impacted on the European systems in the past 20 years, and evaluates new approaches that will change these systems in the future. Private financing is gaining more attention in Italy. Recent legislation has increased the existing co-payments for prescribed drugs, introduced percentage co-payments for clinical tests, and established fixed payment amounts for each prescription.

Mounting criticism in the United States has been leveled at rising costs in the reimbursement system of Medicare and Medicaid. Spending on these programs has risen dramatically in the last few years to an astonishing $85 billion in fiscal year 1984 or 9.3 percent of the federal budget. The financing, benefit, and reimbursement aspects of the two programs have caused expenditures to rise to 2.4 percent of GNP. Carolyne K. Davis (Chapter 5) looks at these mounting costs and suggests specific policy changes to deal with the problem.

Employing over seven million people, with 7,000 hospitals, 19,000 nursing homes, and 450,000 practicing physicians makes health care the third largest industry in the United States. Total spending is projected to reach $756 billion or 12.0 percent of GNP by 1990. Rising health care expenditures in the United States are the result of demographic, technological, and reimbursement factors that cause a major redistribution of economic resources.

There are several structural features of Medicare and Medicaid that fuel rapidly rising expenditures: reasonable cost and charge reimbursement systems; the structure of Medicare's benefit package; "freedom-of-choice" of providers; and open-ended financing. Up until October 1983, higher costs resulted in higher reimbursements, leaving little incentive for price competition. The results have been an inflationary cycle that has spiraled to dizzying heights. Starting in October 1983, the Social Security Amendments require a prospective payment scheme to help lower the rate of increase in Medicare hospital expenses. It is believed that this program will increase productivity and motivate hospitals to specialize in the kinds of care in which they are most efficient.

Physician reimbursement is critical to rising health care costs in the United States since physicians account for over 70 percent of expenditures. Medicare physician expenditures increase from 16 to 20 percent per year. Technically, Davis feels, it is the most difficult to reform and provide incentives for efficiency. To control these rapidly rising expenditures and allow time for basic reforms to be developed, the Reagan Administration is proposing a one year freeze on Medicare physician reimbursement levels. Davis outlines other major policy proposals by the Administration to restrain costs, increase cost awareness, and change historical behavior patterns. For Medicare and Medicaid to survive in the long-run, additional reforms will be needed.

Strategic Planning and Decision Making

Fundamental changes in the health care sector are forcing traditional hospital providers to develop strategies to compete on the basis of cost and convenience. Price and service competition require the hospital administrator to use business planning techniques and analytical tools which might be unfamiliar. Changing environmental forces, such as new reimbursement schemes, increased physician supply, and new models of health care delivery make it difficult to maintain a competitive position without establishing new approaches to the planning process.

Several techniques for business segmentation and economic analysis to assist hospitals in this new competitive environment are explored by Frederick S. Fink (Chapter 6). Hospital segmentation depends on the complexity of the market and its product and service mix. An analysis of the relationships between costs, scale, and experience within business segments indicates certain predictable economic behavior by the hospital. Economic considerations, such as price elasticity and cost position, must be viewed against market coverage, convenience, and quality factors in developing effective strategy. The ability to effectively compete over a broad range of services will lead to a healthier delivery system.

Harry M. Neer (Chapter 7) considers some specific external issues impacting the hospital environment: an increased number of practicing physicians; excess hospital beds through 1990; development of newer forms of health care delivery systems and expansion of existing systems; curtailment of historical sources of capital; renewed governmental pressure to reduce costs; sharp increases in hospital technology due to computer applications; and a growing older population.

Given the increased importance of these external issues, coupled with growing financial pressures, many hospitals have turned to corporate reorganization. Although reorganization has taken place at hospitals of all sizes, it is most prevalent among large hospitals. Planning is an extremely difficult task that cannot take place without an understanding of the marketplace. There are a number of key points within the process such as: corporate philosophy; goals for each entity or department; critical issues facing corporate entities; objectives to satisfy the critical issues; allocation of appropriate resources; use of multi-disciplinary teams of managers; and evaluation and feedback. A successful organization must engage in multi-disciplinary and multi-level corporate planning in order to survive in the future.

Top level managers at hospitals face two important tasks: (1) Deciding what to do in a changing and uncertain external environment in the face of a flood of potentially relevant information; and (2) Being able to get things done through a large and diverse set of people and groups over whom they may have little formal or direct control. Faced with demands and objectives by a variety of groups acting both within the hospital and in its external environment, the role of the administrator often resembles that of a tight-rope walker juggling several balls on the highwire.

Proactive management in this setting is analyzed by John M. Virgo (Chapter 8). Most hospital executives concentrate on the economic and techno-logical environments in developing their plans. Many administrators have a "blind side" for strategic planning from the political-legal and social sides of the external environments in which they must operate. Because change can be turbulent in the health care sector, long-term macro level strategic planning must be conducted by management.

A major impact on the complexity of decision making is the emergence of the regulatory agency. Virgo looks at the changing nature of regulation, its effect on management and develops a power-structure model for decision-making in the hospital. Several groups impact on decisions and balancing these competing demands is the challenge facing hospital management.

Increased awareness of social responsibility must also be regarded as a manageable part of running the hospital. Society, to the administrator, is composed of those sets of common interest groups in the power-structure model, with each group expecting some level of satisfaction of its personal objectives. Although measuring social performance is difficult, Virgo suggests the establishment of a management information system to aid the institu-tionalization of external social values.

A good example of macro-level forecasting is given by Arthur M. Randall in Chapter 9. He attempts to look into the future to examine outside in-fluences affecting health care. Analysis of demographic factors shows that there will be an aging of the population, which will be better informed, and have a greater demand for quality health care.

Computers will play an ever increasing role in patient medical care. Patient monitoring will increase substantially by the 1990's and extend beyond intensive care units to other units, and to outpatient care. The health care computers of tomorrow will have greater memory, storage, and reporting capabilities. They will be smaller, faster, and less expensive.

Randall predicts that regulatory agencies will become streamlined, have permanent funding, and enjoy increased power and authority. Regional health care agencies will maintain an extensive data base of health care information. A national database will be able to provide patient records and histories through a nationwide computer network from terminals in hospitals and physicians' offices. Microelectronics will dramatically change the storage of health care information. A complete medical history will be able to be stored in a ring, watch, or a tooth filling so the individual would always have the information in time of emergency.

With increased computerization throughout the health care system, the role of hospital management will change dramatically. Information available to the executive will likely quadruple, according to Randall. Planning will require cross-disciplinary expertise and greater sophistication, accuracy, and direction by highly specialized management teams.

Cost Control in Health Care

A fundamental problem faced by the United States and European health care systems is the spiraling increase in costs. Carolyne K. Davis and Alfonso D. Esposito (Chapter 10) provide a historical description of research into the problem.

Research directed by Congress in 1967 showed that Medicare provided little incentive for hospitals to control costs. In 1972, Congress authorized research into different reimbursement methods in an attempt to find a way to determine rates paid to hospitals for services provided. By 1975, several state demonstration projects were underway to test budget review systems and hospital payment methodology. The result was the identification of 317 diagnosis related groups of hospital patients and the development of costing techniques. Since 1975, several other demonstration projects refined the prospective reimbursement system and improved the techniques for treating case mix.

In 1982, the Tax Equity and Fiscal Responsibility Act (TEFRA) became law and formally established a prospective payment system to limit Medicare inpatient operating costs. It also set target rates to limit the amount by which hospital reimbursement could be increased each year. TEFRA, however, was designed as an interim measure and did not provide sufficient incentives for hospital cost control.

The Social Security Amendments of 1983 are designed to offer such incentives to hospitals. As of October 1, 1983, hospitals are no longer reimbursed for their actual expenditures. A nationwide schedule of rates set payment levels hospitals receive for services performed. Separate schedules are applied to hospitals in different geographical areas, with hospitals in the same area paid a similar rate for the same service. Only short-term general hospitals are included under the program.

This dramatic change in hospital reimbursement is designed to alter hospital behavior in a number of areas: new accounting systems to measure costs; increased use of efficient business techniques; increased attention to the nursing function, increased specialization in services based upon efficiency; management from a clinical cost perspective, and a reassessment of the need and use of current facilities.

The new reimbursement system is an extension of the diagnosis related groups (DRG's) developed in 1975. Robert B. Fetter, one of the original developers of DRG's, and Jean L. Freeman, explain the underlying conceptual framework of them in Chapter 11. Basic productivity measurements applied in manufacturing are now being applied to health care.

Hospital outputs are the specific goods and services received by the patient. Inputs are those labor, material, and equipment resources from which patient services are derived. The hospital can be equated to a multiproduct firm, with each product made up of multiple outputs. A production function for each service can be developed to show the relationship between inputs and outputs. Research results have established 467 DRG's, each defined by one or more variables, representing a multivariable system classifying hospital discharges. The output of the hospital is defined by classes of patients using similar sets of services.

Fetter and Freeman have been able to extend the input-output technique to other countries. Data from France, the Netherlands, and the United States are compared to hospital case mix and productivity among the three countries. The importance of international comparison of DRG's is that it allows examination of hospital resource utilization by different health care systems.

New Productivity Techniques

Historically, the cost for health care was determined by an average rate per patient, per day or per occupied bed. Charles T. Wood (Chapter 12) feels that in today's more sophisticated health care setting, per diem rates must give way to alternative pricing systems. Current health care pricing averages cost of services, thus one does not know what individual actual costs are. Hospitals cannot be competitive and efficient unless reliable cost data are established.

Cost accounting, budgeting, and identifying cost of production unit measured by resource output should be, according to Wood, the new approach to health care management. Individual service units should have regular management audits to measure and control productivity. A monitoring system also needs to be established to test resource utilization by diagnosis, by physician, and by units within a hospital or among hospitals.

To demonstrate this new approach, Wood applies it to the operating room, nursing services, and cost per patient day at Massachusetts Eye and Ear Infirmary, where he serves as General Director. He concludes that a more organized management information system needs to be developed to measure differences between hospital cost centers and hospitals. All resources that go into caring for a specific disease need to be monitored by doctor and by hospital.

Employee relations can also have an important impact on productivity. Hospital management in this area is undergoing rapid change due to reductions in financial resource allocation, new personnel management theories (such as Ouchi's Theory Z), and new employee values and expectations. These changes, coupled with the need for increased productivity, lead John E. Baird (Chapter 13) to suggest that hospitals should engage in Quality Circles. Employees in the same work unit come together in a group to identify, analyze, and solve quality and efficiency problems in their particular area. Applied correctly, Quality Circles can be highly successful in enhancing productivity and in improving the economic viability of the hospital. Baird applies the Quality Circle concept by outlining the procedures through which Quality Circles are implemented in the hospital setting.

Quality Circles in hospitals are just beginning to be implemented, with the first ones in the United States established in 1980. To date, nearly 100 hospitals have implemented such a system. Detailed results are just starting to emerge. Overall, these systems seem to result in cost savings, reduced errors, increased efficiency, reduced absenteeism, reduced turnover, lower numbers of grievances, improved employee morale, and greater employee cooperation. The future potential for Quality Circles is substantial, and will continue to spread throughout hospitals, not only in the United States, but worldwide.

The Changing Role of Nurses

The multitude of changes in health care have also impacted on the nursing profession. For example, the establishment of the Clinical Specialist and the Nurse Practitioner has changed the clinical practice of nursing. Both have improved access to health care and helped in reducing cost. Through these and many other positive programs, Gloria S. Hope (Chapter 14) feels that nursing has responded well to the changing environment of recent years.

However, she feels that the profession has not yet gained autonomy because of the bureaucratic organization of most hospitals. Since nurses serve as agents of the hospital and also carry out physicians' orders, a nurse's contributions are often overlooked. This has resulted in dissatisfaction, as evidenced by attempts to unionize, high turnover, and decreasing professionalism. In the future, nurses will be recognized as a separate power group rather than being controlled by the institutional environment of the hospital. They will more actively participate in group decision-making efforts in solving common problems. Hope analyzes the role of nursing in the changing environment through the year 2000. Its future is now brighter than ever since the profession is beginning to speak out and is becoming actively involved in designing health care programs.

To be an active participant in the decision-making process, however, requires nurses to participate in strategic planning, along with the hospital administrator. The nursing administrator must effectively apply strategic management concepts to the nursing component. Lyndsey Stone (Chapter 15) feels that the nursing executive must establish long range plans in the areas of product, technology, production, and marketing.

The nurse executive must be able to work within the framework of the business functions of hospital management. More frequently, he or she is brought into the long range strategic planning process, since nurses often occupy vice presidential level positions in the organizational structure. The nurse administrator is increasingly expected to develop plans which fit into the overall goals and objectives of the hospital.

Stone lists a number of points needed to make a nurse executive an effective strategic planner; similar goals, philosophies, and competencies; an understanding of the parameters of a top level decision maker; ability to make corporate level contributions in decision-making; and the ability to judge proposals on factual and complete information.

It is important for the CEO to realize that the nursing function represents an important power group in the hospital setting. As such, nursing must be viewed as an executive area of managerial expertise. Only when the nurse administrator actively accepts this strategic management role will nursing receive the level of recognition that it deserves.

The nurse administrator who is involved in formal strategic planning will establish higher performance standards for his or her staff. Acting as a key executive in the planning process can serve to motivate nursing personnel whose ideas and concerns are taken into consideration. Dorothy and Richard Fox (Chapter 16) feel that over time, active participation in the planning process provides a sense of direction to the nursing staff. One can expect a significant improvement in performance when the nurse administrator is involved in systematic strategic planning. Besides providing a sense of direction to the department, planning is a control mechanism that sets limits and monitors movement away from stated goals and objectives. It also provides a source of professional satisfaction for nurses involved in the process.

In addition to strategic planning concerns by nurses, economic and employment issues will also be important future considerations. In recent years, average salaries have increased to nearly $20,000 per year. However, because of a relatively flat life cycle earnings pattern, newly hired nurses earn only slightly less than nurses with many years of experience. This creates frustration, dissatisfaction, and a demand for a more equitable salary scale. Because of this and other economic and welfare factors, unionization of nurses has increased, especially since 1974 when the National Labor Relations Act was amended to cover private, nonprofit hospitals.

In addition to unionization and its impact on nursing salaries, Richard C. McKibbin (Chapter 17) analyzes the demand and supply of nurses, nursing education, problems in the work setting, the political-economic role of nurses, and the impact of changing hospital organizational patterns. He concludes that the challenge facing the nursing profession in the future will be to develop the ability to adapt to a changing environment of larger, more bureaucratized hospitals. Nurses will have a more difficult time establishing themselves as a separate autonomous group in the decision-making process.

Consumer Preferences and Health Care Accessibility

Health care planning has, for the most part, largely ignored the planning processes used in other sectors of the economy. Other sectors use leading indicators to identify changes in market behavior. The consumer of health care has incorrectly been assumed to be a passive responder to the system. Consumers do have definite preferences and the failure to evaluate and incorporate consumer preferences has led to sub-optimal decision making in hospitals.

Research by Kevin G. Halpern, Trevor A. Fisk, and James Sobel (Chapter 18) shows strong consumer preferences in health care, distinctly segmented into different psychographic groups, similar to preferences in other marketplaces. The health care planner and provider must be aware of this relationship to determine the need for services, paralleled by sensitivity to consumer attitudes. Planning must take place only after consumer preferences have been taken into consideration. The consumer can no longer be viewed as passive and incompetent, to be manipulated in an array of artificial restrictions affecting demand and supply. If consumer preferences and demands are not met, consumers may turn outside the system.

A "medical counter-system" may develop which would include "wellness" spending on services designed to lower the use of conventional health care, growth of self-diagnosis, and use of alternative treatment providers. The result may be the existence of two parallel systems—one unresponsive to consumer demand and the other highly responsive. A systematic analysis of consumer attitudes, preferences, and satisfaction levels must be incorporated into the present system to prevent this from occurring.

Since consumer preferences have been largely ignored, hospital management often wrongly perceives the needs or desires of the patient. Where marketing does exist in hospitals, it is usually relegated to a middle-management staff function with little allocation of resources. Research by Algin B. King (Chapter 19) points to the fact that many hospitals do not recognize the nature and role of the marketing function.

A hospital, to be financially viable, must cover costs and operate at least at the break-even occupancy level. To do this successfully in the long run, requires attention to the demands of the patients and the admitting physicians by using modern marketing concepts. Many hospitals skirt financial disaster through their lack of marketing techniques to identify and meet, not only the needs of the patient, but also those of the physician.

Since hospitals compete among each other and are similar to businesses in the private sector, management must recognize and understand that the offering of health care services should be made on a competitive basis. Modern, competitive marketing techniques need to be utilized to find consumer preferences to facilitate the hospital in providing appropriate services.

An underlying, fundamental social issue must be considered when discussing consumer preferences, especially in light of the cited international emphasis on the lowering of health care costs: What will be the impact of changing policy on quality of life issues? Cost-benefit analysis must be viewed within the context of its social impact on the consumer of health services.

European and U.S. systems have, at varying levels, been based upon health care as a right rather than a privilege. The degree of government involvement varies between countries, however. Medicare and Medicaid have attempted to provide a "safety net" in the United States compared to more comprehensive public intervention in some other countries. Martha Albert (Chapter 20) examines the size of the holes in the net to see how many people fall through. She finds that people are excluded from the system and that current attempts to reduce expenditures will increase those numbers.

Changing social attitudes and moral and ethical questions are affecting the accessibility of health care. Abortion, environmental health, organ transplants, kidney dialysis, and a host of other issues are the center of current debate over who should receive care and who should pay for it. Will esoteric services be made available only to those who have the capability of paying?

If rationing is to take place, who will make these life and death decisions: the patient, the physician, the family, the hospital, or the government? Albert feels that the current social environment has changed within the last few years to a mixture of utilitarian and social approaches to health care delivery with a deemphasis on unilateral availability of health care.

Part Two

International Evolvement of
Health Care

Chapter Two

Philosophy and Cost of Health Care in France

CLAUDE E. AMELINE*

The health care system in France is two-fold: it combines economic liberalism and governmental intervention.

Liberalism is first of all a philosophy which is at the root of the French medical practice: the physician has the freedom to choose where to practice, what to prescribe, and how much to charge for his services. The patient has the freedom to choose his physician or the hospital where he wishes to be treated, and can change his choice as he pleases.

Liberalism also means the existence of a large and independent private sector. Sixty-eight percent of French physicians have either a full or part-time private practice outside hospitals. Thirty percent of all hospital beds are located in private clinics. Among these private establishments, 18 percent are profit-making and 12 percent are non profit-making. They play a particularly important role in obstetrics and simple surgery. They charge for the day in addition to professional fees.

The intervention of government is demonstrated by both the existence of public hospitals and a comprehensive system of health insurance. Public hospitals account for 70 percent of the beds. These hospitals are mainly predominant in medical research, general medicine, and psychiatry. They are financed by a global per diem price which covers their overall expenses.

Health insurance is mandatory and covers almost 100 percent of the population. It is divided into professional schemes: business and industry, agriculture, mining, and the like. Hence, the type of insurance will vary from one profession to another; but generally these variations are quite small. This health insurance is financed by premiums which amount to 18 percent of the salary for the majority of employed people; of the 18 percent, three-fourths is paid by the employer and one-fourth by the employee. Subscribers pay on their own the local physician and for the medicine prescribed. Later, they receive a partial reimbursement of their expenses (generally 75 percent of the physician's fee and 70 percent of the prescription bill). If they choose

*Translated by Veronique Zaytzeff, Professor of Foreign Languages and Literature, Southern Illinois University at Edwardsville.

17

to go to a public or a private hospital they pay only 20 percent for stays shorter than a month and for minor surgery; they pay nothing for longer stays or for major surgery. The amount which is billed to the subscriber is called "the balance" (*ticket modérateur*).

For approximately half of the population this system is complemented by non-profit optional insurance coverages (mutuals) which reimburse the "balance" to the subscriber. Finally, there is a system of assistance for the poverty-stricken—the medical aid—which makes an advance on all expenses and can also pay the "balance."

In this system, the state is responsible for regulation and control. The implementation (collecting of premiums, payment of allowances, and reimbursements) is entrusted to autonomous organizations, in particular to the health insurance offices which are jointly administered by representatives of unions and employers.

What are the results of such a system? They rank France in an average level among other developed countries:

a) In terms of health indicators, with a life expectancy of 70.1 years for men and 78.3 for women in 1980, France lags behind the Scandinavian countries, the Netherlands, Switzerland, and Japan, but is ahead of countries such as the United States, Great Britain, Germany, and Italy. The same is true as far as prenatal or infant mortality are concerned.

b) In terms of health expenses, with a proportion of 8 percent of the Gross National Product (*Produit Intérieur Brut*) in 1981, France is ranked seventh among the 24 countries of the Organization for Economic Cooperation and Development (OECD).

As in all industrialized countries, the share of the national wealth given to health care has greatly increased in the past 30 years: it has almost tripled since 1950. The average rate of increase has been 7.5 percent per year from 1950 to 1975. Since then, it has clearly diminished thanks to a series of restrictive measures (5.4 percent average); but starting with 1982, it seems to be on the increase again.

For a number of years, due to the world economic situation, the incomes subject to premiums and the number of subscribers have not been able to keep pace with the increase in expenses. As a result, the health insurance system is in deficit. This deficit calls for a periodic increase in premiums and revisions in policies. The government and public opinion are increasingly dissatisfied with this state of affairs and long-lasting measures to reform the system have become necessary.

It would be proper to study the causes for this increase in health costs in greater detail before considering the measures which might lead to better control of the system. *What are the reasons for the increase in cost?* The rapid and continued increase in the cost of health insurance is due to two sets of factors. Some are common to all industralized countries and others are specific to France. In addition to these factors, one needs to emphasize the relative inefficiency of the existing means of control.

Common Factors

Among the general causes of increasing expenses one must mention, first of all, those which are due to an increase in *demand* for medical treatment. Thus, it should be pointed out:

a) Aging of the population. Since the turn of the century the progress made by hygiene and medical science has allowed an increasing number of people to reach an advanced age. This portion of the population in France has increased both in absolute number and in relative number. In France, persons over 65 represented 13.9 percent of the population in 1980 versus 11.1 percent in 1946. The percentage of very old people (over 75) has also increased, rising from 3.4 percent in 1946 to 5 percent in 1980. These people are the ones who require medical attention most: nearly twice the national average.[1]

b) The after-effects of sickness, accidents, and handicaps. Many diseases which formerly caused a quick death are now treated but they require a lengthy care, a long recovery, even a permanent follow-up (grave accidents, chronic deficiencies, severe mental handicaps). For example, each patient requiring renal dialysis in a hospital costs 340,000 Francs per year (approximately $5,000).

c) Pathology due to modern living or working conditions. The number of traffic accidents increased by 125 percent from 1953 to 1981. Certain changes in eating habits (abuse of sugar and fats, irregular eating hours, increase in the use of tobacco) increase the risk of numerous diseases. The increase of production line work, and night shift work in industry seems to have caused the development of various problems (insomnia, anxiety, stomach diseases). These types of work also increase the probability of industrial accidents (accidents are more numerous towards the end of shifts and during the night). The present increase in unemployment has, quite probably, direct and indirect impact on the health of part of the population.

d) The pain and discomfort threshold is lower. As the general standard of living improved benign afflictions became more intolerable. With the help of the physician and of medicine, one now wishes to eliminate or relieve them immediately.

e) Finally, one can observe a tendency to "medicalize" many social or

---

[1] Persons over 70 years of age, representing 8 percent of the French population, account for 15.7 percent of all hospital expenses and 14.4 percent of other health care expenses.

psychological problems. In the absence of family support or social facilities, one "medicalizes" the care of elderly persons, the education of numerous children with problems. Medical science is asked to remedy anxiety, drug addiction, alcoholism, psychosomatic troubles, family or sexual problems. Without realizing it, citizens of developed countries have adopted the famous definition of health as stated by the World Health Organization. Looking for complete physical, mental, and social well-being, people tend more and more to turn toward the physician in order to satisfy their desire for it.[2]

However, the increase in the cost of health insurance does not depend solely on new claims made by the population. It also depends on the *supply* of health care. In this case, in all industrialized countries, the major factor has been the increasing role played by hospitals. The center of gravity of the health care system has shifted. Instead of going to local practioners, people go to hospitals which have at their disposal the most advanced means of diagnosis and health care.[3] For several reasons, the hospital tends to be more and more costly:

a) Charitable institutions which managed many establishments up to the 1950's have progressively disappeared. The religious personnel working in these establishments for a symbolic remuneration, without overtime payments or social security coverage, have been replaced by salaried agents paid through public contributions.

b) The salaries paid to these agents increased faster than the general price index. In fact, they have followed the general movement of salaries. Quite often they have even benefited from preferential measures in favor of low paid workers (since many of the staff were poorly qualified) or of specific measures geared toward the upgrading of certain professions (notably nurses).

c) The development of labor law has also had greater impact on hospitals than on other undertakings. The number of annual working days keeps diminishing (in principle, presently, it is 220 days in France; in fact, it is closer to 200). The same is true of the time spent at work per week (one person at a patient's bedside means employing 5.2 persons, without absenteeism). The increase in the length of paid maternity leaves or leaves for child-raising has also played a role since a large percentage of hospital personnel are young women.

d) The progress of technology has increased the cost of both investment and operation. The purchase of a scanner costs from 6 to 8 million Francs

---

[2] It is understood that a "demedicalization" of the above-mentioned problems would not lower their cost where society is concerned. It would simply shift the cost to other financial sources.

[3] This development has been slower in France than in other countries. However, since 1980, French hospital expenses have surpassed other French health care expenses. In 1981, they increased to 52 percent of the total expenditures.

(approximately $1 million); a nuclear medicine machine, from 1 to 4 million Francs; a radiotherapy machine from 2 to 9 million Francs. In addition, these machines are extremely expensive to maintain and must be serviced by well qualified personnel.

e) The modernization of hospital equipment has also brought higher costs: the elimination of large wards not only implies construction work but also expenses for additional personnel in order to maintain a satisfactory level of patient supervision.

For these reasons, the total number of personnel and their cost continue to increase in hospitals. The number of non-medical staff (private and public sectors) increased 48 percent between 1972 and 1980. The number of physicians in public hospitals (full-time physicians) during the same period increased by 67 percent. The combination of personnel costs and medical fees represents approximately 75 percent of the running costs of hospitals today.

French Factors

The general factors just mentioned are reinforced by several factors specific to France: the increasing number of physicians, the extension of health insurance, and the methods of payment.

The increasing number of physicians. The number of practicing physicians in France has increased 66 percent in the last 10 years, going from 65,000 in 1971 to 108,000 in 1982. As we have already seen, hospitals largely gained by this increase. It allowed them to expand their services. By the same token, it strongly contributed to increase hospital expenses, since hospital physicians are better placed than others to make costly decisions.

As for non-hospital doctors, one has to make a distinction between the general practitioner and the specialist. When the number of general practitioners is on the rise, the practice of each one tends to decrease while the total volume of their practice remains stable. Each new specialist, on the contrary, tends to create a new field of activity comparable to that of his already established colleagues; thus, causing an increase not only in the number of consultations but also in the number of prescriptions. Since the number of specialists has increased by almost 40 percent in the last ten years, this has resulted in rather considerable additional expenses.

Growth of health insurance. In 1955, the various health insurance plans covered 28.8 million persons, today, they cover 53 million. Such an increase was a major social improvement, since it guaranteed a real right to health care to the entire population. It is probable—and conceivable—that it contributed to an increase in the amount of medical expenditures, although one cannot say to what extent.

Methods of payment for health care. The financing of French health care is traditionally based upon the payment of individual consultations, visits, examinations, treatments, hospitalizations, and the like. This method of payment, associated wtih an extremely decentralized organization, has a structurally inflationary character, as it ties the resources of private physicians and those of health institutions to the volume of their activity. Therefore, it may lead to abuse. One can also add that the present nomenclature favors the technical aspect too much, to the detriment of the clinical one, which in turn, is much against the whole philosophy of the patients' needs.

Generally speaking, one must notice that the greater part of the people involved in the health system have an interest, one way or another, in seeing that expenses increase:

a) The physicians who receive their professional fees;

b) The directors of establishments for whom an increase in the number of hospital days means additional resources, therefore, easier administration (the status of the directors is, by the way, dependent upon the number of beds they manage);

c) The unions representing the hospital personnel are naturally interested in the improvement of working conditions and in the increase in the number of staff; and

d) Finally, the locally elected politicians sitting on the board of directors. As a matter of fact, the hospital is often the main employer of its sector and local communities finance only a small part of it.

Inefficient Control

In order to put an end to increasing costs, some regulatory measures have been implemented. However, they do not yield sufficient results.

The Health Services Map. The fragmentation of the French system between public and private, autonomous establishments makes true health care planning difficult. However, the hospital law of December 31, 1970, requires submission of all introductions, extensions, transformations, or transfers of beds or of major technical equipment for approval or authorization. The decisions are made on the basis of a "map" which divides the territory into health districts and defines for each of them the needs to be satisfied. In addition to this, a law of December 1979 entitles the Minister for Health to close down unnecessary facilities in public hospitals.

The law has effectively avoided the purchase of unjustified equipment. For example, 154 requests for scanners have been rejected so far, against 96 requests granted. In 1981, only 56 percent of the additional beds requested by the private sector were authorized. However, while it was possible to reduce the number of new additions, it proved impossible to enforce the elimination of unnecessary equipment in public institutions. Several reasons explain this failure: the imperfection of health services maps which are sometimes based on questionable data; the unfairness of treating the private and the public sectors differently; and professional or political pressures. Undoubtedly, during a period of unemployment it is difficult to eliminate existing services on the basis of theoretical norms. No wonder that, even allowing for the needs which remain to be satisfied in some sectors, the number of beds continues to increase in public establishments (1.9 percent from 1974 to 1981) and in private establishments (9 percent from 1974 to 1981).

Medical Profiles. In 1971, following an agreement between the National Health Insurance Fund and physicians organizations, "statistical charts of professional activity" were instituted. These charts are more often called "medical profiles."

This system was to alert and, if necessary, sanction physicians whose volumes of activity or prescriptions would far exceed a national average. However, it had the inconvenience of not being qualitative enough. Furthermore, if it singled out individual aberrant behavior, it could not influence the behavior of the entire profession. Finally, there was a lack of political drive to enforce these medical profiles.

The statistical charts of professional activity have been introduced very slowly and they have not shown visible results on the level of expenses. Therefore, there is no system of information which would allow physicians really to measure the financial consequences of their decisions. It is even more regrettable since their training, up to very recent years, has not made them at all sensitive to the economic dimension of their activity.

Limitation in the number of physicians. In 1971, the government decided to impose a *numerus clausus* on the number of students entering their second year of medical studies. The aim was to diminish the annual number of new graduates by one-third. This measure will not produce any visible results before the end of the 1980's and the number of practicing physicians will continue to grow rapidly. It will go from 1 physician per 500 inhabitants as it is at the present time, to 1 per 330 in the year 2000.

These are the principal reasons which explain the rapid and continuing rise in the cost of health expenses for the last 30 years. One ought to add that the people involved in the system notice the consequences of their behavior only after a long period. In case of a deficit of the health insurance scheme, the collecting of extra premiums and other adjustments take place many months later: the feedback comes too late to influence the growth of expenses.

Has France, then, succeeded in setting an acceptable limit to health care costs in relation to the national wealth? Of course, nobody can claim to define an ideal level for the efforts made in favor of health care improvement. One could also point out that certain other expenses have increased even more rapidly between 1970 and 1978. While medical expenditures increased by 78 percent, other expenditures such as housing, automobiles, and home equipment increased by 87 percent, and insurance increased by 163 percent.

However, an essential difference exists between these expenditures. Only health care is financed socially and based on mandatory contributions. This is the reason why its growth is much more noticeable and cannot be allowed to go on at the same pace for very long. The expenses will only continue to grow unless real control is introduced. In the current period of slow economic growth, they would result in an intolerable burden for the economy or would call for unacceptable sacrifices in other sectors.

In most countries, governments and public opinion have awakened to that fact. We also know that progress in health care is not always proportional to the additional monies which are allocated to it.

Bringing Health Care under Better Control

Many different ways can be considered to bring health care under better control. I shall first mention some ways which do not seem to provide a real solution. Then, I shall turn to those which seem to be more promising.

False expectations. These include prevention, progress in technology, and a total revamping of the French system of health care.

Prevention. It is known that prevention can take numerous forms. Not all forms come under the health care system and its financing.

a) Primary prevention (actually trying to prevent diseases); secondary prevention (aiming at detecting and treating them at an early stage); and tertiary prevention (trying to avoid or minimize the after-effects).

b) Passive prevention (based solely on the action of governmental authorities) or active prevention (which requires the participation of the citizens themselves).

Prevention, in any form, if applied with discrimination, is invaluable. It has yielded substantial results against infectious diseases. More recently, it has been quite successful in the field of perinatology, traffic accidents, and industrial accidents. In addition to its obvious advantages for individuals (better quality of life, longer life), prevention is very important for the economy since it contributes to the global preservation of the work force, hence, to the financing of public expenses. Consequently, it must be pursued and developed, and the French Government intends to do so.

One, nevertheless, should not expect a decrease in health costs from it. In lowering the death rate of people who are still rather young, prevention contributes to the aging of the population. It thus leads to an increase in degenerative diseases (cancers, cardio-vascular diseases, etc.) which science does not know how to treat effectively and which are the most costly. Presently, most diseases in France are chronic diseases, characteristic of an aging population. Consequently, prevention shifts, rather than solves, the problem of health costs.

Progress in medical technology. In industry, as well as in a portion of the service sector, technical progress reduces costs because man is replaced by the machine. It is not the same in the medical sector. The use of the extremely costly equipment mentioned above is not accompanied by a reduction in personnel. Quite the contrary. Hospitals used to be an industry based on manpower. Nowadays, they need both capital and manpower with manpower becoming more and more qualified.

Furthermore, one rarely sees new techniques eliminating older ones completely. True, there have been some examples: vaccinations replaced sanatoria, protheses can replace external equipments. More often than not, however, one witnesses new and more expensive additional techniques (radiology, scanners, nuclear medicine).

Anything which decreases the price-tag of technical intervention, the pain or the discomfort it causes, or makes it more available, increases the demand for it. Therefore, the fields in which expenditures increase most are those where numerous technical innovations appeared recently (non-aggressive explorations, automatized analyses): a 7.5 percent average increase per year in the volume of radiology; a 12 percent increase in the volume of laboratory analyses.

Revamping the health care system.

a) One could entertain the idea of increasing competition and the choices offered to the consumer in developing networks of health care facilities similar to the American "health maintenance organizations." This system, in fact, seems to reduce the health expenses of affiliated members.

It presupposes, however, the existence or the development of additional hospitals, each of which would offer most types of treatments. Failing this, patients would have to undertake long trips in order to reach the hospital they have decided upon. This seems incompatible with the planning which, for the last ten years, has been trying to limit gaps as well as double use, all over our territory. It is also incompatible with the organization of France's health insurance (uniform rate premiums, one single organization for all subscribers located in the same zone). Finally, it is difficult to imagine a public town hospital free to decide which organization it should join.

b) It could also be decided strictly to limit the amount of monies allocated to health care.

This type of system exists in countries such as Great Britain and Sweden. Every year, Parliament or, as the case may be, regional assemblies vote on resources which will cover all public health costs. These resources are then distributed by zone and by establishment, service, or function. They cover investment on the one hand and running costs on the other, therefore introducing cash-limits.

This system allows an excellent control of expenses. It forces national and local politicians to take interest in health management. It increases geographic flexibility by taking into account the specific health care needs of a region.

The system, however, is too restrictive. It presupposes a detailed knowledge and a total control over all health care facilities, like in a national health service. Such a reform would doubtless provoke extreme opposition on the part of physicians, private establishments, certain local communities, unions, and health insurance institutions. Probably, a very strong consensus to preserve the diversified system of health care exists in France.

Possible Alternatives. As I mentioned before, the French health system is based on doctors' complete freedom to prescribe and on the individual reimbursement of incurred expenses. In such a system, each prescription automatically results in an undertaking to reimburse expenses. For this reason, an immediate decrease in public health expenses could take place by simply transferring part of these expenses to different financial sources. One can also go a step further by looking for ways to control overall health care expenditures, be they private or public.

Reducing health insurance expenditures. The financing of medical care, is at present, as follows: 72 percent is paid by health insurance premiums; 25 percent is paid by households (of these, 21 percent is paid directly by members and 4 percent is paid by mutuals) and only 3 percent is paid by the state and local communities. If a change were to be made, it would consist in increasing the amount paid by households, increasing the amount paid by the state or local communities, or a combination of both.

Increase in household share. Such an increase can be obtained in several ways: by raising the existing "balance" (the patient pays a percentage of the cost of the treatment) or by resorting to various alternatives. An all inclusive participation could be established (similar to a tour package), the "balance" being calculated on the basis of the household's income. Another option would require the members of a household to pay all of the expenses, up to a certain amount, an amount which would vary according to total income. In each alternative, households would be free whether or not to subscribe to additional insurance coverage with mutuals.

All these formulas raise technical, political, and economic questions.

– Technical (what would be the cost of administration; delay in reimbursement if one takes into consideration the household's income or their total amount of expenses over a certain period of time?)
– Political (is it appropriate to redistribute incomes within the frame of the health policies, to step back from the principles of insurance, to limit the

role of mutuals?)
- Economic (what would their impact be on health costs and on the economy in general?)

Without attempting to answer all these questions, I should like to note that:

a) The "balance," under any form, is only applicable to and can have an effect solely on "petty risks": by raising the prices of coffins one cannot prevent people from dying! In fact, 73 percent of the expenses do not include a "balance" (90 percent in the case of hospitalization costs). One observes, in the same vein, that 70 percent of the expenses are due to 10 percent of the cases. These figures demonstrate that the crux of the problem does not come from the "petty risks" but from serious cases. Furthermore, it is notoriously difficult to tell where the "petty risks" end. Therefore, the "balance" finds its limitations very quickly from the point of view of health care demand. It does have, however, a mechanical effect on health costs covered by health insurance.

b) To resort increasingly to mutuals, would not necessarily increase demand (taking into account the above-mentioned observations) but it may result in discrimination. Low paid workers would have limited access to this type of protection and would, therefore, be at a disadvantage.

Increasing the state's or local communities' participation. The state or local communities would be able to finance a greater part of the costs, either by increasing traditional taxes such as income tax, VAT (value-added tax), etc., or by resorting to other formulas such as taxing certain consumer goods considered as superfluous or hazardous to health. The technical aspects here are less important than in the case of the "balance." Political and economic questions are, on the contrary, just as difficult. They would imply the possible redistribution of incomes, a greater role for local government versus trade unions and employers and uncertain effects on the economy. Each solution presents advantages and drawbacks in relation to the levels of domestic prices, international competition, investment, and the job market.

The French Government is considering all these options, however, it has not yet made its decision.

Overall health expenditures control. There is no panacea for achieving satisfactory control of all health care costs. Instead, there is a body of measures which can be combined and which can complement each other. Four such measures are:

a) Improving hospital organization and management. The present mode of hospital financing, as already mentioned, presents inflationary risks. Certain aspects of their organization (such as their fragmentation between individual, independent services) can also impair their economic efficiency. These structural factors will disappear, to a large extent, in public hospitals, thanks to the phasing out of per diem resources and introduction of new departments. Implementation will take place in the beginning of 1984. These two reforms will be complemented by an improvement in internal systems of information.

b) Evaluating the quality of medical treatments. Society owes its citizens health care which is at the same time *necessary, efficient,* and *as cheap as possible.* Serious research needs to be conducted in order to find out whether the treatments provided satisfy all three conditions. Naturally, it is the responsibility of the medical profession to determine this. However, physicians need to have systems of continuous information which would link together pathology, methods of treatment, and results. It is necessary to group problems together in meaningful aggregates, to compile all possible types of answers, to compare their effectiveness and recommend the most cost-effective ones.[4] These suggestions could be implemented in several ways:

- By setting up medical profiles which would be more qualitative and put to better use;
- By a systematic evaluation of medical equipment according to the field of utilization, performance, reliability, durability, operating costs and influence on exterior trade; and
- By developing new systems of information within the hospital, (a project known as "medicalization of information systems").

This calls for the collecting of basic data describing medical and hospital activities, comparing them to the range of cases treated (diagnosis related groups or groups of similar treatments). These new management and health care aids will be based on a new, specially devised nomenclature of medical and other interventions.

c) Alternative forms of medical treatment. The methods of analysis indicated above might result in new forms of health care: out-patient treatment, dialysis at home, transfer to other types of establishments, etc. However, these recommendations can be implemented only if a real choice is possible between the different formulas. All too often, institutional or financial factors tends to prevent it.

An official report has shown that in many cases it is not the nature of the disease which determines the type of treatment and its cost but rather the initially prescribed treatment or the type of institution involved. Abolishing per diem resources will allow an easier choice within the general hospital (for example, the choice between hospitalization or ambulatory care). But it would be necessary to take a further step in order to facilitate alternative care and the transfer between different institutions: acute care hospitals,

---

[4] It is true that this kind of approach will, in certain cases, reveal that some hospitals are not properly equiped and, therefore, will result in an effort to modernize them.

long-stay establishments, foster care, etc. All of this implies a unified system for allocating resources.

d) The reform of health care planning. As a result of studies conducted in three regions, the French Ministry of Health is considering a reform of health care planning. Parliament will soon discuss a bill which calls for:

   i) Greater uniformity in the rules of planning applicable to the private and public sectors; and

   ii) New health services maps drawn up at the regional level within overall limits and guidelines issued by the Ministry. These new maps will be based on finer data than the present ones. They will take into account the distribution of the population by age and by sex and its state of health (statistics showing the rates of morbidity and mortality). Thanks to a more realistic analysis of the needs, government authorities will be able to make better informed and, therefore, more efficient planning decisions.

■ ■ ■ ■ ■

The above enumeration is not limitative but it is a minimum. The objective, one should stress, is not to reduce health care expenses or even completely stabilize them in real value. This would presuppose a restraint which would be difficult to bear, considering the structural factors of growth which will continue to exist, and would automatically lead to not treating some pathologies.

The number of physicians will, in fact, continue to increase. This will raise the overall amount of their fees to a certain extent and will also increase the induced demand. The general decrease in the number of working days will also have financial consequences for hospitals, although these consequences will not be exactly proportional. Geographic inequalities will have to be reduced in terms of equipment, personnel, and working conditions. Lastly, many establishments still need to be renovated since they are in poor condition, and the entire system will always have to move forward in order to keep pace with the progress in medical and hospital technologies. The number of hospital personnel per bed will have to increase since it is still low (approximately one employee per bed while in the United States there are 2.5 employees per bed).

Thus, there is no simple solution to limit the increase in health care expenses. This increase constitutes a general and long-lasting trend of modern developed societies, and results from a fundamental need for security and well-being spurred by apparently limitless promises of technical progress.

In the absence of an ideal solution, France, as any other country, will have to use all the means compatible with her institutions and her own values. It will be difficult, without a doubt, but it is necessary to act quickly: an uncontrolled drift of the system could eventually call into question its principles and some of its most positive aspects.

Chapter Three

Health Care Planning: Past Experience and Future Directions

ROBERT J. MAXWELL

Planning in the British National Health Service

Planning in the NHS in its present form dates from June 1976 when the Department of Health issued a guide called *The NHS Planning System* [June 1976]. The genesis of that guide lies in the reorganization of the National Health Service in 1974. The health authorities then created were responsible for *all* health services for the first time, so that there was a potential opportunity to consider the full spectrum of services for a defined population (e.g., a District of, say, 250,000 people, and a Region of 1 to 5 million). Moreover the emphasis behind the 1974 reorganization was rational and managerial, which led naturally to a planning system in the same mold. "Delegation downwards" (from Central Government to Region to Area to District) was to be matched by "accountability upwards" [*Management Arrangements for the Reorganised National Health Service,* 1972]. The planning system formed a systems component that was a natural corollary to major organization change: the only illogicality was that the planning guide should be issued two years after the reorganization, rather than a year before it.

Of course planning has a longer history than that in the NHS. For example *The Hospital Plan* of 1962 published a ten year rolling plan of hospital construction for England and Wales and tried to lay down planning norms and guidelines for hospital provision throughout the country. The construction program thus begun, developed quite detailed systems of hospital construction planning and control, known as Capricode. Nor was planning solely about physical structures, although that was where the main emphasis lay. Manpower planning and control had a place too, in the regional and specialty distribution of hospital medical appointments and in the distribution of general practitioners. During the 1960's also there was increasing government concern about such strategic planning issues as the treatment of chronic renal failure; the improvement of conditions in hospitals for the mentally ill and mentally handicapped; and the adjustment of historical inequities in regional funding.

31

The NHS Planning System

Nevertheless the 1976 planning guide was in its day a major innovation: the introduction of a national system for the comprehensive planning of services, as distinct from construction planning or manpower planning or the tackling of individual strategic issues.

The NHS planning system was conceived in a rational, comprehensive mold. Planning was a five step sequence:

- *Taking stock,* with an emphasis on statistical and other information about all major services
- *Objective-setting,* influenced by (among other things) national and regional policy guidelines
- *Developing strategy,* based on a detailed examination of options, by the planners and by health care planning teams.
- *Developing detailed implementation plans,* covering finance, staffing and other implications
- *Monitoring implementation* and thus preparing for the next planning round

All planning was to have the characteristics of relevance to needs; relevance to supply; realism; consultation; compatibility and flexibility. Something of its flavor appears in Figures I to IV from *The NHS Planning System,* 1976.

Like other rational, comprehensive systems of analysis this one has strengths and weaknesses. The strength is that it can provide a documented and orderly means of changing health services over a period of time. The weaknesses are:

- *The growth of a planning industry* with the generation of masses of paper; holding of many meetings; the development of a specialized, arcane language; and the production of plans that are read mainly by the planners and have relatively modest impact on real life.
- *A degree of rigidity.* Planners (and those they work for) can be understandably reluctant to change plans in which they and others have invested so much effort. The planning timetable can become a hectic steeplechase, in which plans have to be prepared to very tight deadlines each year. People who voice objections late in the day or suggest new options for investigation are by no means popular. The plan once prepared has a life of its own.
- *A degree of frustration.* If over a lengthy period plans do not seem to result in the improvements hoped for, those who have invested effort in them may well become frustrated and discouraged.

The Present Position

The NHS planning system described above constitutes the existing orthodoxy. With more or less enthusiasm, plans along the lines prescribed are prepared each year, reviewed, adopted and passed to higher levels. Health authorities have a few specialist planners. The planning methodology is described and refined.

Nevertheless it is time to take a long hard look and consider some of the misgivings about this approach to the planning of health services, and some ideas for new approaches.

A major problem for the NHS planning system (apart from its inherent characteristics) is the drastic change in economic, social and political climate which coincided closely with its birth. In particular, the system fitted better with a period of predictable, if slow, growth of resources in real terms. The emphasis was on adjustment through differential rates of growth, and on reallocation of resources at the margin. Planning for retrenchment, or for major changes within a static budget, is a very different matter, which makes the expansionist tendencies of the NHS planning system seem irrelevant.

Ideas for New Approaches

It is not my intention to prescribe a new planning system but to welcome an exchange of ideas about a range of approaches that have something worthwhile to offer. We may need to draw on several such approaches, which are not necessarily mutually exclusive, and to promote a variety of experiments. Here I will do no more than sketch some of the approaches that seem to me interesting and relevant. Among these are:

- *A mixed-scanning approach to analysis.* Etzioni's attempt [1967] to synthesize the incremental view of problem-solving, with the rational, comprehensive view, is no longer new. Its implications for health care planning are still very well worth thinking about.

- *Planning for uncertainty.* By this I mean an idea that is well illustrated by an approach taken by the Ottawa-Carleton District Health Council in Canada [1978]. The Council used a modified Delphi technique to develop a range of plausible scenarios about the future environment, and tested a range of planning proposals to see which proposals stood up best in these very different possible futures.

- *Planning as a forum for the public exchange of information and ideas.* The emphasis here is not on backroom analysis, preceded and followed by public consultation, but on planning as a form of structured public debate. One example was the threatened closure of a London medical school [Miller and Norris, 1980]: the type of "wicked" problem on which there is a strong likelihood of differences of opinion.

- *Planning with an emphasis on cost-saving and on identifying which services should if necessary be reduced.* I am not aware of much co-

herent planning along these lines. It would provide the reverse of planning for growth, and would be a logical reaction to financial retrenchment. A few steps along these lines by the Oxford RHA have aroused
some public and political controversy. One could well argue that this
is what this approach should do.

- *Planning as a means of developing and debating a few guiding strategic
  ideas.* The thought, well voiced by Harlan Cleveland of the Hubert
  Humphrey Institute at the University of Minnesota, is that "Planning
  has to be improvisation by the many on a general sense of direction
  which is announced by 'leaders' only after genuine consultation with
  those who will have to improvise on it" [Cleveland, 1980].

■ ■ ■

These ideas are not mutually exclusive. Nor am I suggesting that the present
NHS planning system should be scrapped root and branch. I do believe, however, that it is time we examined these and other ideas of what planning
should be about, and sought to make health care planning more intelligent and
more useful than it has yet been. In the world of public decision-making
about health care, the need for some form of planning is inescapable. We
must simply learn to do it much better.

FIGURE I
A MAP OF PLANNING ACTIVITIES

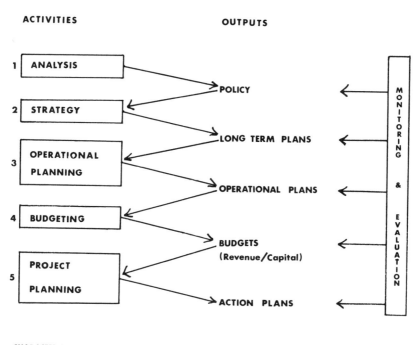

ACTIVITIES

1 ANALYSIS

2 STRATEGY

3 OPERATIONAL PLANNING

4 BUDGETING

5 PROJECT PLANNING

OUTPUTS

POLICY

LONG TERM PLANS

OPERATIONAL PLANS

BUDGETS (Revenue/Capital)

ACTION PLANS

MONITORING & EVALUATION

CHARACTERISTICS OF ACTIVITIES

1	2	3	4	5
• Continuous	• Relatively long term (up to 10-15 years)	•Relatively short term (1 to 3 years)	• Concerned with financial allocations generally firm for one year, open to revision thereafter	• Identifies specific steps and and responsibilities for implementation of approved project
• May lead to policy changes at any time, but not necessarily to immediate implementation	• Relatively broad in approach	• Intensely concerned with the feasible rather than the ideal		• Only required selectively (i.e., for some projects)
	• Needs revision only in light of major policy changes	• Needs revision annually		• Varied information

FIGURE II

BASIC QUESTIONS UNDERLYING THE NHS
PLANNING PROCESS

1.   WHERE ARE WE NOW?

Planning teams and service managers will be supplied with a variety of background information which will help them to take stock of the present situation.

2.   WHERE DO WE WANT TO BE?

This will involve objective-setting and the mapping out of strategy which will take place within the framework of guidelines.

3.   HOW DO WE GET THERE?

The means of achieving aims and objectives will be spelt out in strategic and operational plans.

4.   HOW ARE WE DOING?

Some form of monitoring will be necessary to ensure that the intended results of the planning process are being achieved.

FIGURE III

NHS PLANNING IS A LEARNING PROCESS − − − −

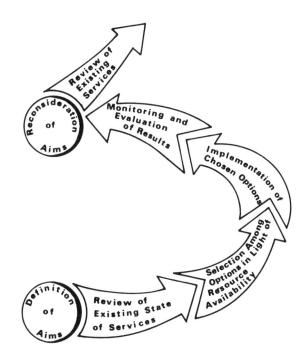

FIGURE IV
THE FLOW OF GUIDELINES AND PLANS IN THE NHS

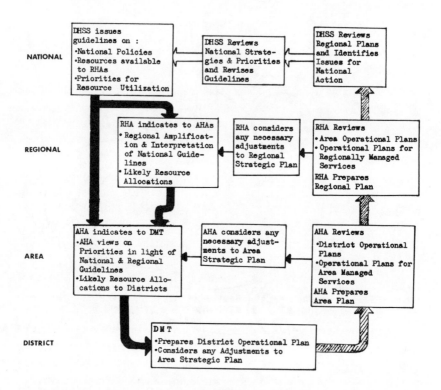

REFERENCES

The NHS Planning System, DHSS, June 1976. See also Kenneth Lee and Anne Mills, *Policy-Making and Planning the the Health Sector.* Croom-Helm, London, 1982 and Michael Butts, Doreen Iriving and Christopher Witt, *Principles to Practice,* Nuffield Provincial Hospitals Trust, London, 1981.

Management Arrangements for the Reorganised National Health Service, HMSO, London, 1972, p. 10.

The Hospital Plan for England and Wales, HMSO, London, 1962.

Amitai Etzioni, *Mixed-scanning: A "Third" Approach to Decision-making,* Public Administration Review, December 1967.

Ottawa-Carleton Regional District Health Council Planning Programme, *Planning Health Services in Ottawa-Carleton,* Ottawa, OCRDHC, 1978.

Eric Miller and Michael Norris, *Planning Processes for Medical Education and the Health Services in London,* The Lancet, October 18, 1980.

Harlan Cleveland, *Into the Eighties—Together,* Aspen Institute for Humanistic Studies, 1980.

Chapter Four

Old Beliefs and New Doubts in Health Care Policy in Europe

GILBERTO MURARO

Introduction

The evolution of health care systems in most European countries from the beginning of this century up to a few years ago, seemed to follow a very definite pattern: from private medicine (private supply and private demand, with price discrimination and charity) to public insurance (that is, public support for demand within some compulsory insurance schemes, with private supply) and, finally, to full public financing and supply (i.e., with the public authority assuming strict control also on the quantity, quality, and prices of supply, following the seminal model of the British National Health Service). The creation of the national health service in Italy, starting from January 1, 1979, and modelled exactly on the British system, seemed an additional proof of that evolutionary law.

In the last few years, however, there appeared symptoms which have led many people to doubt that full public financing and supply will be the stable structure of the health sector.

In order to assess correctly how likely a reverse in trend is, we will first recall briefly the theoretical reasons in favor of public medicine; next the evolution of European health systems in the last twenty years will be mentioned, and finally comments will be made on some new developments that are at the origin of the present doubts about the future of the European health care systems.

From Private to Public Systems of Health Care

1. The reasons in theory

The essential reasons in favor of public medicine may be described as follows:

   a) Health care is a "merit good" and society can neither accept that an income constraint forbids poor people from getting the necessary care, nor can it fully rely on private charity and doctors' benevolence;
   b) The health care sector is far away from the competitive model and it cannot become competitive because of its structure and of consumers'

ignorance; so, public support of demand risks being jeopardized by suppliers through an increase in prices without any significant growth of the real supply;

c) Since a bilateral monopoly is better than a one-sided monopoly, public interference on the supply side, at least for fixing prices, is correct; but then, organizational reasons and various social goals may well lead the public authority to take full responsibility for the supply [Arrow, 1963; Muraro, 1979].

2. Evolution in Europe, 1962-1974

The good theoretical grounds of the model of public supply may explain the widespread approval of academic students towards the rapid growth of public medicine that has taken place in Europe in the last few decades.

Of course, the general term public medicine covers many different national schemes. Consider, for instance, the financing of the services. On one hand, there is tax-based financing, which may rely mainly on national taxation (as in Ireland and the United Kingdom), or on local taxation (as in the Scandinavian countries); and on the other hand, there is insurance-based financing as in South and Central Europe, which may also be based on few national schemes as in France or on many independent sickness funds under government regulation as in Germany and in Benelux. There are in addition many other combinations and variations of the fundamental systems [W.H.O., 1981, Chapter 7].

On the other hand, the difference must not be overemphasized, because the insurance contributions are commonly a percentage of salary, paid by employers and employees, usually up to a maximum ceiling, that is, effectively an earmarked payroll tax.

Something similar can be said for the organization of the health care system, where the role of central and local government and of other collective institutions may differ between countries; but that does not prevent us from making a clearcut distinction between public and private organizations.

With this in mind, let us look then at some figures. An accurate study of the O.E.C.D. [1977] allows us to follow the growth of public medicine between 1960/63 and 1972/75 through the ratio between current expenditure on health and trend-GNP.

As shown in Table 1, the European average of that ratio was:

	1960/63	1972/75	Increase
Total	4.0	5.9	1.9
Public	2.9	5.0	2.1
Public/Total	72.5%	84.7%	12.2%

TABLE 1

Current Expenditure for Health as % of Trend-GNP

	% of Trend-GNP 1972/75		1960/63–1972/75 Growth (Income Points on GNP)		Income Elasticity of Current Public Expenditure
	Total	Public	Total	Public	
Austria	5.7	3.7	1.1	0.8	1.27
Belgium (1965/74)	5.0	4.2	0.7	1.1	1.37
Denmark	–	6.5	–	2.7	1.73
Finland (1962/75)	5.8	5.5	1.9	3.0	2.19
France	6.9	5.3	2.2	2.2	1.72
Germany (Fed.) (1960/74)	6.7	5.2	2.2	2.7	2.09
Greece (1962/75)	3.5	2.3	0.7	0.5	1.28
Ireland	6.2	5.4	2.4	2.6	1.90
Italy	6.0	5.2	2.1	2.3	1.78
Netherlands (1963/72)	7.3	5.1	2.9	2.3	1.85
Norway (1962/73)	5.6	5.3	2.3	2.9	1.38
Sweden (1963/74)	7.3	6.7	2.6	3.1	1.85
United Kingdom (1962/75)	5.2	4.6	1.3	1.4	1.24
AVERAGE	5.9	5.0	1.9	2.1	1.67
U.S.A. (1960/74)	7.4	3.0	2.4	1.8	2.54

Source: O.E.C.D., *Public Expenditure on Health*, Paris, 1977.

In other words, the share of resources devoted to health care increased considerably in the period observed, and the increase is almost entirely due to public medicine which extended greatly both the share of population covered and the share of health services provided, and thus accounted at the end of the period for 85 percent of the total health expenditure.

It is also worthwhile recalling that current expenditure for health was, in the same period, the most dynamic item within current public expenditure, notwithstanding the great increase of the latter. Health expenditure showed indeed an income elasticity of 1.7, much higher than the corresponding values for social public expenditure (health, education, and income maintenance) and for total public expenditure, which amounted, respectively, to 1.4 and 1.2 [O.C.D.E., 1978].

It is amazing to note that—in comparison with the European average figures—in the United States the income elasticity of public health expenditure was, in the same period, remarkably higher (2.5 against 1.7), the increase of the ratio between that expenditure and the GNP was less (1.8 against 2.1), the value of that ratio at the end of the period was considerably smaller (3.0 against 5.0), and, finally, the ratio of total health expenditure to GNP was higher (7.4 against 5.9).

The meaning of such a comparison is two-fold: first, in the United States, even with quick growth in public interest in health, private expenditure rose even more quickly, so that the health sector in 1974 was still predominantly financed and organized on a private basis; second, the share of GNP devoted to health in the United States was, in 1974, the highest among the O.E.C.D. countries. The final remark is that most Europeans, including experts and politicians, did not give the highest score to the performance of the United States health care as seen from the point of view of the common citizen (which is compatible with the highest rank recognized to the quality of care given by top-level institutions in the United States). And that was an additional reason for believing in the rationale of the European model of health care, directed towards almost complete public supply.

The Recent Troubles of Public Health Care in Europe

In the second half of the 1970's, however, things started to change, and from then onwards, there has been an increasing number of criticisms on the excessive burden of public health expenditure.

Leaving aside the peculiarities of the various countries, one can detect two common and essential reasons for that change: the first is the critical economic situation which exacerbates both competition between public and private in the share of the national product and competition among the various items of expenditure within the public budget; the second is the increasing concern about the rationing problem posed by the positive and increasing price elasticity of demand for medical care, which, in some countries, is further aggravated by the perspective of an "over-supply" of doctors within the public service.

As far as the first reason is concerned, it is well known, both in America and in Europe, that taxpayers exert increasing resistance towards supporting the expansion or even the constancy of the high ratio of public expenditure to GNP reached in the first half of the 1970's: a resistance which has led in various countries to a change in government and has everywhere created a crisis of the welfare state. The paradox is that the economic crisis brings with it the necessity for increasing some components of public expenditure, namely, those directly linked with the bad performance of the economy, such as unemployment subsidies, support for retraining programs, incentives for work mobility, and aid for companies undergoing changes in activity. Thus, the traditional items, like health care, are under pressure from both sides.

As for the second reason it is worthwhile recalling that, following many convincing testimonials, the architects of public medicine in Great Britain—and their fellows in other European countries—sincerely believed that the demand for health care was almost rigid to prices up to the point which caused an income constraint, so that public health care—once the income constraint had been eliminated—would face a once-only explosion of the formerly repressed demand; but, after that, there would not be any menace of an ongoing expansion of the demand. Therefore, after the first period of social medicine, the possible excess of demand would have been easily eliminated by a socially and technically acceptable rationing device, namely, by the judgement of the doctor who would decide only on the basis of the comparative real needs of his patients.

After a few decades, all these generous beliefs have appeared utopic. Thanks to the success of medical science against many serious illnesses and thanks to increasing wealth, nowadays a large part of demand for health care has a positive and increasing price elasticity. On the other hand, it has been demonstrated that in the utility function of doctors—as for any other people—money plays an important role. Finally, account must be taken of the fact that the expansion of health care brings advantages to the pharmaceutical industry, hospital equipment industry, and bureaucracy, not to speak of political interests connected wtih a highly labor-intensive industry like health care.

In such a framework there is no satisfactory device for rationing. The patients push their autonomous demand for the services of family doctors up to the point of zero marginal utility, since zero is the price they pay;

on the other hand, the family doctor who must decide the rest of the story—
in order to appease the patient, to reduce the time for visits, to become
morally a creditor towards the generous pharmaceutical industry—will never
deny the prescription of some drugs or some specialized analysis. From that,
it is a short step to congestion in laboratories and hospitals and to systematic
rationing through waiting time and quality deterioration.

All this means that there is continual pressure for increasing public expenditure without ever fully satisfying demand. It is the basic "inconsistency"
that James Buchanan already underlined in 1965 in relation to the British
National Health Service and that seems to apply to most European health
care systems in the 1970's: on one hand, citizens, as taxpayers who act
collectively in the political area, are not willing to approve unlimited public
expenditure for health, because they have to think of competing social
goals; on the other hand, citizens, as patients who act individually, push
their demands far beyond the limits implicit in the original endowment
given to public medicine.

The perspective outlined above is aggravated in some countries by the
menace of overmanning in the medical profession. Worry in this regard is often
voiced, for instance, in Germany and Belgium; but it is in Italy that the
phenomenon has already assumed dramatic proportions. For many years,
Italy had had the highest relative endownment of doctors. In 1975, for instance, the number of doctors per 10,000 population was 20.5, just a little
higher than the German figure of 19.9, but considerably higher than the
European Community average of 16.0 [Abel-Smith & Maynard, 1979; Maynard, 1981]. After 1975, however, Germany put more restrictions on entry
into the medical faculties, but Italy did not. Thus, the forecast is that, in
1988, only five years from now, Italy will have 42.3 doctors per 10,000
population. That will bring inevitably the following consequences: 1) decrease of doctors in the social-economic scale; 2) enlarged enrollment of
young doctors within the public service who will, however, be kept in relatively low professional and economic positions, thus creating dissatisfaction
and conflict; 3) squeeze of the expenditure for investment and consumption
within the public service, in order to make room for the enlarged expenditure for manpower, given the difficulties of enlarging the total public budget
for health; 4) as a consequence of greater conflict and fewer resources, we
may also forecast a decrease in quality of treatment, at least at the level of
subjective perception by the patients, which will induce some of them to
look for private medicine. In conclusion, overmanning is definitely bringing
enlarged expenditure, without assuring better medical care.

Contemporary Cost Containment

The rising expenditure for public medicine and the decreasing willingness of taxpayers to pay for it have induced all European countries to strengthen cost containment measures. Following a recent review made by the European Regional Office of the World Health Organization [W.H.O., 1981], these measures may be grouped under three headings:

a) Planning. Directed, on one hand, to determining the level and distribution of regional investment, and sometimes to fixing the future supply of medical and paramedical staff, and, on the other hand, to exploring cheaper strategies of care, such as expanded community care and cheaper institutional services (for instance, nursing homes in Denmark, France, Germany, Netherlands, and houses for the elderly in Belgium and France) to avoid prolonged and unjustified stays in acute hospitals;

b) Demand and Control. For instance, by imposing referral rules to patients as far as the access of specialists is concerned (Ireland and United Kingdom) or by providing guidelines and indicators to administrators and clinicians, in order to improve the cost-efficiency and cost-effectiveness of daily decisions;

c) Financial Control. This is the most effective, at least in the short run, given the technical lag of the effects of planning and given the widespread resistance of the medical profession towards use control or whatever may limit doctors' clinical freedom.

The financial measures include, first of all, cuts in capital spending, which is the least politically damaging option in the short term, but may create serious long-term problems.

As for the larger current expenditure, in the countries with closed-end budgets like Denmark, United Kingdom and Italy, the cuts derive from unilateral decisions by the government, like cuts in capital spending though with greater political reaction. For countries with open-end budgets, the control must in some way be negotiated between the parties involved in order to avoid that a delay in updating fee schedules be compensated by increasing use levels which are decided by doctors. As a matter of fact, such voluntary agreements between the public authority and doctors' associations, for instance, on the permissible growth of total fee payments, seem to work well in Germany and Switzerland. Instead, Italy has preferred to switch to a system of capitation payments for ambulatory care.

Finally, in most countries, there is a growing interest in private finance within public medicine. In this regard, let us look at the picture of some years ago given by the already-mentioned survey [W.H.O., 1981, pp. 41-2]:

> The most widespread, wholly private, direct payments are for over-the-counter (non-prescribed) drugs. This is the case in all countries. Wholly private payments for health services *per se* are mainly for services not covered by public funds, and for which private cover is limited or ex-

pensive (e.g., dentistry and opthalmic services) or payments by the un-
insured who have opted out or are not entitled to cover (for example,
maternity cases insured less than 270 days in Switzerland). Direct part
payment (co-payment or co-insurance) for services and products otherwise covered is widespread and varied. The main forms include: co-payment of a fixed amount per item of service or claim (e.g., prescription
drug charges in the Federal Republic of Germany and the United Kingdom), direct payment of a percentage of the bill as used for a wide range
of services in France, and direct payment of a given deductible amount
per claim or per year, only the remainder being covered by the sickness
fund or health service (as in Switzerland or with the *ticket modérateur*
in France). The commonest incidence of direct part payments is for
services such as ambulatory medical care, laboratory tests and prescriptions drugs. Where part payment is required, the proportion or amount
varies (e.g., 10 percent ambulatory care costs and all costs above the insured ceiling in Switzerland; 60 percent of less important drugs in France;
a nominal fee for hospital care in Finland).

Now, we are not able to update exactly the picture, but from much partial
information we have derived a firm belief that private financing in Europe is
increasing its role: both as a result of the development of private medicine in
consequence of budget constraints in public supply, and of the changing pattern of financing within public medicine.

For the latter aspect, Italy may again be a good case-study. A recent law
has increased the existing co-payments for prescribed drugs, both increasing
the level and coverage of fees and reducing the social groups exempted; and
in addition it has introduced percentage co-payments for clinical tests and
also a fixed sum for each prescription. There is a widespread forecast that,
in the near future, a co-payment for each day in the hospital may also be
introduced. This is advocated on two good grounds: 1) that the co-payment
system must be as broad as possible, in order to reduce the switch to free-of-
charge forms of care; 2) that it is worthwhile putting some co-payments even
on the segments of health care whose price elasticity is considered low, such
as hosptial stays, because in any case it reduces the political burden of general
taxation.

Co-payments, i.e., private financing within public medicine, are by themselves an incentive to private medicine. In addition, a policy of developing
private medicine may explicitly be pursued: this seems to be the case of
Great Britain and will probably be the case of Italy too, where the government is trying to enlarge the percentage of doctors enrolled on a part-time
basis, as a device to reduce public expenditure.

Perspectives

Now, how shall we judge such developments in health policy? At one
extreme, there are those who consider the welfare state already dead, and
that we are in Europe at the beginning of a reverse in trend which will sharply

reduce the scope and methods of public intervention in health care. At the other extreme are those who consider the recent deviation from the path followed in the past as a temporary adjustment to the adverse economic cycle, so that, after the recovery of the economy, the social forces will once again push towards public medicine. One can also put the European Office of the W.H.O. in this second group, at least judging by the conclusions of the above-mentioned survey [W.H.O., 1981, p. 85].

One would prefer to take an intermediate position. We do not think that we are going back to private medicine coupled with state intervention limited to lower-income social groups. But we do not think either that the present adjustments will disappear after the economic recovery of Western countries: we forecast that they will stay and further develop, so that we are going towards a new permanent equilibrium, with more space for competition and private financing but always within the fundamental model of public supply.

REFERENCES

B. Abel-Smith and A. Maynard, *The Organization, Financing, and Cost of Health Care in the European Community,* Commission of the European Communities, Social Policy Series, No . 36, Brussels, 1979.

K. J. Arrow, "Uncertainty and the Welfare Economics of Medical Care," *American Economic Review,* December 1963.

J. Buchanan, *The Inconsistencies of the National Health Service,* J.E.A., Occasional Papers, London, 1965.

A. Maynard, "The Inefficiency and Inequalities of the Health Care Systems of Western Europe," *Social Policy and Administration,* No. 2, Summer 1981, pp. 145-63.

G. Muraro, "Sistemi alternativi di organizzazione e finanziamento del settore sanitario e loro effetti sul benessere sociale," *Rivista Internazionale di Scienze Sociali,* 1969, pp. 439-508.

_____ , "La crescita della spesa sanitaria pubblica," *Rivista di Diritto Finanziario e Scienza delle Finanze,* XLI, No. 1, March 1982.

O.C.D.E., *Evolution des dépenses publiques,* Paris, 1978.

O.E.C.D., *Public Expenditure on Health,* Paris, 1977.

W.H.O., World Health Organization, Regional Office for Europe, *Health Services in Europe,* Third Edition, Copenhagen, 1981.

Chapter Five

Reforming the U.S. Health Care Financing System

CAROLYNE K. DAVIS

Introduction

This paper examines the basic structural problems facing the Federal health care financing programs of Medicare and Medicaid. In FY 1984 Federal spending on these programs will total $85 billion, 9.3 percent of the Federal Budget and 2.4 percent of the Gross National Product.

This paper analyzes the causes of these increases in the context of the underlying financing, benefit, and reimbursement features of the Medicare and Medicaid programs, and the overall U.S. health sector. The difficult social and policy choices underlying solutions to the health care cost problem are discussed and potential policy measures are analyzed. The paper is organized into four parts. First, the underlying structural characteristics of the U.S. health care industry are discussed. Second, the Federal financing programs of Medicare and Medicaid are described. Third, the factors responsible for increases in Medicare and Medicaid expenditures are enumerated, and their impacts on program financing are discussed. Fourth, both conceptual and basic policy approaches for dealing with the Federal health care financing problems are outlined.

The Health Care Industry

Health care is this country's third largest industry. It employs over seven million people and its resources include 7,000 hospitals, 19,000 nursing homes, and 450,000 practicing physicians. Health care spending has increased rapidly over the past 30 years and in FY 1981 represented 9.8 percent of gross national product and 12.2 percent of the Federal budget. In 1981, the nation spent $287 billion, or $1,225 per person, on health care. By 1990, total spending is projected to increase to $756 billion and comprise 12.0 percent of GNP.

In 1980, some 197 to 207 million individuals, 87 to 91 percent of the civilian U.S. population had some type of public or private health insurance coverage. Private insurance covered more than 174 million or 78 percent of the population. About 140 million of these individuals received coverage through employment based policies with employer contributions for premiums. About 96 percent of the elderly and about half of the poor were covered by Medicare and/or Medicaid.

In 1981 public (43 percent) and private (25 percent) insurance payments account for 68 percent of all health expenditures. However, the proportion of hospital costs paid by third parties is much larger than for nursing home or physician services. In 1980, 89 percent of hospital spending was paid for by third parties compared to 57 percent for nursing homes and 62 percent for physicians.

Health care expenditures are expected to continue their rapid rise because: (1) the population as a whole is aging and will consequently use more health care; (2) health care technologies are becoming increasingly sophisticated and expensive; and (3) health delivery and reimbursement systems provide few incentives for efficiency.

The rapid rise in health care expenditures has had a major economic impact on business, government, and the American public. These large increases have created financial hardships for individuals, raised taxes, and diverted funds from other economic uses.

Several characteristics of the health care industry insulate it from normal market forces and contribute to the rapid rise in health care expenditures. Widespread and often first-dollar insurance coverage from public and private sources reduces cost-consciousness by consumers and providers. The reimbursement procedures of both public and private insurers discourage the efficient use of resources. Provisions of the tax code distort normal demand and supply forces. Rapid technological advances, coupled with the medical ethic to preserve life at virtually any cost and generous reimbursement from public and private insurers, have led to the overutilization of new and expensive medical technologies. Consumer ignorance about health and medicine, bans on advertising, and the unavailability of price and quality information have made the consumer highly dependent on the decisions of medical care providers. Although the consumer of health care services generally makes initial contact with a provider, the amount of service that a patient receives is usually determined by the provider.

Medicare and Medicaid

Largely in response to an inability of private health insurance markets to provide affordable coverage to the aged and the poor, in 1965 Congress enacted the Medicare and Medicaid programs. Implicit in these programs was the need for Federal subsidization of the costs of care for these groups of individuals.

Medicare is a Federal health insurance program for the aged and disabled. It covers approximately 26 million aged, 96 percent of all elderly, and 3 million disabled individuals. Medicare consists of two parts, a Hospital Insurance Program (Part A) and a Supplementary Medical Insurance Program (Part B).

All persons aged 65 or over who qualify for Social Security cash benefits and, (as of 1972) individuals who have been receiving Social Security disability benefits for 24 months or more, are automatically enrolled in Part A. Part A is financed by a 2.6 percent payroll tax shared equally by employers and employees. It covers 90 days of hospital care per spell-of-illness and allows an additional 60 days to be used over the beneficiary's lifetime. Part A also covers 100 skilled nursing facility days per spell-of-illness and an unlimited number of home health visits. Hospital services are subject to a deductible ($304 in CY 83) per hospital spell-of-illness and coinsurance for: days 61-90 of hospital care (one-fourth of the deductible); each of the 60 lifetime reserve days (one-half of the deductible); and for days 21-100 of skilled nursing facility care (one-eighth of the deductible). Part A providers of services are reimbursed directly by the program and generally cannot bill beneficiaries other than for applicable cost-sharing. Effective October 1, 1983, hospitals will be reimbursed on a prospectively established rate per case. Other Part A providers are reimbursed on the basis of their reasonable costs. Medicare Part A benefit payments in FY 1984 will be $44 billion.

Part B benefits are available on a voluntary basis to the disabled enrolled in Part A and to all individuals over 65 by payment of a monthly premium ($12.20 in CY 83). Premiums finance about 25 percent of program costs, with the remaining 75 percent coming from general revenues. Part B covers physician and other outpatient services, subject to a $75 annual deductible and 20 percent coinsurance. Part B practitioners are reimbursed on the basis of their reasonable charges. However, practitioners can bill beneficiaries for amounts in excess of the program-determined reasonable charges. Medicare Part B benefit payments in 1984 will be $20 billion.

Private insurance companies act as fiscal agents, performing most claims processing and administrative functions for both Parts A and B. Fiscal agents are reimbursed for their reasonable costs incurred in providing these administrative services. Medicare expenditures for administrative costs will be $1.4 billion in 1984.

Medicaid is a State-administered, Federal matching grant program that finances medical services for certain categories of low-income individuals, primarily those eligible to receive cash payments under (1) the Aid to Families with Dependent Children (AFDC) program and (2) the Supplemental Security Income (SSI) program for the aged, blind, and disabled. In addition, 30 States have exercised the option to extend coverage to "medically needy" individuals who meet the SSI or AFDC categorical criteria but whose incomes are slightly above the welfare standards or who have incurred substantial medical expenses. An estimated 22.5 million individuals are Medicaid recipients. The Federal share of program costs averages 56 percent, is financed from general revenues, and ranges from 50 percent in the highest per capita income States to 77 percent in the lowest per capita income states.

Federal law mandates that states cover hospital, physician, skilled nursing facility, family planning, home health, laboratory, x-ray, rural health clinic, and nurse midwife services for all eligible recipients, and early and periodic screening, diagnosis, and treatment (EPSDT) services for children under 21. States may also provide a variety of optional services, including intermediate care facility services and prescription drugs. States may limit the amount, duration, and scope of services. Coinsurance may be imposed only in limited instances and the amounts must be nominal. States have considerable discretion in setting reimbursement rates for medical care providers. Providers who participate in the program must accept Medicaid-determined reimbursements as payment in full and cannot bill beneficiaries. Federal and State Medicaid benefit payments will be an estimated $36.4 billion in 1984, of which $20 billion is Federal.

States may process claims themselves or contract with private organizations. Nearly half of the states currently contract out all or part of the claims processing functions. Medicaid administrative expense will be over $1 billion in 1984.

In 1981, while spending by all levels of government accounted for 40 percent of all personal health care spending, Medicare and Medicaid expenditures represented 29 percent. The market share that Medicare and Medicaid expenditures represent varies considerably by type of service. Medicare and Medicaid accounted for 36 percent of all hospital spending, 23 percent of all physician spending, 51 percent of all nursing home spending, and 8 percent of all spending on drugs and sundries for patients outside institutions.

The type of services paid for by Medicare and Medicaid differ greatly. Medicare primarily pays for acute care services, with 72 percent of Medicare spending going for hospital services, 22 percent for physician services, and 1 percent for skilled nursing facilities. Currently, the largest component of Medicaid is long term care with 40 percent for nursing home services, 36 percent for hospital services, and 9 percent for physician services. The bulk of both Medicare and Medicaid spending is for institutional services.

Medicare and Medicaid Expenditures

Medicare and Medicaid expenditures have been increasing at rapid rates. Medicare spending increased from $14.8 billion in FY 75 to $66.3 billion in FY 84, a 17.6 percent compound annual rate. Similarly, Federal Medicaid spending increased from $7.1 billion in FY 75 to $21.2 billion in FY 84, a 12.6 percent compound annual rate. In real per capita terms, between

1975 and 1984, Medicare expenditures increased at a 4.4 percent compound annual rate and Medicaid expenditures increased at a 3.2 percent compound annual rate.

In order to design appropriate policies to deal with the root causes of the current expenditure problem, it is important to know the extent to which the current levels of spending for particular services are due to: (1) changes in the number of people eligible to receive services (population), (2) changes in the amount and type of services received per person (utilization and intensity), and (3) changes in the cost per unit of service (price). This information is useful in evaluating whether reimbursement limitations for particular medical care providers, utilization review of particular services, specific benefit reductions, and/or eligibility limitations for particular beneficiary groups would be the most appropriate way to deal with the current expenditure problem. In general, between 1975-1984 price increases accounted for about half of the increases in Medicare and Medicaid spending. Increases in utilization/intensity of services accounted for another 30 to 40 percent, and population increases accounted for the remainder.

Several structural features of Medicare and Medicaid contribute to these rapid expenditure increases. These same characteristics are also inherent in most private health insurance policies. They include the reasonable cost and reasonable charge reimbursement systems, the structure of the Medicare Part A benefit package, beneficiaries' complete "freedom-of-choice" of providers, and the open-ended nature of Medicare and Medicaid financing.

Prior to October 1983, hospitals were reimbursed under Medicare and Medicaid on the basis of reasonable costs. Physicians under Medicare (and about half of the State Medicaid programs) are reimbursed on the basis of reasonable charges. Under these reimbursement systems, the higher the costs or charges, the higher program reimbursements. In other words, there are no incentives for price competition. These methods have proven to be highly inflationary, since increases in medical care prices and increased utilization/intensity of services have been almost fully reflected in Medicare and Medicaid hospital and Medicare physician payments. The Social Security Amendments of 1983 require the Medicare program to pay hospitals on a prospective rate per case basis starting in October 1983. This system should mitigate future inflationary "price" effects on Medicare hospital outlays. However, the system does create incentives for hospitals to increase admissions, and hence the impact of prospective payment on utilization/intensity will have to be closely monitored.

The structure of the Medicare Part A benefit package does not encourage efficient utilization of hospital services on the part of either beneficiaries or providers. Once the hospital deductible is met, there is no cost-sharing until the 61st day of hospitalization, when heavy cost-sharing is imposed. Thus, there are no financial incentives for efficient utilization of services during short stays. At the same time, beneficiaries do not have catastrophic protection during long hospitalizations.

Under both Medicare and Medicaid, beneficiaries can receive services from any participating hospital or physician, regardless of the cost of that provider. Since Medicare and Medicaid generally pay most providers' costs and charges and beneficiary cost-sharing is limited, there are few financial incentives for beneficiaries to choose lower cost, more efficient providers.

Medicare and Medicaid expenditures are essentially open-ended. Medicare is basically an insurance program which pays for all covered services rendered to beneficiaries. Payments flow out of trust funds financed by payroll taxes on the working population, premium contributions of the elderly, and general revenues.

Medicaid financing is also open-ended. The Federal government matches State Medicaid funds with no overall limit. This financing system, coupled with state discretion on income eligibility standards, groups covered, and benefits, has resulted in tremendous variation in eligibility standards and benefits among states. Some states have elected to provide generous benefits, while others have provided only minimal benefits.

The Medicare and Medicaid programs have had a significant impact in terms of the locus of financing of health care. While Medicare and Medicaid are credited with significantly improving access to health care for the poor and elderly, these successes have been achieved as a result of substantial increases in the funding commitments of Federal, state, and local governments. In 1965, 70 percent of health expenditures for the elderly were financed by private sources, while 30 percent was from public sources. By 1981, these percentages had been completely reversed with public payments accounting for 64 percent (Medicare 45, Medicaid 14, and other public programs 5), while private payments accounted for 36 percent. In real per capita terms, health expenditures for the elderly have doubled, while real per capita private payments for the elderly (excluding Part B premium payments) have increased by about 4 percent. In other words, the elderly are getting twice as many services but paying about the same amount for them as they did in 1965.

An alternative way of measuring the value of Medicare insurance benefits is to compare the value of the benefits relative to the beneficiary's contributions. In the case of Medicare Part A benefits for a male reaching age 65 in 1982 who has paid in the maximum possible payroll tax contributions since the inception of the program in 1966, the present value of the future health benefits stream is 7.5 times his interest compounded payroll tax contributions. If this individual has a non-working wife, the return is 17 times his contribution level. Assuming the employer's equal payroll tax contribution is shifted onto the employee, these returns are halved. Nevertheless, Medicare Part A is an extremely good investment.

A similar situation occurs under the premium and general revenue financed Supplementary Medical Insurance Trust Fund. The share of premium costs has shifted significantly since the inception of the program. Part B premiums were originally designed to cover half of the costs of the program with general revenues covering the other 50 percent. However, due to limitations on annual premium increases, inadvertent premium freezes, and coverage of the disabled in 1972, the current Part B premium covers only 25 percent of program costs for the aged and 22 percent of total program costs including the disabled.

The high rates of increase in Medicare and Medicaid benefits and the financing shifts to Federal and state governments are severely affecting the financing bases of these programs. For Medicare, the Hospital Insurance Trust Fund, financed largely by payroll taxes, is under severe pressure as expenditure increases engendered by the aging of the population, increased utilization/intensity of services, and inflationary increases in medical care costs far outstrip the revenues generated by the current payroll tax structure and relatively smaller working population. By 1984, expenditures will exceed revenues, and under the most plausible economic assumptions, the Medicare Hospital Insurance Trust Fund will be unable to meet its obligations in 1990. The financing picture is even worse over the 25 year period 1983-2008. To maintain solvency of the Hospital Insurance Trust Fund over this period, payroll taxes revenues will need to increase by 43 percent or expenditures will need to be reduced by 30 percent. Similarly, the Federal general revenue contribution to finance Part B will increase from its current level of 75 percent. This will occur because future beneficiary premium increases are limited to Social Security cash benefit increases while program costs increase at higher rates based on medical care inflation and utilization/intensity changes.

While historical 15 percent increases in Medicaid spending have recently been reduced to less than 10 percent, states are facing problems both in terms of reduced revenues to finance their programs and increased demand for services provided by such programs.

Federal Financing Issues

Basic policy reforms to insure an appropriate allocation and distribution of health care resources need to focus on both the Federal programs as well as the overall delivery system. The Federal health programs must provide for reimbursement arrangements and benefit structures that encourage efficient use and provision of services. Financing mechanisms must assure sufficient revenue to cover program costs. At the same time, impediments to private markets' working should be removed. The Reagan Administration has developed a series of proposals to encourage efficient consumer and provider behavior and to promote the working of market forces to contain costs.

Basic approaches to reducing expenditures include limiting prices paid for services, reducing utilization, and reducing program benefits or the number of individuals eligible for benefits. Revenues can be increased through various financing mechanisms.

With regard to reimbursement reforms, the 1983 Social Security Amendments made a fundamental change in the way Medicare will reimburse hospitals. Starting in October 1983, Medicare will reimburse hospitals on the basis of a prospectively established rate per case. For each of 467 diagnosis related groups, a prospectively established price will be determined. More complex diagnoses will have higher prices. Thus hospitals treating sicker patients will receive higher reimbursements. Since hospitals will be paid the prospective rate irrespective of their costs, hospitals which provide services in a cost-effective manner will earn financial rewards, while those that are inefficient will incur losses. Hospitals will have incentives to specialize in the kinds of care they can provide efficiently and by knowing in advance their Medicare reimbursements, they will be able to plan efficiently. Currently, some eight state Medicaid programs reimburse hospitals on a prospective basis.

While prospective payment to hospitals will provide efficiency in the hospital sector, inefficient reimbursement methods in the physician sector are a significant problem. While services by physicians are only 20 percent of all health spending, physicians account for over 70 percent of expenditures. Physicians' decisions on use of hospital services, diagnostic testing, etc., are critical determinants of overall health expenditures. Medicare, many private insurers, and about half of the state Medicaid programs reimburse physicians on the basis of their customary, prevailing, and reasonable charges. Under this system, program reimbursements are based on individual and collective physician charging patterns. This system has proven to be inflationary and resulted in urban-rural, specialty, and cognitive versus procedural payment imbalances. This system also encouraged inpatient over outpatient treatment, is complex to administer, and is confusing to beneficiaries and providers. Moreover, current Medicare participation rules allow those physicians who are not willing to accept Medicare physician payment rates as payment in full, to "extra-bill" beneficiaries for differences between Medicare reimbursement levels and physicians' actual charges.

While the physician reimbursement area is perhaps the most critical in terms of controlling health care costs, it is technically the most difficult to reform. First, there are some 450,000 physicians and, there are no complete data on physician practice patterns and billing. Second, behavioral information on physician responses to alternative reimbursement and participation systems is extremely limited. Third, from a governmental perspective, the Federal impact on overall physician spending is quite limited, since Medicare accounts for only about 17 percent of all physician spending and Medicaid is 5 percent. Fourth, physicians can circumvent Medicare reimbursement limitations by directly billing patients. Fifth, physicians can offset price constraints by increasing utilization of their services. Thus, while alternative physician payment reforms, such as fee schedules, and various physician participation systems are possible, for the reasons outlined above it is difficult to assure that such system can assure access, control costs, and provide incentives for efficiency. Nevertheless, in order to get a handle on the 16 to 20 percent annual increases in Medicare physician expenditures, the Reagan Administration is proposing a one year freeze in Medicare physician reimbursement levels while basic reforms are developed.

Utilization reductions are a second method for containing health care costs. Since increases in utilization/intensity of services account for over 30 percent of the increases in Medicare and Medicaid expenditures and since physician and hospital price controls provide incentives for increased services, utilization controls are an essential ingredient of any cost containment strategy. Utilization reductions can be achieved by promoting beneficiary cost-sharing and increasing enrollments in alternative delivery systems.

The current Medicare cost-sharing structure does not promote efficient use of resources since once the Part A deductible is met, there is no cost-sharing until the 61st day of hospitalization. On the other hand, there is no catastrophic protection for beneficiaries with long hospital stays. Cost-sharing can reduce health care costs by reducing utilization and does so without any regulatory intervention. The Reagan Administration has developed a proposal to require cost-sharing for short stays while providing catastrophic protection for individuals with long hospitalizations. This proposal will provide incentives for efficient utilization of services while at the same time providing beneficiaries with coverage for unbudgetable catastrophic expenses.

The Reagan Administration has also proposed to require nominal copayments, $1-2, for use of hospital and physician services by Medicaid beneficiaries. Currently there are no copayments on these services. The level of the payments is nominal in recognition of the limited ability of Medicaid beneficiaries to pay. The proposal is designed to provide Medicaid beneficiaries with the correct incentives for appropriate use of services.

Alternative health delivery systems, organized systems of care that compete with fee-for-service practices, are another means of controlling health care costs both through the utilization and price side. Health maintenance organizations (HMO's) are the most familiar alternative delivery arrangement. Such plans place providers at financial risk for excess program costs. They have been effective largely by reducing hospital use. The Reagan Administration is attempting to foster use of alternative delivery systems through its Medicare voucher proposal. Under this proposal, the Medicare program will pay 95 percent of the costs under the normal fee-for-service system to an organization which provides the Medicare benefit package and meets certain other standards established by the Secretary. If the organization's costs are less than the 95 percent Medicare payment, the organization and/or beneficiary can keep the difference. This proposal provides incentives for cost-effective alternative delivery arrangements, promotes competition, and relies on private market forces to control costs.

State Medicaid programs are attempting to control utilization through authorities provided in the 1982 Tax Equity and Fiscal Responsibility Act. In particular, states can apply for waivers of Federal requirements on beneficiary freedom-of-choice and can obtain Federal waivers which allow them to provide normally uncovered home and community-based services. Over 13 states have been granted waivers of beneficiary freedom-of-choice and 33 states have been granted home and community-based service waivers. Such waivers promote effective case management systems, use of lower cost facilities, and provide incentives for substitution of non-institutional for more expensive nursing home care.

A third method of containing program costs is to reduce benefits or to change eligibility rules. Given the basic nature of many Medicare and Medicaid services, benefit reductions are difficult to design. However, given the current government fiscal crisis, reductions in over-used or less important services could be considered. Eligibility for services could be delayed, or groups entitled to coverage could be narrowed. Given the vulnerable populations covered by Medicare and Medicaid, eligibility and benefit reductions for those truly in need of services are not desirable choices. Since such changes do virtually nothing to restructure incentives or reform the health care delivery system, utilization and reimbursement options which encourage efficiency and financing options which have the potential for more equitable sharing of program costs are preferable choices.

A fourth method of dealing with increasing health care costs is through financing changes. Such changes can apply to both private and public programs. The current tax treatment of employer contributions for private health insurance, in which employer contributions for employee health insurance are tax deductible business expenses but do not count as income to the employee, will cost the Federal government over $20 billion in FY 1984 in lost tax revenues. This is the second largest Federal health program, and its benefits are regressively distributed. Moreover, by subsidizing the cost of health insurance, tax subsidies create incentives for first dollar coverage, over-insurance, etc. They also insulate individuals from the impacts of rising health costs on insurance premiums. The Reagan Administration has proposed legislation to limit the amount of such contributions. Employer contributions in excess of the limits, $175 per month for family policies and $70 for individual policies, will be treated as earned income and subject to Social Security, income, and unemployment compensation taxes. This proposal is designed to promote overall health systems reform by reducing the current incentives for excessive insurance.

Financing changes can also be employed to improve the solvency of the Federal financing programs. Increased Federal revenues can be obtained through tax or premium increases. Revenue enhancements for Medicare could include increasing payroll, income, or Federal excise taxes. The Administration has proposed increasing the Medicare Part B premium from the current 25 percent of program costs for an aged individual to 35 percent through 2.5 percentage point increases in the premium between 1985 and 1988. Premium or tax changes have the advantage of spreading the additional financial burden over all beneficiaries or all income earning individuals, whereas cost-sharing changes impact on only users of services.

Since Medicaid recipients have low incomes, it is difficult to design premiums that produce significant revenues. Given the Federal-state nature of the program, tax changes need to be carefully designed. Similarly, changes in the matching formula have substantial effects on individual states, and hold harmless features tend to be quite expensive. Lastly, Medicaid financing could be substantially altered by the Federal government taking over complete responsibility for the program. However, the enormous differences in state Medicaid programs make federalization a very difficult undertaking.

The Administration's reforms are complimentary efforts to restrain costs through behavior changes and cost awareness for all parties in the health care system—providers, patients, and third-party payors. Nevertheless, it is apparent that the financing problems underlying Medicare in the long-run are so severe that additional reforms will be needed. The ultimate solution will require balancing equity, allocational, and basic political concerns. With regard to Medicaid, the Federal-state matching requirements, the new flexibilities given the states, and possible additional state flexibilities may be sufficient to finance the program at its currently relatively lower rates of growth. Nevertheless, the health care cost problem is far from solved, the solutions will not be easy.

Part Three

Strategic Planning and
Decision Making

Chapter Six

Business Segmentation and Competitive Economic Analysis

FREDERICK S. FINK

Introduction

The U.S. health care delivery system is undergoing fundamental change. Changing supply factors, the emergence of new delivery sites, and changing methods of reimbursement are forcing the traditional hospital to rethink its approach to health care delivery as well as the factors that drive a successful strategy. What was once an organization focused essentially on physician and community needs is becoming a price and service competitive business. In the future, the economics of service delivery can be expected to drive competitive advantage and success.

The emergence of price and service competition will require business planning techniques and analytical tools that are unfamiliar to most of the hospital industry today. The value of effective business segmentation and economic analysis of competitive position has been well established in the commercial sector. This paper reviews the environmental factors driving industry change, and explores several techniques for business segmentation and economic analysis that can assist hospitals to maintain their competitive position in the future. Examples are drawn from recent client assignments to support the suggested approaches to segmentation, economic analysis and strategy.

Environmental Developments

Environmental changes are forcing traditional hospital providers to develop strategies to compete on the basis of cost and convenience. While a number of factors influence the hospital sector, changing methods of reimbursement, physician supply factors, and new delivery entities are three key forces that will shape the future industry structure. These forces can be expected to lead to a more cost competitive industry. Failure to understand and respond to these changes could seriously threaten the viability of the hospital as we know it today.

Changing Reimbursement

Fundamental reimbursement changes are occurring in the amount, basis,

and source of payment. Budgeted funds available for Medicare and Medicaid
programs as well as the level of benefits provided will be cut substantially
in the future, as forewarned by the Tax Equity and Fiscal Responsibility
Act of 1982 (TEFRA, P.L. 97-248). Simply put, the government cannot
afford the continued growth in the share of GNP consumed by health care,
in excess of $280 billion and over 9.5 percent of GNP in 1981 (see Table 1).

TABLE 1
COMPARISON OF MAJOR COMPONENTS OF GNP — 1981

INDUSTRY SECTOR	1981 REVENUES (Dollars in Billions)	PERCENTAGE 1981 GNP	REAL GROWTH 1972 - 1981 (Constant 1972 Dollars in Billions)
HEALTH CARE	$283.8	9.5%	$61.7
FOOD	$275.8	9.2%	$33.3
CONSTRUCTION	$236.7	7.9%	$ 2.9
CHEMICALS	$180.0	6.0%	$39.4
TRANSPORTATION	$158.0	5.3%	$ 5.7

1981 Gross National Product = $2,995.1 Billion

Federal and state governments, in an effort to curtail ever-increasing costs,
are finally considering altering the payment basis, from a retrospective to
prospective system. For example, recently implemented changes in California's Medi-Cal program provide for direct contracts with selected area hospitals for all Medi-Cal eligible patients. Contract selection is based on price per
patient day bids submitted by interested hospitals. Legislation will also allow
commercial insurers in California to negotiate flat per-diem rate contracts
with selected hospitals within the next year.

On a national level, TEFRA mandates the department of Health and
Human Services to design and implement a new Medicare payment system
that eliminates cost-based retrospective reimbursement and promotes cost
efficiency. A prespective scheme based on pre-established rates for 356
diagnosis-related groups (DRG's) has been announced as the anticipated
approach, although the details of the program remain unresolved.

Whatever the eventual design of the Medicare program, Federal, state
and commercial reimbursers appear intent on purchasing services based
more on price and service rather than historical costs. The new system should
favor more efficient, lower cost providers and require hospitals to become
more cost competitive.

The implications of the new reimbursement procedures will be significant.

Failure to respond could be disastrous as witnessed by one San Francisco hospital that estimated it would lose 35 percent of its medical staff if it was not awarded a Medi-Cal contract [*Modern Health Care,* January 1983, p. 21].

Cost competition is also being driven by the other major purchaser of health services, the industrial employer. Through the support of HMO's and direct discount purchasing (Preferred-Provider Organizations) employers are taking an increasing interest in controlling health care costs by using their market and purchasing leverage. Over the next decade, the share of services purchased through traditional insurance mechanisms is likely to decline, substituted for by direct purchase contracting (HMO's and PPO's) on the part of major employers. In metropolitan markets, contract purchase of health services by HMO's and PPO's is expected to account for 15 percent or more of the total health market by 1990 [see Figure I].

FIGURE I
PROJECTED CHANGES IN PAYMENT SOURCES
HOUSTON, TEXAS
1980 – 1990

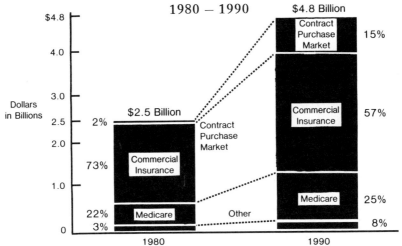

SOURCE: DHHS, Rice Center, BA&H

Physician Supply

Increases in physician supply across the U.S. are resulting in fundamental shifts in delivery settings and competition for the control of the value added structure.

As shown in Figure II, the supply of physicians is projected to continue to increase through the next decade at a rate exceeding the general population growth rate, resulting in a declining volume of patients per physician or market share over the next decade. As a result of this rapid increase in physician

FIGURE II
HISTORICAL AND PROJECTED CHANGE IN PHYSICIAN SUPPLY AND VISITS
1970 − 1990

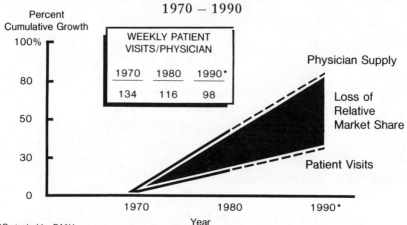

*Projected by BA&H
SOURCE: Profiles of Medical Practice, AMA; DHHS

FIGURE III
CHANGES IN PHYSICIAN SUPPLY AND REAL INCOME
1971 − 1990

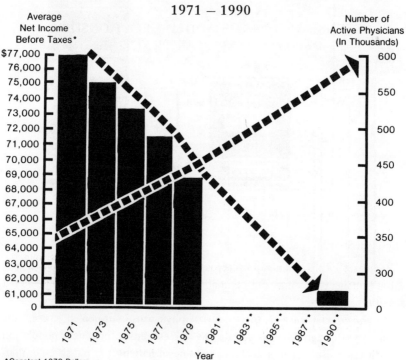

*Constant 1979 Dollars
**Projected by BA&H
SOURCE: Periodic Survey of Physicians, 1970 - 1980, AMA; U.S. DHHS

supply, a decline in real income per physician has been taking place over the last decade and is projected to continue [see Figure III].

The combination of increasing supply and declining real income is forcing physicians to consolidate into larger group practices that offer economic advantages both in terms of the expense of running a physician practice and advantages in terms of the value added per physician within a group [see Figures IV and V]. As these physician groups form, they represent significant economic entities that increasingly are competing with the traditional hospital for both diagnostic and therapeutic services that can be provided outside of the hospital. Because physicians groups are not subject to the same regulations as hospitals, they can develop services more rapidly, and usually provide them at a lower cost, giving them a significant competitive advantage in the delivery of diagnostic and therapeutic services.

Physicians are also developing urgent care centers and off-hour care facilities to capture patient volume that has traditionally been provided in the hospital emergency room. Priced below the cost of an emergency room but above the cost of a physician office visit, the urgent care centers provide an attractive and convenient setting for the consumer who does not have a strong primary physician relationship.

FIGURE IV
EXPENSE AND VALUE ADDED RELATIONSHIPS
IN PHYSICIAN GROUP PRACTICE

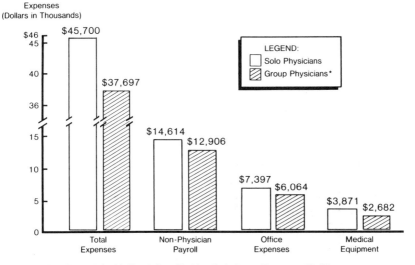

*Group Practice Defined As Three to Seven Physicians Sharing Income, Expenses, and Facilities
SOURCE: Periodic Survey of Physicians, 1978, AMA

FIGURE V

EXPENSE AND VALUE ADDED RELATIONSHIPS
IN PHYSICIAN GROUP PRACTICE

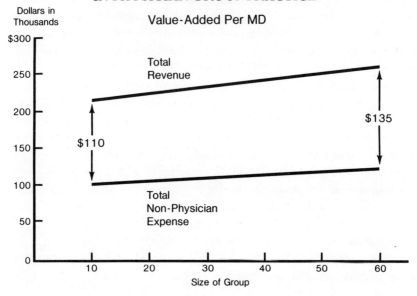

SOURCE: MGMA

New Delivery Mechanisms

The final major environmental factor influencing hospitals is the development of new modes of health care delivery that respond to consumer preference for convenient, low cost health services. A variety of new delivery settings are developing that offer lower cost, highly convenient medical care in direct competition with the traditional hospital. Most rapid growth has occurred in outpatient diagnostic and therapeutic services, typically delivered in a free-standing, easily-accessible, high traffic location such as a shopping center. Growth in these alternate delivery settings has been dramatic and is expected to continue over the next decade [see Figure VI and Table 2].

In some markets, the penetration of alternate delivery settings such as urgent care centers is considerable, as observed in the map in Figure VII for the Greater Houston area which already has over 70 free standing urgent care centers in the community.

In summary, an increasingly complex and fragmented delivery system has changed from the fairly simple physician's office, public clinic and hospital of the 1960's [see Figure VIII] to a complex, highly competitive delivery structure with numerous competitors targeting convenience or price niches that the traditional hospital has been unable or unwilling to serve [see Figure IX]. As this competition intensifies, traditional hospitals could be damaged without sound strategy formulation. As competition increases for routine, high volume, low cost procedures that can move outside of the hospital into the free-standing environment, hospitals will be left only with high cost, low volume, inpatient services that do not generate enough revenue to support the high fixed cost investment in the typical hospital. Unless hospitals learn to compete more effectively in the changing environment, we can anticipate a continuing erosion of their volume, capital base, and ability to deliver quality health care in the United States.

TABLE 2
HISTORICAL AND PROJECTED GROWTH
IN FREE-STANDING FACILITIES

	1979	1981	1983	1986	CAGR
Emergi-Centers	100	335	950	N/A	76%
Surgi-Centers	N/A	90	N/A	270	25%

SOURCE: National Association of Free-Standing Emergency Centers, 1982; **Same Day Surgery** November 1981.

FIGURE VI
HIGH GROWTH NON-HOSPITAL BUSINESS SEGMENTS

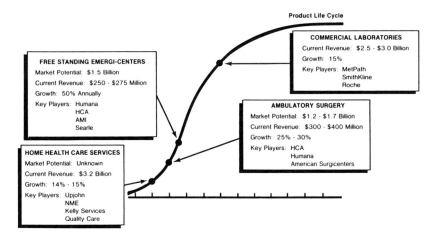

FIGURE VII
FREE-STANDING URGENT CARE CENTERS
IN HOUSTON, TEXAS
1982

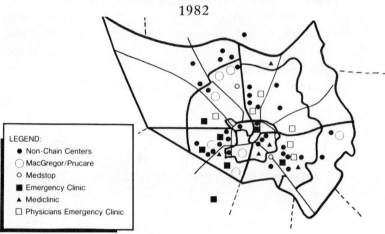

LEGEND:
- ● Non-Chain Centers
- ◯ MacGregor/Prucare
- ○ Medstop
- ■ Emergency Clinic
- ▲ Mediclinic
- □ Physicians Emergency Clinic

Strategic Planning Considerations

In order to compete effectively hospitals need to understand how to segment their businesses and the economics of delivery within each segment.
Given a more competitive and price sensitive industry in the future, hospitals need to begin to evaluate their activities using for-profit business concepts such as business segmentation, portfolio and economic analysis and

FIGURE VIII
U.S. HEALTH CARE DELIVERY STRUCTURE
1960

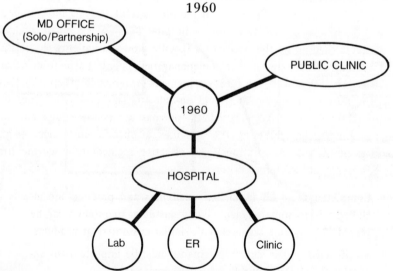

FIGURE IX

U.S. HEALTH CARE DELIVERY STRUCTURE
1980

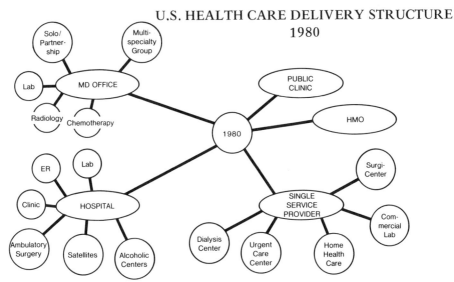

market coverage analysis. Although other unique industry factors will continue to drive demand for health services, utilization of appropriate analytical techniques can assist in the determination of which business segments to pursue and how to maintain a competitive advantage. The remainder of this paper focuses on selected valuable techniques for strategic planning in hospitals.

Business Segmentation

Business definition or segmentation is the first step in strategy formulation and may be the most difficult. It requires careful analysis and common sense. In terms of formal definition, a hospital business is a set of services or products that meets the needs of a specific group of patients/physicians with economics that are distinct and managerially controllable from other businesses. In other words, a business segment represents a group of activities that hospital management should be able to significantly influence or control through recruiting physicians, purchasing special equipment or other resources, or marketing the activities to specific customers (e.g., patients, physicians, corporations). An effective segmentation scheme for any business must fulfill three criteria:

- **Completeness** — All important customers and products are included within some segment. Every customer or product can be placed in only one segment with similar customers or products.

- **Significance** — The defined segments must be important for answering the strategic questions under consideration.

- **Practicality** — Each segment can be identified and analyzed in some practical manner at a reasonable cost and can be accessed through selective use of controllable resources.

As a general rule, hospital business segments fall into three broad categories:

- **Inpatient Services** — The bundled set of services (laboratory, nursing, surgery, radiology) that together treat specific clinical diagnoses requiring an inpatient stay.
- **Outpatient Services** — Those unbundled services within specific departments (laboratory, radiology, surgery) that can be provided on an outpatient basis.
- **Non-Patient Services** — Those activities such as laundry services, purchasing services or other commercial activities which a hospital can sell to other institutions to provide additional revenue.

Proper segmentation for any hospital will vary with the complexity of its markets and its product/service mix. Businesses should be identified based on a variety of factors including patient diagnosis, physician specialty, procedures performed, assets utilized, and payment source. Figure X presents possible business segments for three different types of institutions.

FIGURE X

HOSPITAL BUSINESS SEGMENTATION SCHEMES BY INSTITUTIONAL SIZE

SMALL COMMUNITY HOSPITAL	LARGE, DIFFERENTIATED COMMUNITY HOSPITAL	ACADEMIC MEDICAL CENTER
Generally Undifferentiable Clinical Resources	A Few Organized Clinical Departments With Differentiable Resources	Many Organized Clinical Departments With Differentiable Resources

Inpatient:
• General Acute Care — Medicine
• General Acute Care — Surgery
• Obstetrics
• Pediatrics
	Inpatient:
	• General Acute Care — Medicine
	• General Acute Care — Surgery
	• Routine Obstetrics
	• High Risk Obstetrics
	• Pediatrics
	• Cardiac Care
	• Oncology
	• Orthopedics
		Inpatient:
		• General Internal Medicine
		• Pulmonary
		• Endocrinology
		• Neurology
		• General Surgery
		• Gastroenterology
		• Neurosurgery
		• Vascular Surgery
		• Cardiac Care
		• Oncology
		  — Hematology
		  — Other
		• Burn Care
		• Others

Outpatient: Emergency Room Radiology Lab	Outpatient: Emergency Room Radiology Lab Ambulatory Surgery Physical Therapy Others	Outpatient: Emergency Room Ambulatory Surgery Specialty Clinics (e.g. pre-natal, oncology) Reference Lab
	Non-Patient Services: Laundry Shared Service Business	Non-Patient Services: Laundry EDP

Once an institution develops an effective business segmentation scheme, the hospital can then evaluate its portfolio of businesses along a variety of dimensions to assess its internal capabilities and its external competitive position. This step requires an effective cost finding and allocation system that allows the institution to determine the costs and profitability of services delivered by each production function or department within the hospital [see Figure XI]. These analyses can be of immediate value to the hospital administrator in identifying opportunities for greater price realization of productivity improvement.

Once departmental costs and profitability have been identified, these costs must be allocated to each of the business segments within the institution. For instance, if cardiac services represents an appropriate business segment, then all of the costs and revenues related to treating cardiac patients generated within the laboratory or radiology departments need to be allocated to that business segment. It should be noted that this type of cost accounting goes well beyond the level of sophistication of most cost accounting systems in the hospital today. Further, as we will discuss, cost analyses need to be developed based on true or actual costs, not cost as determined by the Medicare reimbursement methodology, which is manipulated to maximize reimbursement.

FIGURE XI
DEPARTMENTAL CONTRIBUTION

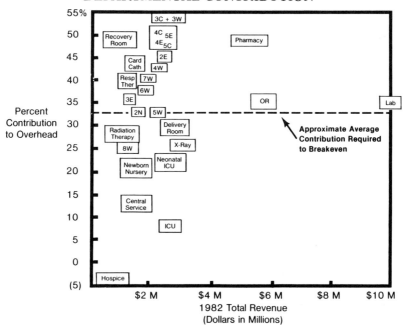

NOTE: Contribution = Total Department Revenues Minus Total Identifiable Department Expenses
SOURCE: BA&H

Once costs and revenues have been allocated to each business segment, the segments can then be analyzed along a number of key strategic variables. Possible variables to include in the assessment include growth versus percentage of cost based revenue [see Figure XII] or growth versus profitability by program [see Figure XIII]. Other key variables to assess in terms of each business segment include the volume of services, demographic characteristics of the market served, physician specialty requirements, potential barriers to entry, intensity of competition, and price/service/convenience/quality tradeoffs in terms of the purchase decision. Examples of how business segmentation analysis can assist the hospital in strategy include:

- Determination of which businesses to curtail or increase based on profitability and market outlook in order to relieve overall capacity constraints.

- Determination of a bid for a contractual volume of services based on the actual costs of providing a specific service.

- Establishing a hospital-wide capital allocation system based on business attractiveness.

- Assessment of the implications of a major change in reimbursement on desired case mix.

FIGURE XII
PROGRAM SIZE AND PERFORMANCE CHARACTERISTICS

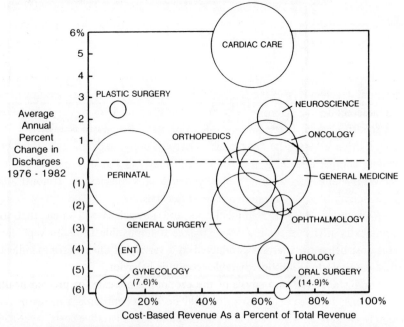

NOTE: Circle Size Indicates Relative Amounts of Revenue, 1982

FIGURE XIII

GROWTH AND PROFITABILITY BY PROGRAM

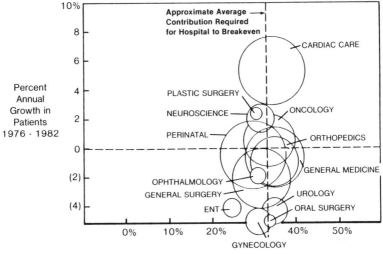

Percent Contribution to Corporate Overhead

NOTE: Contribution = Gross Program Charges Minus Expenses Associated With the Program
       Corporate Overhead = All Expenses Not Directly Associated With a Program Such As EDP Department,
       Finance, Materials Management, Interest on Bonds, etc.

Competitive Cost Position Analysis

Once the cost and profitability of the hospital's business segments have been assessed, they can then compare their cost position to their competitors and begin to reach conclusions about possible competitive advantage. This requires an understanding of cost and economic behavior in hospitals.

Analysis of the relationships between costs, scale and experience within hospital business segments indicates that hospital businesses exhibit predictable economic behavior that can be utilized to drive strategy. In a cost competitive arena, determination of a hospital's cost position relative to its competition is essential. Assuming relatively minor technology differences among competitors, relative cost position may be primarily determined by delivery volume or accumulated experience of a business as demonstrated by economy of scale or experience curve analysis.

While many hospital administrators and physicians will argue that the complexity of health care delivery makes it impossible to identify predictable cost behavior, analyses conducted in a variety of client settings indicate that hospitals do exhibit predictable economic behavior.

For instance, in an analysis of the economies of scale for prepaid health care plans, total costs per member year decline as enrollment increases due almost entirely to scale economies achieved in administrative costs. As shown in Figure XIV, medical costs and hospital costs tend to level out above en-

FIGURE XIV
ECONOMIES OF SCALE FOR PREPAID PLANS

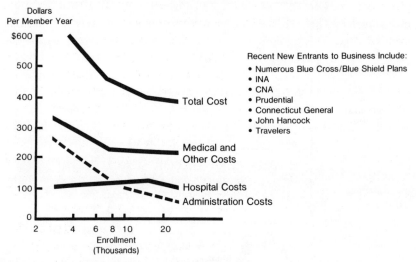

FIGURE XV
COMPARISON OF KAISER PLAN ADMINISTRATION
COSTS TO TYPICAL SMALL PLAN

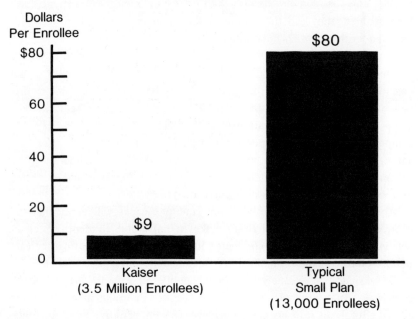

rollment of 10,000 but continuing economies exist for administrative costs. By spreading administrative costs per enrollee over a larger base, the Kaiser plan has a cost advantage of almost 9 to 1 over a typical small plan as shown in Figure XV. This suggests that economies of scale will favor the development of large, national HMO's, and that most small, community based prepaid plans are doomed to failure.

Similarly, scale effects can be demonstrated with respect to institutional size and hospital chaining or multi-hospital system development. Figure XVI compares labor costs per occupied bed versus bed size in not-for-profit and for-profit hospitals in the United States.

FIGURE XVI

COMPARISON OF LABOR SCALE ECONOMIES IN FOR-PROFIT AND NOT-FOR-PROFIT HOSPITALS

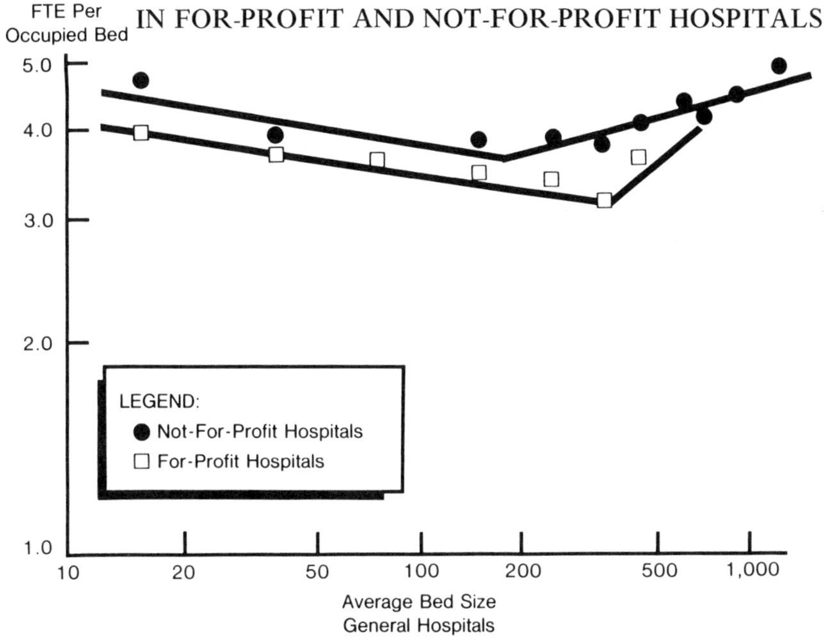

SOURCE: AHA Hospital Statistics, 1982 Edition

As the two curves indicate, scale economies can be realized up to the 200 to 400 bed size after which larger hospitals become less efficient, higher-cost providers. This results essentially from increased departmentalization and specialization and loss of scale economies in larger hospitals. It should be noted that the for-profit hospitals in the United States tend to have a significant labor cost advantage versus not-for-profit hospitals, suggesting that proper economic incentives can lead to improved productivity. The curve also suggests that for-profit hospitals are slower in fragmenting and departmentalizing their activities and therefore achieve scale economies in larger hospitals than the not-for-profits.

The development of hospital chains or multi-hospital systems can also lead to significant cost economies in health care delivery. Figure XVII compares corporate cost versus total patient volume in seven major not-for-profit hospital systems. Significant scale economies are realized as total patient volume managed by the system increases.

These systemwide economies can be translated into specific competitive advantage within a local market as well. Figure XVIII compares fixed cost per patient day versus total patient volume for hospitals in the Albuquerque hospital market.

The ability to spread fixed costs over a larger patient volume and other scale factors give the institutions that are members of a multi-hospital system significant cost advantages. Even when adjusted for differences in the intensity of care provided, multi-hospital system institutions have a significant cost advantage over the other institutions in the market [see Figure XIX].

FIGURE XVII

COMPARATIVE ECONOMIES OF SCALE IN CORPORATE
COSTS SELECTED NOT-FOR-PROFIT SYSTEMS
1980

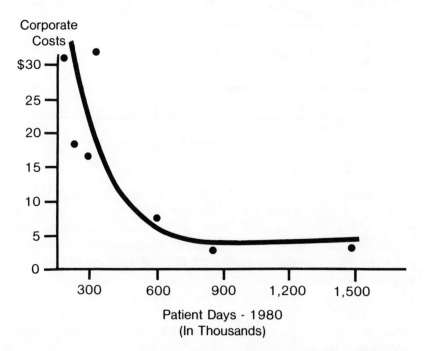

Patient Days - 1980
(In Thousands)

Scale and experience advantages can also be demonstrated in specific business segments. Comparing departmental operating costs for a group of California hospitals operating within the same market indicates that direct costs per day for obstetrics, critical care, and medical/surgical services all demonstrate positive scale effects [see Figures XX, XXI and XXII]. In the same group of hospitals, scale effects are also apparent within individual anciallary departments such as radiology and laboratory [see Figures XXIII and XXIV]. This suggests that institutions that are able to focus their business activities within specific business segments can potentially drive down their costs and increase market share in a competitive environment.

FIGURE XVIII
COMPARATIVE ECONOMIES OF SCALE
FOR SELECTED ALBUQUERQUE HOSPITALS

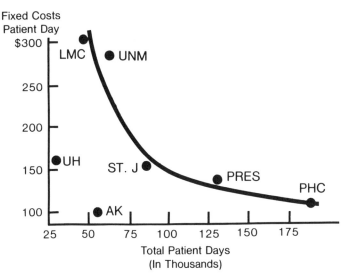

*Fixed Costs Include Capital and Overhead Assigned As "Other Costs" on Institutional Reports

SOURCE: Hospitals Costs Reports, 1981

FIGURE XIX
RELATIVE COST AND SERVICE INTENSITY FOR
SELECTED ALBUQUERQUE HOSPITALS

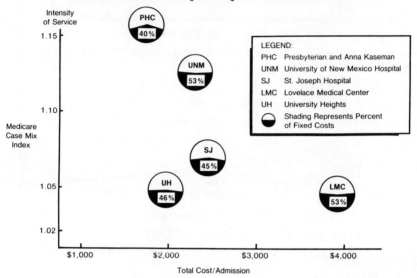

FIGURE XX
COMPARISON OF TRENDS IN DIRECT DEPARTMENTAL
OPERATIONS COSTS[1] WITH UTILIZATION

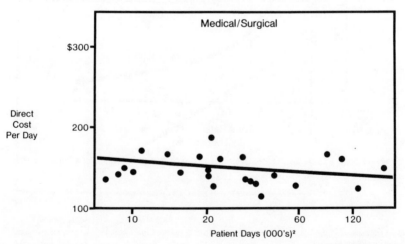

[1]Direct Departmental Costs Include Room, Dietary, Nursing, Minor Supplies & Equipment, But Excludes Ancillary Services
[2]Based on a Logarithmic Scale
SOURCE: California Health Facilities Commission

FIGURE XXI

COMPARISON OF TRENDS IN DIRECT DEPARTMENTAL OPERATIONS COSTS[1] WITH UTILIZATION

1980

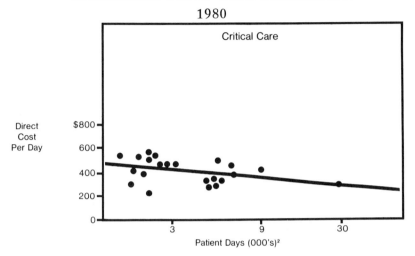

[1]Direct Departmental Costs Include Room, Dietary, Nursing, Minor Supplies & Equipment, But Excludes Ancillary Services
[2]Based on a Logarithmic Scale
SOURCE: California Health Facilities Commission

FIGURE XXII

COMPARISON OF TRENDS IN DIRECT DEPARTMENTAL OPERATIONS COSTS[1] WITH UTILIZATION

1980

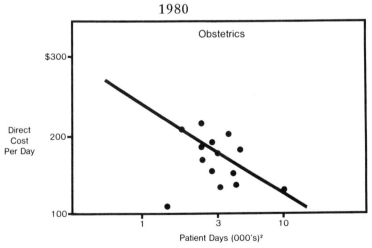

[1]Direct Departmental Costs Include Room, Dietary, Nursing, Minor Supplies & Equipment, But Excludes Ancillary Services
[2]Based on a Logarithmic Scale
SOURCE: California Health Facilities Commission

FIGURE XXIII

COMPARISON OF TRENDS IN SELECT ANCILLARY
DEPARTMENTAL COSTS[1] WITH UTILIZATION
1980

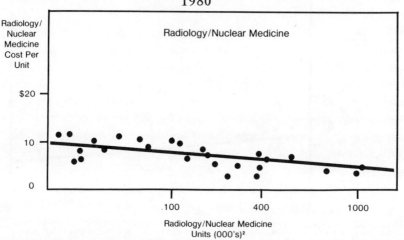

[1]Diagnostic or Therapeutic Services Performed by Specific Facility Departments
[2]Based on a Logarithmic Scale
SOURCE: California Health Facilities Commission

FIGURE XXIV

COMPARISON OF TRENDS IN SELECT ANCILLARY
DEPARTMENTAL COSTS[1] WITH UTILIZATION
1980

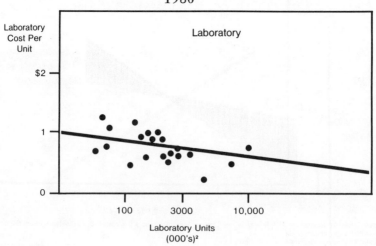

[1]Diagnostic or Therapeutic Services Performed by Specific Facility Departments
[2]Based on a Logarithmic Scale
SOURCE: California Health Facilities Commission

The importance of rigorous business segmentation and cost position analysis cannot be underestimated. For instance, in order to remain competitive in general medical services in the future, a large teaching hospital may need to eliminate departmentalization in order to reduce overhead and take advantage of its potential scale advantages.

Furthermore, good economic analysis may indicate potential advantages in a business where traditional assessments would indicate otherwise. With the appropriate segmentation, individual business cost curves may differ considerably from the average cost curve of a major hospital service, which could lead to entirely different conclusions about competitive position.

However, in order to effectively utilize cost analysis for strategy it is important to understand the differences between true cost and reimburseable cost within a business segment. Because current cost reimbursement requires allocations that average costs within and across departments, they may distort the CEO's view of the profitability of a business and lead to a suboptimal strategy decision. Figure XXV depicts the typical difference between actual and reimburseable costs within a hospital laboratory. Reimbursement allocations tend to load higher costs per unit on simpler procedures and understate the cost of more complex procedures.

Failure to understand actual costs in developing pricing strategies for the department leads to creation of a price umbrella for simple procedures

FIGURE XXV

EXAMPLE OF IMPACT OF CURRENT COST REIMBURSEMENT METHODS ON HOSPITAL DECISIONS

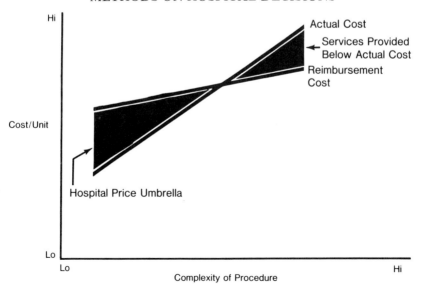

and undercharging for low volume, complex procedures. In one instance, a client found himself unable to compete with a local reference laboratory that priced services well below the hospital's reimburseable cost for routine procedures. When the reference laboratory received requests for complex procedures, they would purchase the service directly from the hospital at a rate above the hospital's perceived or reimburseable cost but below the actual cost of providing the service.

A similar example can be shown in the case of Ambulatory Surgery. In the hypothetical price/cost curve shown in Figure XXVI, because of reimbursement cost allocations, a hospital may not be exploiting (or even aware of!) its favorable cost position in delivering outpatient surgical services. While the hospital's larger surgical volume could lead to a true cost position below that of a local ambulatory surgery center, its reimbursement determined cost position suggests a higher cost and price due to cost allocations to the surgery department to maximize inpatient reimbursement.

FIGURE XXVI

HYPOTHETICAL PRICE AND COST CURVES AMBULATORY SURGERY

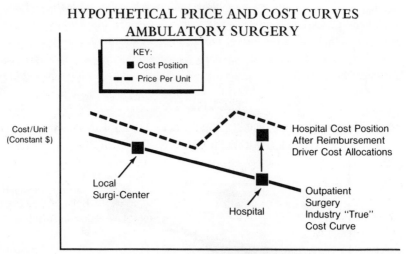

In this situation cost reimbursement incentives may price the hospital out of the market for ambulatory surgery when it in fact is the low cost provider. It also encourages increased capital investment in the total health system to develop the local surgery center and drives up total systemwide costs of health services.

Effective business segmentation and economic analysis can enable strategy conclusions such as these to be drawn and permits sound decision-making, such as a decision to lower prices for ambulatory surgery in order to generate additional volume and prevent competition from entering the market and moving down the cost curve.

Market and Other Factors

While economic considerations are critical in developing hospital strategy, they must be weighed against market coverage, convenience and quality factors in developing effective strategies. As shown in Figure XXVII, the importance of cost and price position may vary in strategic importance in different business segments.

While certain services with a relatively low level of acuity or perceived concern to the patient may be driven by price and convenience factors, diseases of a more critical nature can be expected to be less price elastic in their demand and driven more by quality and technological capabilities. It therefore becomes critical to determine in which relative arena a specific business segment is competing. In highly price and convenience elastic markets the ability to gain share and move down the cost curve to maintain competitive advantage can be critical. In other services the ability to build a strong image based on the quality of services or technological capabilities of the institution may drive success.

However, analysis of highly competitive markets suggests that price and convenience are becoming increasingly important except in the most sub-specialized market niches. This can be demonstrated in the Houston market, where the hospital system with the most distribution points has been able to translate effective market coverage (defined here in terms of the percentage of total population within a given distance of each facility) into a significant market share advantage [see Figure XVIII].

In other words, by developing more numerous and convenient facilities that blanket the market instead of centralizing all of its capacity, the system has been able to capture significant market share and develop a sustainable advantage in terms of its overall cost position.

While most health care businesses are entering stages where price cost competition is becoming a major driver, many other factors contribute to effective strategy and performance including:

- Quality and service
- Level of patient anxiety associated with the medical procedure
- Patient convenience
- Technology
- Level and type of reimbursement

In the future, hospital strategists will be required to project the influence of these factors on individual businesses and identify which success factors are critical to a particular mix of activities.

FIGURE XXVII

KEY SUCCESS FACTORS IN HEALTH SERVICE BUSINESS SEGMENTS

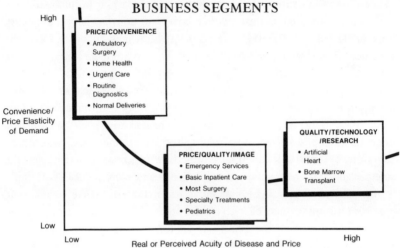

FIGURE XXVIII

CORRELATION BETWEEN MARKET COVERAGE AND MARKET SHARE, HOUSTON, TEXAS
1982

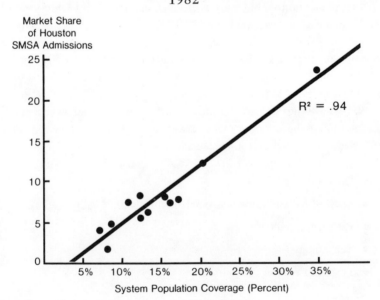

SOURCE: Bureau of the Census, Texas Association of Hospitals, BA&H

Conclusions

Hospitals have traditionally been able to compete and be successful by serving their community and meeting the needs of their medical staff. However, today the environment is forcing hospitals to behave more like commercial economic entities in their approaches to the services they provide and how they compete within them.

An exploration of the utilization of business segmentation and economic cost analysis techniques within the hospital environment indicates that most services do demonstrate predictable cost behaviors and scale effects. This suggests that hospital strategies can be improved by effective segmentation and cost analysis within those segments. In order to accomplish this hospitals need to develop cost accounting systems that provide the necessary information base in terms of the actual costs of delivery of services.

Finally, changes in the reimbursement system which provide incentives for hospitals to understand their true costs and to behave in a rational economic fashion could potentially reduce the proliferation of unnecessary free-standing facilities and reduce the total level of capital investment in the health care system without compromising the quality or price of services offered. While some proliferation of facilities will be driven solely by convenience factors, the ability of hospitals to learn to compete on an actual costs basis across a broader range of services could lead to a healthier and more cost effective health care delivery system in the United States.

REFERENCES

Modern Health Care, January 1983, p. 21.

Chapter Seven

Not-For-Profit Corporate Reorganization

HARRY M. NEER

I. Introduction

This presentation attempts to discuss briefly a process which will assist an organization in continuing to achieve success in the midst of a rapidly changing environment. Further, this presentation briefly discusses corporate reorganization, since many are promoting these new forms of organizations as a means to success. However, prior to launching into the presentation, we must have a common understanding of several key words and phrases. Among these words and their definitions are:

- Corporate Philosophy and Goals — philosophy, general mission of the corporation — goals, general guidelines and direction that provide the pathway for orderly development of the corporation.
- Corporate Objectives — specific strategies for the development of the corporation which are measurable and have a completion date.
- Success — the business will continue to grow and satisfy its goals.
- Corporate Strategic Planning — involves a process of establishing, implementing, monitoring and evaluating strategies to satisfy a goal or an objective which involves multi-levels of the management staff.

What challenges are we facing in the hospital industry? My comments will rest upon the experiences in Oklahoma; however, many of these external environmental pressures are found throughout the United States. We have dramatic external environmental changes occurring, which if not addressed by a corporation, one or more will minimize the opportunity for the corporation to have continued success—maybe survival.

II. External Environmental Pressures on Hospitals Will Intensify in the 1980's

The external environmental pressures on hospitals and their medical staffs will increase, thereby modifying physician practice styles, increasing physician competition for patients and impacting patient volumes for hospitals and physicians. Among the identified external issues facing hospitals and their medical staffs are:

1. The Continued Increase in the Number of Practicing Physicians in the State
of Oklahoma Will Result in Greater Competition for Patients and Physicians

The 1970's gave Oklahoma City and Tulsa an overbedding condition in its
hospital communities, while physician supply, mix and distribution were considered inadequate. The 1980's will give Oklahoma an oversupply of physicians serving the residents of Oklahoma. Competition for patients by physicians will increase in metro areas. There are several potential consequences
resulting from an increased competition for patients.

- Ethical standards will continue to change, even to the point of physician
  advertising.
- Greater pressure will be exerted on hospitals by some physicians to
  "promote" their services.
- Physicians in the subspecialties will continue to move into rural communities; therefore, impacting referrals to Oklahoma City and Tulsa.
- The increased number of doctors of osteopathy with their continued
  move to subspecialties will become a greater threat to the M.D. in the
  state.
- New "gimmicks" will be invented by some physicians to promote their
  services and increase their economic position.
- Physicians will continue to be polarized into geographical and hospital
  groups.
- Organizations and hospitals will find it easier to provide physician man-
  power for:
  - HMO development
  - Minor emergency clinics
  - Industrial clinics
- Medical specialty territorial disputes will increase, i.e., thyroid surgery,
  facial plastic work, etc.
- The distribution of physicians in rural Oklahoma will improve markedly.

It appears the population will not absorb this increased number of physicians. The growth in population in Oklahoma will not keep pace with the increased physician numbers.

The hospitals in the metro areas of the state will be negatively impacted
as a result of the oversupply in the physician population. Among the negative
impacts are:

- Decline in the total referrals from communities outside the metro areas;
  therefore, a reduction in patient admissions.
- Increased competition from physicians with hospitals by developing
  revenue services to maintain their economic status, i.e., ambulatory
  surgical units, birthing centers, laboratory and x-ray support services,

free-standing emergency services, etc.

- Severely compromise the hospital in securing sufficient financial resources to maintain its facilities and equipment.

2. Oklahoma and Oklahoma City Will Continue to Have Excess Beds Through the Year 1990.

Low occupancies, beds closed and financial difficulties will have significant impacts on hospitals throughout the state with serious consequences in Oklahoma City and Tulsa. There are a number of potential consequences from the current overbedding conditions, worsening however in the future.

- Greater competition will result among the hospitals in Oklahoma City.
- Selected hospitals out of desperation will modify the ethical standards position by advertising, developing services for promotion, etc. Hospitals will be spending large sums of money in an attempt to seduce the public.
- Shared services and multi-institutional arrangement will be developed with the primary motive of securing patients.
- Hospitals will attempt to compete with physicians in the delivery of selected primary care programs.
- Industry will be targeted for free programs—health oriented—to secure a relationship to funnel patients into their hospital system.
- Hospitals will attempt to polarize physicians into institutional relationships, therefore making the physician more dependent upon the hospital.
- Opportunities for cooperation among the hospitals will not be taken advantage of; therefore, hospitals will continue to operate in secret. Sharing of information among metro hospitals will parallel closely with the dinosaur—extinction.

3. New Forms of Health Delivery Systems Will Develop while Existing Systems Will Grow in Number and Size.

Hospitals will opt to join multi-institutional arrangements; therefore, the hospital industry will move from a cottage industry to multi-lithic institutional structures.

- Oklahoma is targeted by the major proprietary chains as fertile ground with acquisition as their primary mode.
  - HCA-HAI
  - Humana
  - AMI
  - Advanced Health Systems
  - Lifemark
  - Hyatt Medical Enterprises
  - National Medical Enterprises

- Not-for-profit systems are developing in Oklahoma, while several systems outside Oklahoma are attempting to penetrate the market.
  - Baptist Medical Center – ProHealth
  - Baptist system
  - St. Francis Hospital
  - Wesley Medical Center
  - Presbyterian Hospital – IHP Corp
- PruCare, the first HMO, has developed and will succeed. PruCare will capture 100,000 persons in Oklahoma City by 1990. We expect a second HMO developing in the Oklahoma City area by 1990.
- There will be an increase in the free-standing minor emergency clinics, industrial clinics and surgery centers developed by physicians and hospitals in Oklahoma City.
- Hospitals will develop community centers to capture primary care patients, therefore referring to their physicians.

Several results and impacts will be felt by hospitals in Oklahoma City.

- Selected hospitals will become an acquisition of the proprietary chains, i.e., Edmond Memorial Hospital.
- Selected hospitals will merge, be managed or acquired by a not-for-profit system.
- Hospitals will diversify their services, therefore compete directly with the medical community.
- Full-time and hospital based physicians in medical specialties will become more common. We may see a hospital-based group practice develop.
- A hospital-sponsored HMO may become a reality.
- Feeder institutions will be developed by hospitals competing in suburban areas for patients—feeding specialties at hospitals.

4. The 1970's Sources of Capital May Not Be Available and/or Sufficient for Hospitals to Modernize, Expand, Replace Equipment and Purchase New Technology in the 1980's

In the 1960's philanthropic, depreciation and earned income provided the funds for equipment and modernization. The tax-exempt bond market of the 1970's enabled hospitals to expand, modernize and purchase new equipment. It appears in the 1980's the tax-exempt bonds will not be a favorable means for hospitals' capital requirements. Among the significant impacts upon hospitals are:

- Many hospitals are highly leveraged with significant limitations imposed by hospitals continuing to debt finance.
- Hospitals currently have capital needs in excess of their ability to raise

funds from operations and philanthropy.

- Hospitals' undercapitalization condition will continue the stress upon working capital.

5. The Debate on National Health Policy Has Shifted from a Focus on Regulation to One of Price Competition. Governmental Pressures and Actions will be Intensified toward Hospitals in Order to Reduce the Federal Share of Health Care Expenditures.

Federal, state and local governments continue to pass laws, add and modify regulations in an attempt to reduce their share of the health care expenditures. These reductions have generally shifted these costs of hospital care to the private sector. Many have called this action of the federal government "indirect taxation." There are several important facts illustrating that the 1980's will be more of the same—reduction of federal government participation in paying for the poor and the elderly. Among these are:

- Federal expenditure in health services has increased 358 percent in ten years, 1970-1980, from $27.8 billion to $99.6 billion.
- Total expenditure in health services has increased 185 percent in the same ten-year period, from $133 billion to $247.2 billion.
- Factors effecting this increase:

  - General inflation (utilizing GNP deflator)   52.8%
  - Hospital inflation (utilizing GNP deflator)   9.9%
  - Utilization (admission/population)   8.5%
  - Population changes (aging growth)   7.9%
  - Quality (intensity/admission)   20.9%

                                                     ———
                                                    100.0%

- 1980 expenditures $247.2 billion:

  - 68 percent paid by third parties (government included)
  - 42 percent paid by federal and state governments
  - 29 percent paid by individuals
  - 3 percent other (mostly philanthropy)

- The amount of services paid by out-of-pocket funds has reduced by one-half in the past thirty years from 66 percent out-of-pocket in 1950 to 33 percent in 1980. The result has been almost total price inelastic responses in the health services marketplace. An exception to that is expenditures for pharmaceuticals which is the most price elastic item in health services. From 1960-1978, the increase in cost and expenditures for drugs increased 10 percent while dental costs, the next most price elastic, increased 150 percent, physician fees 210 percent and hospital costs 500 percent. Because of price insensitivity and capital capabilities, many items which might have developed outside the hospital have become hospital services contributing to this large increase in hospital expenditures.

- Critical health issues that are faced by Congress:
  - Spiraling costs up 20 percent over 1980.
  - Medicare/Medicaid will exceed FY 81 budget by one billion dollars.
  - Significant new rate increases because of cost shifting to rate payor forced by regulation.
  - Major change in planning regulations, the results of which are speculative.
  - Lack of available capital in bond market for tax exempt financing of hospital capital needs.
  - Myriad of introduced legislation recommending restructuring and reform of the medical care reimbursement methodologies.
  - A general pattern of continued, steady growth of medical and health care unit prices and aggregate costs during a period when other major sectors of the economy exhibit reduced inflationary and cost pressures.
  - The interfund borrowing from Social Security trust funds by Congress to support Social Security system through 1988 will be effective in holding the continued trust funds above the safe levels only until 1984.
  - Some Blue Cross Blue Shield plans are in financial difficulty.
- The Office of Management and Budget projects that under current federal health policy, costs will continue to increase and that Medicare and Medicaid alone will reach $67 billion in 1982, or it will be 86 percent of federal government outlays for health services and will be 16.5 percent of total federal budget.
- Two ominous messages surface from this data:
  - Major efforts may be expected in the area of reducing federal expenditures. The President is requesting a $115 billion cut for FY 83. With 16.5 percent of total budget in health care, that is a fairly large target.
  - The only readily apparent target for cuts is the 20.9 percent categorized by government as intensity and categorized by health services professionals as quality (see increase factors).
- HHS has submitted a budget for FY 83 (legislation currently being considered by Congress) which projects cuts of $2,547,000,000.
  - Extend limits on federal payment under Section 223 for Medicare laboratory tests, drugs, and other ancillary hospital services— $528 million.

- Reduce reimbursement to hospital-based physicians from 100 percent to 80 percent of charges — $100 million.
- Specify that interest and other income earned by institutions on funded depreciation be offset against interest expense on capital indebtedness — $60 million.
- Raise Part B premium under Medicare to equal 34 percent of current program cost by 1985 instead of 24 percent — $458 million.
- Eliminate nursing differential — $98 million.
- Reduce the rate of return on equity capital for proprietary providers to the rate of either short-term treasury bills or long-term government bonds, whichever is lower — $90 million.
- Medicaid reductions are set at savings to the government through long-term block grants and reduction in the matching rate for Part B buy-in by 50 percent — $604 million.
- Elimination of utilization review requirements — $99 million.
- Eliminate End-Stage Renal Disease Network — $5 million.
- Eliminate PSRO program — $5 million.
- Savings through a health care competition proposal — $500 million.
- Total of $2,547,000,000.

6. Dramatic Changes Will Occur in Hospital Technology as a Result of Computer Applications.

Computerization of tomography was the beginning of the explosion of this technology and its applications in radiology, nuclear medicine and other hospital technology. Radiological equipment with a life of ten years is a past phenomena until the application of computerized diagnostic equipment is matured. Immediately available to the hospital industry are equipment advances which must be acquired in order to remain in a competitive position. Among the results of these developments are:

- In order for Presbyterian Hospital to remain competitive and offer the state of the art to its patients, capital will be required to acquire:
  - Laser technology
  - Digital subtraction angiography
  - Computerized axial tomography
  - Computerized ultrasound tied into CAT scanners
  - Others
- The acquisition of the new non-invasive technologies will reduce and/or possibly eliminate existing invasive techniques for the future. These will lower income levels in several of the ancillary services.

7. An Aging Population will Result in Greater Utilization of Health Care Services while this Group will have Greater Difficulty in Paying Their Medical and Hospital Bills.

The 1980's will result in a greater proportion and number of persons aged 65 years and over. This group has traditionally utilized greater medical and hospital services. Among the potential impacts are:

- Hospitals will have a growing number and proportion of its patients 65 and over. Hospitals' allowance for discounts will rise since Medicare and Medicaid are cost reimbursement which does not meet the cost of caring for these patients.

III. Corporate Reorganization

Corporate reorganization, or the legal rearranging of a hospital and its related components, has become increasingly popular because of growing financial pressures, increased competition and the need to protect assets and maximize reimbursements. Many hospitals in the United States have viewed corporate reorganization as a means to the end, survival for some and insured success for others.

Ernst & Whinney surveyed hospitals in the United States in an attempt to determine the state of the art of corporate reorganization and published and distributed the results in September 1982. Early 1982 a letter surveyed over 7,000 hospitals with 500 responding and agreeing to participate. A total of 155 met the criteria where the corporation was operating under the new corporate structure or the board had approved and the management was in the process of implementation. Basically, Ernst & Whinney found the following:

- All sizes of hospitals were involved with corporate reorganization with urban representing close to 50 percent.
- It was most prevalent among large hospitals.
- Hospitals gaining most immediate satisfaction from reorganization were smaller hospitals and those less dependent upon cost reimbursements.
- Greatest problems in studying and planning for reorganization were lack of support of the board, management and medical staff.
- After reorganization, the greatest executive challenges were managing the new structure and maintaining good communications.

The survey indicated 26 percent of the respondents felt corporate reorganization solved its problems, 62 percent said it solved some, and 12 percent said it was too early.

External pressures, capital requirements, preservation or protection of income are among a number of reasons given for corporate reorganization. The most significant and maybe fatal negative given to corporate reorganization—how can you manage it when you are through? Planning is an extremely difficult process at best. Corporate reorganization must facilitate the planning process, take advantage of the marketplace and ease the management problems. We have seen a number of concepts seized upon by the hospital industry for "survival"—health promotion, marketing, long-range planning, advertising, diversification, etc. Conditions have and will change impacting our industry—solutions and new words will continue to be the answers to our problems. For some corporate reorganization will position the institution in the marketplace—for some only a fade.

The solution lies in corporate business planning with an understanding of the marketplace.

IV. Strategic Business Planning

Corporate strategic business planning involves a process of establishing, implementing, monitoring and evaluating strategies to satisfy a goal or an objective which involves multi-levels of the management staff. There are a number of elements to the process of corporate strategic business planning which must be present in order to achieve the desired results. Among these are:

- Parent corporate philosophy, mission and goals.
- Philosophy and goals for each corporate entity and/or department.
- Each fiscal year establish the critical issues facing the corporations.
- Establish corporate objectives to satisfy these critical issues.
- Develop a budget to allocate the appropriate resources to address and satisfy these corporate objectives.
- Establish multi-discipline teams of managers to develop tactics (steps) to accomplish the objective. These planning teams have been entitled Tactical Planning Teams (TPT).
- Corporate officers will monitor the implementation of the tactics for each TPT. An evaluation of the results will be accomplished by each TPT and the corporate officers. Table 1 describes the process graphically.

The following discussion will attempt to summarize the process and highlight the key points within the process. A thorough understanding of the history is essential to maximize the benefits from this process. Further, the planning teams and line officers must know where their business activities are situated in the marketplace.

1. Parent Corporation Philosophy and Goals.

Corporate philosophy broadly defines the mission of the corporation or corporations. The philosophy statement must include a description of the general nature of the products sold, services rendered, markets to be served and required resources for accomplishing its mission. A corporate goal is a general guideline which defines corporate direction or pathway for the orderly development of the corporation. Among the criteria for establishing successful and meaningful goals are:

- A general and broad definition of the products and services rendered by the corporation.
- Define expectations of achievement for the mission.
- Broadly define the markets to be serviced.
- Define resource support and requirements.
- Define expected quality levels in performance of corporate activities.

TABLE 1

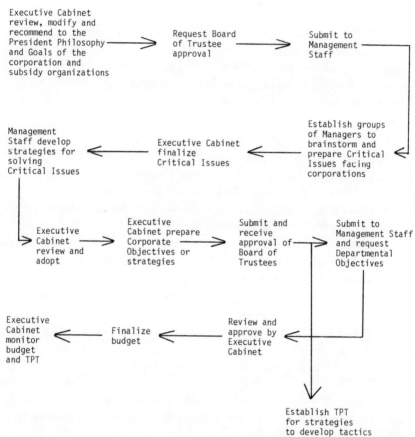

2. Philosophy and Goals for Each Corporate Entity and/or Department.
Essential to the health and continued growth of the corporations are clear guidelines for the development of the departments and subsidiary corporations. These guidelines should be in the form of philosophy and goals and should be consistent with the mission of the parent corporation.

3 Establish the Critical Issues Facing the Corporate Entities.

A critical issue can be defined as a critical problem, circumstance, expected event and/or condition which would significantly alter the immediate or future success of a hospital. Success is defined as a hospital will continue to grow in business, continue to maintain and/or increase its market share, continue to have a well-staffed institution, have cash to pay its expenses, maintain a high quality of care, appropriately meet the demands of its consumers and experience a minimum 5 percent net income.

A critical issue can be a barrier and/or an opportunity affecting success; therefore, it may be a negative or positive influence. These critical issues should be segregated by corporation, with primary attention to overall critical issues facing the corporations.

4. Establish Corporate Objectives or Strategies to Satisfy these Critical Issues.

A corporate objective is measurable with a specific time for implementation and completion. These strategies entail a series of specific tactics or steps in carrying out the objective or strategy.

5. Develop a Budget to Allocate the Appropriate Resources to Address and Satisfy the Corporate Objectives.

Presbyterian Hospital has prepared a budget manual which provides the guidelines in the preparation of the budget. The budget process should identify the resources necessary to meet the corporate strategies or objectives to satisfy the critical issues facing the corporations.

6. Establish Multi-Discipline Teams of Managers to Develop the Tactics (Steps) to Accomplish Each Strategy.

Corporate planning in a highly diverse, multi-discipline, high technology and specialization environment requires frequently multi-disciplinary approach to establishing the tactics and steps to accomplish its objectives.

7 Monitoring the Progress of the TPT is Essential to the Success of the Overall Process.

The corporate officers must monitor the process and deadlines. Line organization controls the process through the line organization.

V. Conclusions

The key to a successful organization is multi-discipline and multi-level corporate planning. An organization must have clear understanding of its marketplace with strategies to address the corporate position. The changing environment requires an institution to identify the critical issues facing the corporation and then design corporate objectives (strategies) to satisfy the critical issues.

Whether corporate reorganization is a fade for you or not depends upon the success of your planning process and management skills at all levels of the organization.

Chapter Eight

Decision Making in the Regulatory Setting

JOHN M. VIRGO

Introduction

The environment in which a hospital operates is made up of a complex set of interrelationships that are constantly changing. Change takes place slowly at times, but can quickly turn turbulent. Faced with demands and objectives by a variety of groups acting both within the hospital and in its external environment, the role of the administrator often resembles that of a tight-rope walker juggling several balls on the high wire.

The following attempts to place this acrobatic feat of skill, endurance, and ingenuity into a model of strategic management decision making. Social responsibility within this model is also analyzed in an attempt to provide guidelines for the administrator under pressure from a variety of internal and external sources.

The first section of the paper looks at the major tasks facing top level hospital management. It considers strategic management from a long-run proactive viewpoint, given the external environment in which the hospital operates. The second section looks closely at the political-legal environment in light of its potentially turbulent impact on the hospital. The changing nature of regulation in the health care sector is considered next. Strategic management in a pluralistic, power oriented setting is then developed into a model of decision making for the administrator. Once the model is established, the question of social responsiveness is addressed, along with why a hospital needs to be socially responsible. The final section comprises the conclusions of the paper.

Long-Run Strategic Planning

Top level managers at hospitals face two important tasks: (1) Deciding what to do in a changing and uncertain external environment in the face of a flood of potentially relevant information; and (2) being able to get things done through a large and diverse set of people and groups whom they may have little formal or direct control.

There are three ways for the hospital administrator or chief executive officer to look at the future, as depicted in Figure I. First, the short run or micro level emphasizes the near future, up to three years out. Second, most formal plans and managers focus on the medium level of three to five years into the future. Third, leading hospital executives emphasize a much longer cycle by expanding their horizon planning to include the long run or macro level of ten or more years into the future.

FIGURE I

PLANNING FOR THE FUTURE

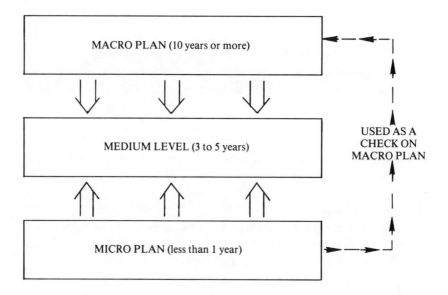

The macro level plan is fed into the data base for the medium level plan. Micro plans are used in two ways. First, they provide guidance in establishing the moderate level plan. Second, they are used as a checkpoint to analyze, verify, and update the macro level plan.

Most hospital executives concentrate on the economic and technological environments in developing these plans. Many administrators have a "blind side" for stategic planning from the political-legal and social sides of the external environments in which they must operate. Figure II shows the hospital surrounded by these four major environments.

The economic environment deals primarily with the external forces that have a direct economic effect on the hospital. For example, high interest rates make it less feasible to expand physical facilities or make large purchases of expensive equipment. The technological environment impacts heavily on the hospital by creating new services and programs that the hospital must adjust to. Administrators pay particular heed to both of these environments in the planning process.

FIGURE II

THE HOSPITAL ENVIRONMENT

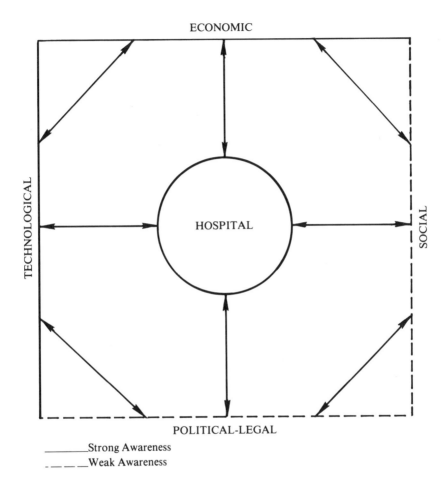

ECONOMIC

TECHNOLOGICAL

HOSPITAL

SOCIAL

POLITICAL-LEGAL

_____Strong Awareness

_ _ _ _ _Weak Awareness

However, the political-legal and social environments are much more diffi-cult for the administrator to grasp because they have a more indirect impact. The political-legal environment can have both a positive and a negative impact on the hospital. From a positive standpoint, there are the regulations that protect the hospital. At the same time, new laws might have a negative effect on the economic welfare of the hospital.

The social environment affects the laws and their level of enforcement. Social changes in the 1960's and 1970's emphasized quality of life issues which in turn caused major medical programs to be developed, such as Medi-care and Medicaid.

Long-term strategic planning becomes even more difficult when one realizes that not only are there four major environments, but they are all changing at a different pace. Because change can take place at a turbulent rate for the hospital, it is imperative that the administrator engage in long-term, macro level strategic planning. The long-term planning process is difficult when the external environment changes rapidly. It is virtually impossible to map out the future. Managers are faced with "whitewater" turbulence, i.e.,how different and at what speeds will change take place. Planning is a learning experience—we literally plan to learn and learn to plan.

The progressive hospital administrator must always have alternatives which lead to contingency planning ("what if" planning). This allows management to take a proactive stance rather than a reactive stance. Management's response is then constructive rather than destructive or dysfunctional.

To be proactive, the administrator needs to do "horizon scanning" to map out trends, evaluate how these will impact on the health care industry, and integrate these into the functional realities of running a hospital. Remember, the hospitals and the industry need a long lead time to analyze, evaluate, and change policy. It is like trying to turn the Queen Mary around in the middle of the ocean. Those hospital executives who can turn it around the fastest will reap the rewards.

Pluralism is a structural change that recently has had a large impact on hospitals. Top executives must answer to numerous semi-autonomous and autonomous groups. Power between these groups is diffused with no one group having overwhelming power over the other groups. What that means to today's hospital executives is that the industry is moving toward individualism and fragmentation where a number of diverse groups are demanding (and getting) more and more of the busy CEO's time and attention. Therefore, the external environment is becoming more and more important.

One of the main functions of the administrator is to carry out the mission of the hospital in an efficient and effective manner. A major challenge in the future will be to increase efficiency without decreasing effectiveness.

Historically, the emphasis by the administrator or CEO has been placed on the coordination of the usual functional aspects internal to the hospital, including physicians, staff members, nursing departments, technical departments, general services, financial departments, and the like.

The goal of the administrator can vary. Is his goal the well-being of patients in the hospital or, as some have argued, the maximization of hospital size to increase personal prestige and salary? [Ward, 1975, p. 56]

Numerof [1982, p. 290] has pointed out that the administrator should strive for a high level of integration. The task is similar to that of an orchestra conductor coordinating different instruments into a melodic performance. As the leader, the conductor must set "the emotional tone, expecting excellence, creativity, and full involvement with each performance."

Today's administrator must also expand his orchestration, however, by including many other groups that are external to the hospital. Such external groups would include third party payers, numerous governmental agencies, suppliers, professional associations, accrediting boards, community groups, and a host of other external forces. The challenge is to balance internal functional demands with external groups demanding the administrator's time and attention.

A proactive hospital administrator, who is "horizon scanning," finds that the formal organizational plans are too limiting. These plans emphasize the micro-to-moderate planning levels and are explicit, rigorous, and especially replete with financial ratios.

The macro planning of the executive, however, tends to be loosely connected and contains goals or plans that are not explicit. Over time, as more information is obtained from the micro planning level, the executive incrementally updates his macro plans, making them more complete and more tightly connected.

To do this, the administrator relies on the development of certain interrelationships with these various pluralistic power groups, which may not necessarily involve people directly within the executive's functional areas. Today's CEO often reacts to the initiatives of others for a variety of reasons. A good deal of the typical CEO's time during the day is unplanned, with time spent on topics that are not on the office agenda. Why is this so, when schools of business teach the rigors of planning, organizing, controlling, directing, staffing, and so on?

The CEO has been trained to be a weight lifter (a specialist) but who is now expected to be a tennis player (a generalist). During his rise to the top, specific functional responsibilities have been added, one on top of the other. This is fine so long as he is interacting internally. But when he reaches the top, he is faced with a variety of problems that often are external to the hospital. And it is these external relationships that many CEO's are least qualified to handle.

The following section attempts to analyze the political-legal environment and the impact of regulatory agencies as an external force affecting strategic decision making by administrators.

The Regulatory Setting

Interrelationships and conflicting social goals among groups within society have increased the complexity of the hospital environment. Rapid advances in technology have required specialists with training and experience to make intelligent decisions in a variety of problem areas. No longer does the hospital operate in a *laissez-faire* environment that can easily resist government attempts to correct social ills. Rather, the government has become a partner in the hospital environment. Quality of life issues, along with the need for benefit-cost analysis of hospital services, have created a myriad of regulatory agencies in recent times.

It has been argued by students of law and political economy that the regulatory agencies are in effect a fourth branch of government. They exercise the powers of the executive, judicial, and legislative functions of government. Figure III shows how this power is derived. One can see that the powers of the three branches of government are given to the regulatory agencies. The checks and balances, however, are still preserved because each branch of government still has direct formal constraints over the agencies. An important point to remember is that the administrative agencies have both quasi-legislative and quasi-judicial powers.

FIGURE III

REGULATORY AGENCIES: A FOURTH BRANCH OF GOVERNMENT

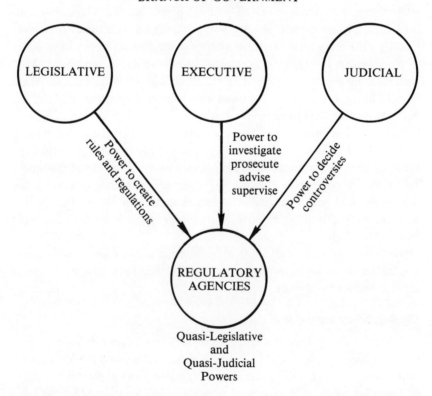

Regulatory agencies are having a growing impact on the entire health care environment. From the 1960's until recently, these agencies have been primarily concerned about quality of life issues and costs have been a secondary factor. It was during this period, for example, that Medicare and Medicaid became an important part of the health care industry. Today, the emphasis has started to shift toward a balance between economic and quality of life issues.

The Impact on Hospitals

There has been a rapid increase in the amount and variety of regulatory agency involvement in hospital decision making. The expansion of government power over hospitals is occurring by use of the operating bureaus of government.

If one attempts to look at the changing hospital-government relationship from the hospital administrator's viewpoint, one finds a very sizable public increase in what historically have been private matters. No hospital, large or small, can operate without following numerous government restrictions and regulations.

Management decisions fundamental to the hospital are increasingly becoming subject to governmental influence, review, or control. Through financing mechanisms and a host of regulations, regulatory agencies have both a direct and indirect impact on the hospital. For example, the new prospective payments legislation, discussed in other sections of this book, will substantially change the way hospitals are paid for treating Medicare patients. Government regulations will increase the control over decisions which heretofore had been made by the CEO.

Every department in the hospital has one or more counterparts in federal, state, or local agencies that have rules and regulations which must be followed in making many decisions. These interrelationships are so extensive that a mirror organizational chart exists outside the hospital's organizational chart.

An example of this extensive array is demonstrated in one metropolitan area where 164 regulatory agencies have some jurisdiction over decisions made in the hospital. There are 40 federal agencies, 96 state agencies, 18 city and county agencies, and ten voluntary and quasipublic groups. All of these groups impact on the functional aspects of decision making and add to the cost of hospitalization. In some cases, it can amount to 25 percent of hospital costs and add $40.00 per day to a patient's bill.

Almost every aspect of hospital activities is thus subject to the impact of government regulations. The end result has been not only an increase in costs, but a change in the internal operations of the hospital to accommodate this mirror organizational chart.

The burden on the hospital administrator is substantially increasing.

Many of these executives are expending from 30 to 75 percent of their time on regulatory problems rather than on the functional decision making process.

Hospitals are quickly approaching a very turbulent stage in this changing external environment. No longer is control over the hospital tripartite among administrators, trustees, and physicians. It is now multipartite to include government regulatory agencies and various pluralistic groups. The challenge of the future is for the CEO to develop mutually acceptable objectives and plans in collaboration with these groups. Such "management by accommodation" may soon lead to a decentralization of power that was once primarily within the domain of the administration.

Changing Nature of Regulation

The changing nature of hospital regulation plays an important role in the understanding of the complex interrelationships the CEO must learn to deal with. Traditional relationships with regulatory agencies which have grown over time emphasize functional aspects of the firm [Wiedenbaum, 1979, p. 14]. New regulatory agencies, however, have come into being in recent years that cut across functional lines and are only interested in specific parts of the organization.

FIGURE IV

**THE CHANGING NATURE OF REGULATION
IN HEALTH CARE**

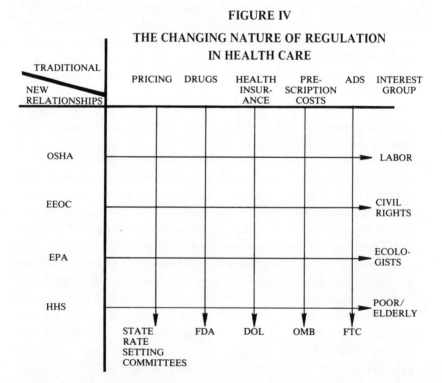

Figure IV illustrates this change in emphasis for the health care industry. The vertical lines are the traditional relationships. Health care pricing has been regulated by state rate setting committees with the federal government taking a somewhat passive role. Drugs have been regulated by the Food and Drug Administration, health insurance by the Department of Labor, prescription costs by the Office of Management and Budget, ads by the Federal Trade Commission.

The horizontal lines, however, cut across these functional areas and represent specific interest groups. These newer forms of regulation are concerned with quality of life issues: Occupational Safety and Health Administration is concerned about labor; Equal Employment Opportunity Commission about civil rights; Environmental Protection Agency about ecology; and Department of Health and Human Services represents the poor and elderly. Recent development of diagnosis related groups by HHS is a prime example of this corss-functional emphasis.

As can be seen from Figure IV, the administrator must respond to a much more compex set of regulations than he faced just a few years ago. He must now reorient his strategy and work closely with the government to guarantee long-run survival of the hospital. Emphasis must change from short-run concerns to a long-term decision making horizon in which the government will play an increasingly prominent role. Decision making will become more complex as government regulators and pluralistic interest groups impact on the administrator's actions. The following section looks at this changing environment and the impact it can have on the decision making process.

A Model for Decision Making

The typical theory dealing with decision making is the organizational chart. The administrator has a chain of command through which orders are issued and carried out. But as noted above, this is a simplistic view of decision making, given the existence of various interest groups and government regulation.

A more realistic model depicts several power groups which either directly or indirectly impact on decisions made by hospital management. Figure V depicts such a power model. At the center is the administrator who serves as a focal point in the process. The model is designed for hospitals with more than 300 beds, but can easily be applied to smaller hospitals. The administrator is at an organizational level where he has the major power to establish policies, prepare budgets, propose programs, and maintain a complex personnel structure. At the same time, he can be focused enough to be in day-to-day contact with details of the programs for which he is responsible. He thus plays a very pivotal role.

FIGURE V

A MODEL FOR DECISION MAKING

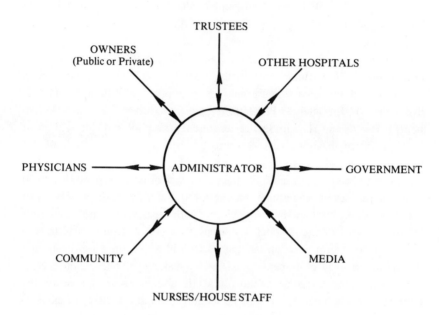

Other power groups include trustees, owners, (private or public), physicians, community, staff, media, government, suppliers, and other hospitals. To work within this power model, the administrator becomes somewhat of a politician. He forms alliances among the different groups, bargains with them, and facilitates compromises among them.

Hospitals of this size often have two or three assistant administrators. As the number of beds increases, the number of assistants usually increases proportionately. The assistants are responsible for the basic functional aspects of the hospital: business or fiscal activities; nursing functions; support services; and professional services [Snook, 1981, p. 20].

The informal organization is shown by the other power groups in Figure V. Historically, the major power groups were limited to the trustees, the administrator, and the physicians. Physicians are included among the major power groups because of their importance as part of the informal organizational structure and because they represent the major clients or customers of the hospital.

Other hospitals are also a major power source because they compete directly for physicians by offering facilities to attract them. Since the physician brings in the patients (and the revenue flow), the ability to attract certain physicians can have an important impact on the economic welfare of the hospital.

One may think of other power groups not identified in the model. The model is for illustrative purposes only. However, one group that will *not* appear in the model is the patient. The patient is not the consumer. Since the physician is the consumer, the patient is, for all practical purposes, not part of the system. The physician instructs the patient as to what type of care he or she needs and what hospital to go to. This point is made by King in another section of this book. Numerof [1983, p. 60] notes that patients "are in the unenviable position of having to negotiate through an obstacle course of buildings and personnel in order to have their needs met." Even if the hospital formally states that its main objective is to serve patients, in reality, the unofficial objective may be to serve the physician.

The responsibility of the administrator is to achieve a high degree of integration in this complex power model. As pluralism continues to grow in importance, the administrator's role becomes more complex. Actions by any internal or external group will impact the others. Balancing these competing demands is the challenge facing hospital management.

To be successful in the long run, management must operate in this power-political setting. Rather than reacting to it, today's administrator must take a proactive stance. Strategic, long-range planning requires embracing the political process so that the two complement each other. The decision making model identified here includes all the constraints and leverages by the power groups, whether that power is used overtly or covertly, and irrespective of the formal place in the organization structure.

Mature hospital management requires a balancing of interests among the various groups and an increased awareness of social responsibility. Administrators must view this responsibility as a manageable part of running the hospital just as they do such functional areas as production, finance, and marketing. The following section looks at how to manage and appraise social responsibility.

Social Responsiveness

The health care field is faced with the challenge of legitimacy. Questoins are now being raised around the country about whether health care satisfies the expectations of society. For example, do hospital costs offer sufficient benefits and rewards for the demand they place on society? The question of social responsibility can easily be seen in the current attempts to establish cost-benefit analysis of hospital activities in light of the demands for social accountability.

Social responsibilities require the administrator to think through the hospital's role and the impact it has on society. To do this requires performance evaluation based upon a balance between economic and social objectives.

Why does a hospital need to be socially responsible? Society, to the administrator, is composed of those sets of common interest groups who have competing demands on the hospital and who contribute to it. The hospital is dependent upon these power groups for survival. Each group contributes to the hospital and at the same time expects some satisfaction of its personal objectives. If the administrator adds together the objectives of each power group, these can be used to assign some value to the social performance of the hospital. A hospital that is socially responsible is one that satisfies in part the personal objectives of its group contributors [Hay and Gray, 1981, pp. 379-80].

Once having identified the groups that make up the hospital's society, it becomes necessary to establish the objectives of each group. It is important that external groups be questioned about their expectations and what "society in general" considers to be socially responsible. What the trustees and the administrator feel are socially responsible actions may not conform to what individual groups think are important. For example, an administrator might devise a program for a community clinic, feeling that this fills a need of the local area, only to find himself in a pitched battle against the physician group which interprets the action as an encroachment into its territory.

The administrator's next task is to select a tool for measuring social responsibility. Measurement devices are still in the embryonic stage of development. A number of different techniques are being tried throughout the country, with no one technique having overwhelming acceptance over any other. Three major techniques for measuring social responsibility are: (1) cost-benefit analysis; (2) inventory evaluation; and (3) survey of performance.

The cost-benefit analysis involves listing the voluntary activities performed by the hospital and attaching a dollar value to the costs and benefits derived. An obvious problem with this technique is that real costs and benefits are difficult to establish. For example, if a hospital hires a group of unskilled minority workers to become nurses' aids and the patient complaint rate substantially increases, what are the costs and benefits? Are the real costs those of advertising, interviewing, selection, and training, or are they broader in scope? How does one apply a cost factor to increased patient complaints? Likewise, how are real benefits measured and whose benefits should be measured—those of the firm, those of the new employees, or those of society? [Hay and Gray, 1981, p. 386]

Inventory evaluation is a listing of socially responsible activities that the hospital is presently engaged in. Each activity on the list is accompanied by an explanation and a subjective evaluationof its importance.

A survey of performance is an evaluation by the different external groups showing how well or how poorly a hospital satisfies its needs. The evaluation can be performed on an annual basis so that comparison can be made over time.

Each of these techniques has as its purpose an attempt to measure how well the hospital is satisfying the different power groups' objectives. It is important to conduct a social evaluation on a periodic basis since objectives of the different groups change over time. What is acceptable hospital performance today may not be acceptable in the future. Central to the whole process is the committment of the administrator, especially in the early stages. This must be communicated in the strongest sense possible to his entire staff to avoid the appearance of a simple public realtions gesture.

The process can be thought of as a management information system for the administrator. It is a creative, dynamic process to assess hospital social performance. To be successful, the results must be turned into hospital objectives and personnel evaluated against these new objectives.

Conclusion

The interrelationships of social, political-legal, and economic issues have turned internal decision making into public concerns. The impact of the health care sector on millions of Americans has made the hospitals of today into public and quasi-public institutions. With the establishment of a pluralistic society, the process of long-run strategic management gives the administrator greater visibility and accountability.

This paper has attempted to analyze the role of the administrator in a rapidly changing setting. Other parts of this book vividly show the public issues that have led to government action and increased demand for social accountability. But hospital-government relations are only one part of the demands placed upon the administrator. Other power groups who contribute to the hospital demand that some of their objectives also be met. The administrator who can anticipate, understand, and deal directly with these competing demands in a socially responsible manner will continue to play an adaptive and vital role in the health care sector.

A collaborative management style will lead to management by accommodation by finding ways of adapting strategic planning to the oftentimes rapidly changing external environment. The complexity of this environment means that the social, political-legal, and economic consequences of management actions are interrelated. Organizational decision making must incorporate external issues in order for the hospital to be a viable economic entity in the long run.

The administrator needs to assume strong leadership in establishing specific policies and procedures to implement managerial action. Greater management accountability must be demanded in all areas where external groups can be affected. Internal decision making should incorporate consideration of the needs and objectives of the groups by institutionalization of external social values. As administrators incorporate social responsibility into the internal decision making process, hospital-government realtions will be strongly improved.

REFERENCES

Robert D. Hay and Edmund R. Gray, eds., *Business & Society,* South-Western Publishing Co., Cincinnati, 1981.

Walter G. Held, *Decisionmaking in the Federal Government,* The Brookings Institution, Washington, D.C., 1979.

Rita E. Numerof, *The Practice of Management for Health Care Professionals,* ANACOM, 1982.

I. Donal Snook, *Hospitals: What They Are And How They Work,* Aspen Systems Corporation, 1981.

Richard A. Ward, *The Economics of Health Resources,* Addison-Wesley Publishing Co., Philippines, 1975.

Murray L. Weidenbaum, "The Changing Nature of Government Regulation of Business," paper presented at a Social and Legal Frmework of Business Conference, 1979.

Chapter Nine

Surviving the '80's and Beyond: Strategic Planning for Health Care Data Processing

ARTHUR M. RANDALL

Planning for the '80's has got to be one of the most challenging subjects in our industry. Not only must those in the computer industry plan for your needs, but we, (and you) must plan for where the many outside influences, including government, computer and other technology, etc. will force us to respond through this decade, and beyond. For those organizations that are successful, they will survive, and those that are not, they will once again fill the graveyards of those organizations that were too late for our fast paced industry.

This presentation will summarize many of the viewpoints and conclusions of my company's effort in developing a strategic plan for health care processing in the 1980's and beyond. We accomplished that task by examining four separate categories. The first and most difficult category was essentially the environment in which the Health Care System will operate in the 80's—or stated another way, where the Health Care Delivery System is going in the remainder of the 20th Century.

We started our examination by simply asking the obvious question: What will the Health Care System look like ten, 20, or 30 years into the future?

Certainly no one can accurately predict future developments, but based on current trends, we believe it is possible to venture an informed opinion. For a five year forecast, we think we are pretty good. Ten, it's only an extrapolated conjecture. Twenty years, at best only an intelligent guess and for 30 years only a guess, and a weak one at that. If we had the ability to look into the future, we might be able to glean a great deal of information. Population characteristics, technology, government involvement, financing, facilities utilization, changes in manpower requirements, and research developments. What else could we discover?

To begin with, we will find that the population of most of the advanced nations would be older, has greater access to health care information and is more active politically, regarding the decisions made pertaining to health care. Somers and Somers indicate that by the year 2030, the elderly will represent

1 in every 6 citizens. This is significantly greater than the current 1 in 8.5 that exists in the U.S. today, and will obviously bring with it a greater emphasis upon care for the elderly, as well as major changes in the socio political environment.

Due to a greater dissemination of medical knowledge through the popular press and formal education, the population of all nations will have a heightened awareness of their own health care condition and needs, and will, as a result, demand better medical care. There will be a greater acceptance of the basic concept that the "individual" must bear the responsibility for his own health, while society will only guarantee: 1) the public health aspects, 2) the education to choose among the various options, and 3) a free access to the system. We do not see a National Health Care System in the U.S. although pressures will continue for such an approach. On the other hand, there appears to be a growing (although small) trend toward private not-for-profit institutions in those countries currently having such a National Health Care System.

With increased knowledge of medical issues, the public will play a larger and more powerful role in the decisions made, relating to health care. The political process always has been, and will continue to be, the avenue of choice for expressing the public's grievances as the citizenry becomes more critical of all health care policies and practices.

The use of computers in the Health Care System will represent major developments in technology. Computer capabilities will expand significantly in the area of diagnostic and treatment programming, as well as in its present expanded role in statistical reporting and financial management.

What are some of the specific computer capabilities we see? First, computers will be far more involved in patient medical care. Direct patient health history information, signs and symptoms and physical examination findings will be only a few of the kinds of information the computers of 1990 will be able to receive and process. Once received, a list of appropriate tests to be performed for the patient will be produced. By entereing those test results into the computer, an elaborate decision tree will be developed to determine probable diagnosis; much like the traditional procedure currently used (mentally) by physicians. Second, a computer, which has an extended patient profile, will produce an appropriate treatment regimen based upon the computer diagnosis.

While this may sound somewhat futuristic, reflect for a moment upon what has already happened to date and then just think for a moment where just that technology will take us in the 80's and 90's. The May 22, 1981 issue of *National Report, Computers and Health,* stated:

> Doctors and nurses in Salt Lake City LDS Hospital are now relying upon a
> computer to alert them to medical conditions that threaten patient's lives.
> 'Alert,' a subprogram of their hospital wide computer system continually

analyzes Admitting, Pharmacy, Lab, and Blood Gas data for each patient. If the data meets specific criteria programmed into the computer, indicating an impending crisis, the computer immediately prints out an 'Alert' along with treatment recommendations. Immediately a nurse clinician contacts the patient's physician and distributes the computer generated treatment protocol. 'Alert,' through the feedback it generates, is modifying the behavior of physicians to act more quickly and appropriately. 'Alert' also helps hospital management to identify areas where physicians need to learn new diagnostic criteria, and treatment schemes, which result in new educational programs for the hospital 'Staff.'

By the beginning of the 1990's we will see that the entire area of patient monitoring will have grown. The monitoring capabilities currently utilized in almost all intensive care units, coronary care units and neonatal units will be far more sophisticated. Monitoring with computers will have expanded to other units, as well as outpatient settings, in the performance of more routine tasks such as temperature, pulse, respiration, blood pressure, etc.

Further, the latter part of this century will see computers operating both internally and externally to the human body, regulating functions for the continuance of life. *Time* Magazine in June 1981 reported that Dr. Jarvik of the University of Utah, had developed an artificial heart, powered by electricity and with further development may reach the level of Wm. Kolfs' artificial kidney. Eighteen months later, in December of 1982, the Jarvik 7, although primitive, was pumping blood throughout the body of a 61 year old patient. Such items will be controlled in the future by small "Sub-Micro Computers" that will constantly monitor the needs of the body and prioritize, initiate and monitor the appropriate action to meet the need. The current pacemaker technology introduced in the late 1950's and expanded in the 60's is an example, although certainly primitive by 21st Century standards, of such technological progress.

Today, implantable defibrillators detect Arrhythmia and if the symptoms last for 10 seconds, the machine waits for an additional 5 seconds to discharge an electrical shock to the heart. Good for 100 such shocks, the implantable device which is powered by Lithium batteries will currently last for 3 years. Twenty-first Century technology may very well be for the natural and remaining life of the patient.

Externally, these micro computers will be able to send "SOS" type alerts and "Calls" for help through high frequency radio triangulation which will allow a hospital crisis center to immediately dispatch mobile emergency vehicles directly to the patient wherever he or she may be. At the same time, through a use of a large scale central computer, both the doctor and emergency crisis center will have a complete medical history available prior to treatment along with a list of potential problems that may occur with this patient as well as detail recommendations.

What about the direction of medical research? Much of the research will be centered on diseases for which no definitive technology was previously available. At the forefront of such research will be the chronic problems of the elderly such as stroke, arthritis, congestive heart failure, diabetes, cancer, arteriosclerosis, as well as the generalized aging process. This will result in many hospitals being closed as acute care facilities to become chronic and extended care facilities for the elderly. Outpatient clinics, primary health centers, health maintenance organizations, and home care services will dominate the delivery of health care not only for the elderly, but for the general population as well.

Regarding the extent of governmental regulation, regulatory agencies will exist but will be more streamlined in appearance. They will be permanently funded and they will command substantial power and authority. Substantial regulations will continue to dominate the decisions regarding equipment acquisition and new service development through wide increases in agency power. However, the organization and control of these regulators may not necessarily be handled strictly through the federal government. Private insurance companies will take on the appearance of the federal regulators as they attempt to protect their pocketbooks and survive under governmentally imposed budget limitations.

Health care institutions will be more cooperative in terms of shared services and facilities. Despite a rapidly increasing population, the number of hospitals in urban and suburban areas will decrease substantially. Those that remain, will, in the main, be in excess of 200 beds, continuing a trend that has been in motion for the last 10 years. However, overall they will become more competitive regarding efficiency, service and cost for services. Physicians will be required to submit, prior to performing any treatment, cost schedules as well as a total "Get Well" proforma health care plan to the patient. Prior to admitting the patient to a hospital, the physician will be required to give the patient a list of all hospitals in the immediate area with facilities adequate for the treatment required, identifying the options such as waiting time, care criteria, costs, etc., so that the patient, rather than the doctor, selects the hospital of choice, based upon known, and competitive fees, and rate structures, and other qualifying criteria. The relatively free hand with which the physicians can essentially and totally control, with little fiscal restraint, patient stay, cost of stay, use of facilities, etc., will be far more restricted, freeing hospitals from much of the "cost responsibility without commensurate authority" for which they have been blamed.

While this may sound difficult today, governmental direction and mandate, accompanied by vast amounts of computer generated case mix and diagnostic related statistics as well as associated costs, will be available via an inquiry from a terminal located in both the physician's office and the hospital.

Merging diagnostic related information with hospital cost information will be a standard for hospital and physician cost evaluation in the future. Management of a hospital will, as a result, be centered upon a whole host of techniques primarily based upon Case Mix Management, utilizing patient care units as the focal point. In addition to the wide use and availability of large and extensive financial and statistical data bases, hospital management will be able to determine cost and service relationships based upon areas of discreet cost influences gained as a result of economies of scale and/or specific cost benefiting specialities.

Both sets of information, diagnostic and cost, on a monthly basis, will be required to be furnished to regional health care regulating commissions by 1990. This system will have grown to a point where all hospitals will be required to submit their combined information to such regional health care agencies which, in turn, will be tied into a National Health Care Data Base, for evaluation.

By 1990, the cost of computer hardware and the relative cost of storing information will have decreased to the point where such medical record data which has been kept on paper so many years will have all but ceased to exist. All patient-related data will be combined and submitted by the hospital to the regional and national data bases. Out of this data base, will come ever increasing controls and constraints over hospitals, other providers, and all practioners. As a result of such controls and financial structure, the health care system will be forced to change radically.

Small non-rural, freestanding, individual, not-for-profit hospitals will have all but ceased to exist. They will be replaced by primary care centers tied into a regional and national financial and statistical data base. The system structure will be geared toward referrals to regional centers, if necessary. However, the need for referrals will be avoided in many cases by immediate access to pertinent diagnostic and treatment information using that National Data Base. Patient records and histories will be available anywhere, anytime. Extensive specialized care such as open heart surgery, neurosurgery and transplant procedures will be confined only to large metropolitan, regional medical centers. How will this change effect the manpower requirements?

We will find, oddly enough, a surplus of physicians existing as a result of increased class sizes of medical schools during the 1970's and 1980's in most parts of the world. The ratio of physicians to population and the changing case mix of the population will have forced a change in the type of physician and their location because of the regionalization of specialized care. More emphasis will be placed on developing general practitioners and family practitioners who, in turn, are incented by economics to practice in rural disadvantaged or less advanced areas. Greater access to consulation and diagnostic assistance (by using the National Medical Data Base) will make practicing in those areas more attractive and productive than currently the case since the practitioner will no longer be isolated from immediate assistance.In turn, general practitioners will spend more time with their patients and, to a degree, will have returned to a system of more personalized care. This movement will have been aided by the fact that physicians will no longer be required to perform frequently tedious, repetitious, or perfunctory work as they do in many routine cases today. Just as self-administered testing kits are now available from most retail pharmacies to determine probability of pregnancy, at a substantially lower cost than a visit to the doctor's office, a whole host of "Do It Yourself Test Kits" will be available for individual self-examination.

Current research has developed such a kit for early warning of several types of cancer. With the advent of such low cost, personally performed, "Medical Checkup" capability, coupled with increasing capabilities for micro computer sophistication, a proliferation of stand-alone computer devices will be located throughout each community to augment the analyses developed by these test kits. Community health testing stations will take the form of the "Blood Pressure for $.50 " systems located in many shopping centers and stores today, and will be, in reality, viable, accurate, and low cost, testing centers to aid, the now more aware individual, of his own health condition. Ranges will be developed by the micro computer so that early warnings will be defined well in advance of the problem that today must surface in the form of either pain or loss of function, which then causes the patient to visit his doctor in later, more acute stages. These stand-alone centers will be available 24 hours a day, 7 days a week, at little or no cost to the patient.

Upon completion of such test, a patient with a real or perceived problem will enter the primary care system through detailed and comprehensive screening clinics where a battery of specific as well as general diagnostic tests will be given, including extensive tree branch logic, history exams, and physicals conducted by a nurse followed by a series of diagnostic tests, suggested by the computers analysis of the extensive personal history files, and data from the physical examination. Computer terminals available at each of these comprehensive centers will utilize the combined information to derive the probable diagnosis in decreasing order of probability. Based on the probable diagnosis, the computer system will then suggest a therapeutic regimen for the patient. The physician's role will then be enhanced and expanded with diagnosis and treatment suggested by the computer which allow the physician to devote more time to patients with more serious or more complicated problems.

Nurses employed by the system will perform many of the technical functions previously reserved for the physician and, as a result, the role of the nurse will be far more expanded than it is today. Gone will be 2- year education programs, having now taken the route of medical training, not unlike the MD he or she will support. New organizational teams will be developed for RN's that will ultimately replace the hospital employed speciality RN's that exist today. Much like medical teams composed of primary care physicians, together with specialty physicians, teamed with anesthesiologists, working with the patient of the 80's specialized nursing teams will emerge for support roles. The nursing field will evolve as a higher paid and, at the same time, lower cost element of the health care delivery system of the 90's and beyond. They will act as clinical practitioners and physicians' assistants and in many remote areas will act as the sole primary source of professional care. Those nurses that continue to work in hospitals will have changed their roles significantly and will relate solely to maintenance, improvement and recuperative, rather than routine and drudging activities.

Extensive nursing notes will be maintained in computer files, but they will be maintained either by the spoken word or by light pen entries, selecting the appropriate comment about the patient's condition. Extensive and detailed, each entry will be codified for rapid (individual or total) massive and immediate cross-sectional analysis of the population as a whole, for research, hospital, and/or individual case requirement purposes. All of the clinical lab data, treatment information, pharmacy profiles, and/or any other data related to the patient's stay will be sorted and organized by the computer. As a result, nurses will no longer be required to perform most of the routine tasks associated with patient care of the 80's. They will finally have the time to give more personalized care to the patient than was ever before possible.

Computers in surgery will be common place in the 80's although such activity is in its infancy today. However, the following is a today reality.

A three-phase research project to aid surgery through advanced CAT Scan technology is being conducted in St. Louis, Missouri, through the cooperation of the Mallinckrodt Institute of Radiology, Washington University School of Medicine, The Cleft Palate and Craniofacial Deformities Institute, and the McDonnell Douglas Corporation. This research project is changing the quality and improving the usefulness of CAT scan images, to the great benefit of surgeons and their patients.

In order to perform a Craniofacial operation successfully the surgeon needs detailed information about the patient's anatomy as well as surgical skill.

In the past, Medical Radiology, the surgeon's best source of information, could only yield some of the answers to his questions. The images provided by conventional skull X-rays, and even by computerized Tomographic (CT) scans, were often large in number, abstract, flat, two-dimensional representations that often failed to show significant elements and relationships of the patient's soft tissue structures, and sometimes of the skull as well.

CT scans are translated into point data using a machine called a Digitizer, then the information is fed into a three dimensional graphics database. The raw data consist of nearly 2,500 points describing the soft tissue and more than 4,200 points defining the bony tissue. The data are retrieved from a 2-dimensional database and displayed on an Evans and Sutherland 3-dimensional display terminal.

The data are placed in the database in the same increments as that of CT scans. The point data, in 3-D space, are curve fitted in both horizontal and vertical directions, providing a model as accurate as the original CT data.

The point data can be interactively manipulated in 3-dimensional space, allowing the surgeon to simulate the effects of surgery on the computer. The 3-dimensional model can be rotated to the left, right, and back to center, or in a complete 180 degree turn. In effect, the patient can also be viewed from inside of the skull outward. Internal features, such as the bony orbits and globes of the eyes, can be viewed with a clarity never before possible, and dimenisons can be added to allow the surgeon to make precise measurements of how far skeletal tissue should be moved.

Administration of the hospital will also be affected. The role of the hospital administrator will be expanded and at the same time contracted. The management acumen necessary to assemble all the information and apply the resources to manage hospitals will require an ever increasing specialization of the management staff. Greater emphasis will be placed upon the ability to develop and understand statistics related to patient care, and the careful application of financial resources, to keep the institution viable.

The administrator will have vast quantities of data graphed, or otherwise culled, so that reams of paper and statistics will no longer require intensive study. At the administrator's fingertips will be the ability to gain quick access to exhaustive information as to the status of the hospital as a whole or its individual parts. To a large extent, hospitals will have very little freedom to operate outside of a rigidly controlled budget determined by case mix, and monitored on a comparative basis by the local, regional, and national level regulating bodies.

Unfortunately, in the real world we are forced to make decisions based on knowledge of the past and, hopefully, an understanding of the present. We do not have, of course, the luxury of knowing, with any reliable degree of certainty, information about the future. We do, however, have an understanding today of the direction, health care technology is taking. That technology includes both the direct delivery of patient care, as well as an increasingly important area of technological improvement in the structuring and manipulation of the patient's database, as well as the manipulation and structuring of all of the financial databases of all of the health care delivery institutions. With this knowledge, we can to some degree predict certain directions in which the technology of health care delivery will proceed. With that in mind, we now will examine more closely the very valuable role computers and computer technology will play in the future of the Health Care Industry.

But, before we do that, I would like you to consider the strides made in the computer industry in just the last 30 years. From this you can see why a weak guess is the best one we can give as to where we will be in the year 2000. This is the second category that we took into consideration when we developed our strategic plan for the "80's and Beyond."

The world's first large-scale automatic computer was the Mark 1, built by Harvard University and IBM some 35 years ago. The Mark 1 weighed five tons and had over 500 miles of wiring, linking in a unit its nearly 4,000 electro-mechanical relays and controls. The first fully electronic computer, Eniac, built by two research scientists, Echert and Mauchly, at the University of Pennsylvania, contained nearly 20,000 vacuum tubes. IBM forecasted that no more than 20 computers would be sold in the succeeding 20 years and it was considered that even that forecast was risky.

Today's technology can pack that same computing power in the space occupied by just one half of one of those vacuum tubes. While the size of computers has decreased, the speed with which they operate has increased phenomenally. Today's computers operate in nanoseconds, and picoseconds.

A nanosecond is to a second what a second is to 30 years. And a picosecond is to a second what a second is to 31,710 years. If you could take a three-foot step every nanosecond (billionth of a second), in one second, you would walk around the world 23 times. The IBM 4341 has switching speeds of 3 to 5 nanoseconds, and circuits have been developed that can switch in 13 picoseconds (trillionths of a second). Now a picosecond is to a second . . . well, you get the idea, it's fast.

Recent developments in the research of the Josephon Junction have produced subnanosecond switching. This is information handling speed that boggles the human mind.

Computer storage devices have taken a technological quantum leap with the development of the magnetic bubble, and other types of memories. A magnetic bubble memory device has been built by IBM scientists that can store the equivalent of about 200 pages of the New York City telephone directory (25 million bits of information) in an area only one inch square. The magnetic bubbles are only a millionth of a meter, or 1/25,000 of an inch in diameter.

Not only have information processing and storage capabilities been greatly increased, the amount and speed with which information can be reported back to the user has also greatly increased. The IBM 3800 Laser Printer, for example, can print up to 450 lines per second. At that rate it can print a

225-page book in 60 seconds. During the same time period, costs for computer processing and information storage have also been greatly reduced.

Twenty-five years ago it cost $1.26 to do 100,000 multiplications by computer. Today it costs less than a penny. If other costs had gone the way computing costs have, you would be able to buy:

- Sirloin steak for about $.01 a pound
- A good suit for $2.00
- A four bedroom house for $1,000
- A standard size car for $80 and gasoline to run it for a penny a gallon
- An around-the-world airplane trip for $9.60

In 1953, one million bytes of information could be stored in about 400 cubic feet of space at a cost of $250,000. An IBM 4341 processor can store the same amount of information in 3/100ths of a cubic foot, a space about the same size as a paperback and the cost for that storage is now about $3,000.

The per second computing power of a $3 hand held calculator is more than the largest IBM computer of just 35 years ago.

Such tremendous strides in computer technology will be greatly utilized, as pointed out earlier, by the Health Care Industry during the remainder of the 20th Century.

The microelectronics revolution that already is transforming virtually every facet of life at breathtaking speed seems bound to continue at least through the end of the 20th Century. Indeed, it is a sure bet that the now-familiar semiconductor chip as well as its successors will become increasingly pervasive.

But the 1980's promise more than just extensions of present trends. New technologies, including optical computers that deal with video images rather than strings of digital codes, supercomputers up to 100 times faster than today's most powerful models, and even new forms of chips, are edging toward the market and will undoubtedly accelerate the computerization of society.

Even though the forces that are driving electronics today will continue to dominate for the rest of this decade, the outcome by 1990 will be no less astonishing. By then, a single chip about the size of a lady bug will hold not 65,000 bits of data but an incredible 1 million bits. Computers will be about the size of a basketball and will do more than today's largest mainframes. With a chip the size of a lady bug, capable of such storage capacity, some forecast that a complete medical history from birth could be disguised and stored magnetically in a ring, watch, or even a tooth filling, always with the individual, ready at any time for an emergency inquiry, and updated upon each visit to a health care institution.

Although the dramatic progress in microelectronics will continue and make future computers smaller, more powerful, and less expensive, these advanced systems still will be no more than dumb—even though incredibly fast—calculating machines. But research in artificial intelligence could change all this, and, in the process, may well have the most sweeping implications for business and society of any technology yet devised, eclipsing even the enormous changes already wrought by computers.

"The construction of artificial intelligences would affect the circumstances of human life profoundly," observes a major new study by the National Research Council. "It would surely create a new economics, a new sociology, and a new history." Adds the study: "If artificial intelligences can be created at all, there is little reason to believe that they could not lead swiftly to the construction of superintelligences able to explore significant medical, mathematical, scientific, or engineering alternatives at a rate far exceeding human ability."

Many researchers believe that such developments are ultimately inevitable. "Intelligence is not a matter of substance—whether protoplasm or glass or wire—but of the forms that substance takes and the processes it undergoes."

Although a solid-state counterpart of the human nervous system, which researchers refer to as a general-intelligence system, may not be built in this century, there already are nearly 10 special-intelligence systems in use by industry, medicine, and academia—and many more are on the way. These so-called expert systems mimic human experts with eerie efficiency.

For example, one such system called Puff (for Pulmonary Function Disease Diagnosis) was developed by a group at Stanford University and is used routinely at Pacific Medical Center in San Francisco to evaluate the lung condition of patients. Edward A. Feigenbaum, Chairman of Stanford's Computer Science Department, noted that 85 percent of Puff's diagnoses are accepted, unchanged, by physicians.

Another system called Mycin (which is no longer in active development) suggests antibiotic treatments for bacterial blood infections, based on a patient's symptoms and laboratory tests. Such diagnoses are especially technical and difficult for all but the most specialized physicians. If a patient's condition is acute, the average doctor is usually forced to prescribe a "Broad Spectrum" antibiotic such as Tetracyclene, instead of a more specific one, simply because he has been unable to explore all of the available evidence.

Mycin was one of the first examples of a so-called expert system, and it is as important for the method used to build it, as for the impressive results it achieved. Platoons of computer science graduate students and professors, who were very familiar with how to talk to computers, interviewed diagnosticians who were experts in blood diseases. The two groups of experts developed a language that made sense to both of them. The doctors were asked to formulate their knowledge into logical steps called "Production Rules" that described the process of elimination they follow when making a specific diagnosis. For example, "if the patient is Black, Asian, or Indian, and the infection is fungal, then rule out Cryptococcus as the infection." Mycin programmers amassed several hundred such rules that progressed from the general to the specific and with them were able to devise a program the diagnostic prowess of which compared favorably with that of nationally recognized human experts.

In another prediction, Earl C. Joseph, resident futurist at Sperry Corporation's Univac Division, suggests in 1990, expert system no larger than a calculator will be serving as "Mind Amplifiers" for architects, attorneys, doctors, and other professionals. "It'll be like an encyclopedia," says Joseph, "But designed so you can talk to it and it'll talk back to you." "If the system's logic cannot find the appropriate information," he adds, "the device plugs itself into a communications link and gets the information from another computer's database just as one doctor would consult with another of his colleagues."

Nearer the realm of possibility than you would think are computers that will utilize artificial nerves made by bacteria. GTE Laboratories, Inc., a subsidiary of General Telephone and Electronics Corporation, is experimenting with polymers modified so that they are able to conduct electricity. Such semi-conductor materials can be produced by genetically engineered bacteria that "act more and more like nerve endings." Thus not only will the computers of tomorrow be able to listen, talk, and think, they will be able to touch and feel.

This brings us to the third category that we took into account when developing our plan—the direction of health care data processing in the 80's and beyond.

The need for a real time on-line interactive archival file of all appropriate data for every discharge that a hospital has had for the last five or ten years is today, staggeringly expensive. The pressures of cost reimbursement and cost containment in health care will make such systems affordable only by the elite well-funded hospitals, until cost for such mass storage declines and reaches the same leveraged levels currently achieved over the last 20 years. Such a cost level would have to be at least 1/126 of the current cost.

The advent of database applications will, in the next ten years, spread to *financial* products, unlike the simple statistical and information files in use today. On-line inquiry into large databases, which is present in very few systems today, will become commonplace in the next decade, as financial managers start to demand some of the same tools enjoyed by their medical and clinical staff counterparts. The ability to retrieve on demand, ad hoc reports will become even more important across the database spectrum in the next ten years. Such databases will be much less expensive than those pioneered in the past and will be affordable so that nearly every hospital will have economical access to them. In fact a data retention decision of the 90's will be: "Is it possible that I may ever have a use for these data in the future?" and if the answer is "Yes," they will be stored . . . forever . . . available on demand. Financial funding techniques will also be streamlined in the 80's and 90's, such that very little interaction will be required by the business office except to monitor the system and follow up on the exceptions.

Eligibility will be determined by immediate access to cross-channeled computer systems linking insurance companies, third party payors and governments or agencies. This is similar to an airline that can schedule a cross-country trip and check for open seats and immediately confirm reservations for Delta, United, and TWA with a few computer entries, automatically. And similar to where all bills paid for such travel are equally cross-linked and settled as a single claim paid for, by you to the airline. A hospital admitting or treating a patient will be able to verify eligibility immediately, through social agencies, employment or insurance company files.

Payment will be equally addressed through claims processing support systems and electronic funds transfer systems. This capability will increase substantially in its importance as the current trend toward higher outpatient services mushrooms in the next ten years and greater emphasis is placed on comprehensive care clinics located throughout the community.

We also foresee an enormous increase in planning applications such as comprehensive statistical and financial modeling. Major systems will be offered, substantially more powerful, than offered today, taking into consideration vast amounts of indigenous and exogenous statistical data, incorporating national, regional, and community aspects as well as patient mix and services for planning purposes. Econometric models will be superimposed and integrated with highly sophisticated and discreet hospital information, including the physical plant, personnel and financial data.

Hospitals will be able to avail themselves of the enormous computing power on large computing systems at costs commensurate with the need. Increasingly sophisticated financial systems will be available through which hospitals will be able to manage on the basis of future expectations and current trending for prevention and corrective measures rather than reacting to what happened about which nothing can be done to avoid.

Energy conservations systems will be even more important as the century closes providing a computer controlled environment consistent with patient needs. Computer systems will be in use that will, for example, upon a patient's discharge from a room, automatically adjust the heat or air conditioning, and turn off all unnecessary lighting. Precise information linked to a control computer will all but eliminate variation in room temperature. It will constantly monitor, forecast and relate the external weather conditions' impact upon internal temperature, not only as it pertains to overall hospital needs but right down to the specific needs of the individual patient and the room in which the patient resides.

Other developments in financial, physical plant and patient care applications will be ongoing, but hardware considerations will be a significant portion of the software development. As the proliferation of such systems increase so will the sharing both directly and indirectly of financial and statistical data. We will see the final delivery of the "distributed data processing systems" concepts which are mainly buzz words today. Intelligent line networks, modular computers, and a true sharing of processing functions between host and mini-based systems will define the architecture of the 1980's and beyond. The software for the various financial products will run on various systems depending on exactly which file is being updated and/or accessed.

By 1990 data communication and patient care systems will become as commonplace in the hospital industry as financial systems are today. An increasing emphasis will gravitate from order/charge and communications, to the results reporting end of the spectrum, recognizing that a hospital is, in reality, a single database, with the patient at its center, around which all hospital functions revolve.

Few hospitals will be able to survive without as a minimum, an automatic order/entry and communications capability, given the very narrow range of cost parameters in which hospitals will be found to operate under more severe and knowledgeable reimbursement authorities.

Labor intensive functions will, when and where possible, be automated, through the advancing technology of robotics, responding to computer control. From rather simplistic computer systems, such as voice recognition, as well as voice response, many patient calls which are now routine and perfunctory nursing duties will be handled by computer. By my making, for example, a simple touch tone instruction of say a "1", a computer audible response of "Water to Room 309, Mr. Randall," will be made and a whole host of activities will occur. With further advanced systems including robotics, a pitcher of water may be directed to my bedside by a computer controlled tracking conveyor. The Friesen concept of computer controlled tracking systems, in its embryonic stages in the 80's will become the basis of an entire industry for hospitals and health care institutions.

With the advancement of computer voice recognition, the initial patient screening process will include a short computer education session whereby the computer will learn to instantly recognize the voice of the "to be" admitted educator/patient. While this may seem to be impersonal, consider for a moment, a constant computer surveillance listening for life threatening indicative sounds, and listening to a patient falling or calling out, "I fell" or stating, "I can't breathe," or "I'm dizzy." Then consider a computer instantly recognizing that a problem exists which in turn alerts all appropriate personnel and then automatically records all initial and subsequent case activities.

Computer diagnostics will also become a reality in the next ten years, although perhaps not at the level envisioned in the early 70's. The many decision making trees by which a physician in his mind eliminates a possible diagnosis, looks at a patient's symptoms and finally comes up with what he concludes are the most probable causes of the patient's illness, lend themselves naturally to computer analysis. One of the major uses will be for paramedic emergencies or small staffed hospitals where an abundance of specialized knowledge is unavailable. On a grander scale this database will represent a composite of all specialists on a national basis, having information on disease of both rare and difficult to define character.

Growth of computers into the medical treatment of a patient will have enormous implications for all facets of hospital data processing requiring computer capability for high reliability, for we are of course, dealing with human lives.

After a patient's diagnosis is determined by the physician, using computer suggestions as an aid, computers will then set up patient profiles for suggested treatment. Regimens can be profiled to include: medication dosages, patient scheduling for each ancillary department, the route of admission, suggested therapy, recommended diet, etc. as well as complete, consistent, and precise nursing care plans. Automatic computer surveillance of the patient 24 hours a day will compile and store information in the form of nursing notes and as a result, will relieve the nurse from much of the subjective, tedious documentation that is required at shift change. With these advances, however, radical new ground will also be broken in areas of liability. Computer programmers themselves will become more intimately involved in patient care and hospitals may be held liable for the results of their action. With today's financial systems, a hospital is usually only exposed to any specific loss that might be posed by an erroneous entry.

Monitoring of patients will be performed by machine to machine interfaces. In the ICU for example, such interfaces will enable a computer file to store the constant monitoring of a patient by electronic digital and analogue devices. Extremely meaningful graphs and charts will be printed by systems to aid a physician in analyzing the masses of data thus generated. This will allow the doctor to concentrate more upon the diagnosis and treatment, than the process of data reduction. Beyond the ICU, routine electronic gathering of temperature, pulse and respiration will, of course, be standard.

All clinical lab data will be stored and organized by a computer, as laboratory information systems become integrated in the overall hospital information system. The many stand-alone systems will be totally merged into the hospital information systems in more than just name. The automatic transferring of ADT activity into the lab system and the automatic reporting of results back to the nursing station, will become the industry standard in the next decade.

Charting will be accomplished by the spoken word and stored in databases. Physicians will be able to dial a central number, and a word processing system will prepare the data, not only for printed reports, but directly into a part of patient history files.

The many statistical reports which hospitals need to produce for the growing number of governmental agencies will become automated as well. Computer links will be made electronically between the federal agency and any data file system operated by a hospital. Report files rquired by these agencies will be scanned on a periodic basis and reports compiled directly by the agency. Thus the massive amount of dollars expended by thousands of individual hospitals to prepare governmental reports will singularly be defined as to the specific file layout required, while the agencies themselves spend their dollars for report generation and computer manipulation electronically against these files.

Information that is authorized by the hospital (or legislated by the law) will automatically be passed to national and regional computerized patient history files. Here, for example, all governmentally required notices of admission, reports of eligibility, and indeed even claims, remittance advice processing and payments will be handled electronically, freeing both hospitals and third parties from the blizzard of paperwork we have today.

Again, using this authorized medical research data, that is passed to these databases at a regional or national level, researchers will be able to analyze millions of case histories to determine potential treatment for various diagnoses. For example, the average length of stay for various diagnoses can be fine-tuned enormously as millions of cases are stored in these files.

As frightening as it may seem, a "big brother" file listing every citizen's medical history might be beneficial. Imagine for a minute if I were admitted unconscious to a hospital while here in Paris and the attending physician is not aware that I developed an allergic reaction to penicillin while I was a patient 13 years ago in a hospital in St. Louis, Missouri. Yet if he could have access to this information immediately some of the fears we all have of George Orwell's 1984 nightmare may go away. If the physician were able to obtain such medical history, the information could save lives and should also overcome fears of the potential abuses of such a giant system.

The fourth category taken into consideration when developing our plan was the direction that health care management was going to take in the latter part of the Twentieth Century. As we see it, one major aspect of health care management will become very critical in the computerized environment of the 80's and beyond. It is simply productivity and here is the primary economic impact potential for computer utilization!

As I mentioned earlier, with the advent of increased computerization and the information that it will provide, the role of the hospital executive and physician will change. The amount of information and statistics that the hospital administrator will have to examine and render decisions upon will no doubt quadruple. Even this information will have already been sorted and sifted through several computers and labeled as necessary reading material for the hospital's CEO of tomorrow. In order to help him use these statistics intelligently, the administrator will have a multitude of trend reports that will show him what decisions have been made in the past and what ramifications these decisions may have for the hospital.

In the final analysis, however, an individual is still going to have to make the decision, and how well and how often we make these decisions will still be a criteria for how well we are doing our jobs. This brings us to a point of contention that is very much in the forefront of the industrialized world today—productivity or lack of it in our industry. How will we maintain our productivity in an environment which seems to stress an over-abundance of depersonalized computer information and particularly in organizations where personnel productivity is so critical and where people cost make up such a large part of the total cost that exists in a hospital? In other words, we must do things more efficiently than we have done in the past.

The answer: We can increase productivity today by concerning ourselves with our employees as individuals and not as members on time cards. That is like motherhood and apple pie, how do we do it? In Japan, where productivity has increased three and a half times faster in the past two decades than it has in the U.S., employees are extremely loyal to their jobs and company. The reason: consensual decision making, collective responsibility, informal control, and holistic concern for the individual worker. This cannot change as we enter the new world of computerization and computer control.

The last category taken into consideration when developing our plan was what kind of company we will have to be, to serve the needs of the health care industry in the 80's and beyond. The answer: We need to be as you, a totally diversified and synergistic organization using our varied technologies and capabilities to provide as many of the needed services we and you can perform well. And as you, our planning will cross many disciplines, and technologies, and therefore long range planning will require an even greater degree of sophistication, accuracy, and direction. During the 70's and 80's we have already developed together many data processing systems including financial, data collection, medical records, and patient care systems. But tomorrow the plans, yours and ours, must relate to the needs of the hospital industry we both serve and the systems you will require now and in the future.

For example as a computer manufacturer (Microdata) our plans must relate to the hardware industry and the hospitals requiring such hardware and the direction you will take in the 80's and beyond. That's standard data processing technology. But, for example we are also at work on an earth-circling pharmaceuticals laboratory that will use a process called continuous flow electrophoresis. A process that separates materials in fluids by means of electrical charges, which is far more efficient in the microgravity of outer space.

Flights for this laboratory process are planned for the space shuttle, to determine whether space processing can improve upon earth processing for drugs either in short supply or not pure. And these plans must related to the space effort and the direction it takes in the next 20 years.

Our development of the Automicrobic system for the National Aeronautics and Space Administration pinpoints infectious microbes 50 percent to 80 percent faster than conventional testing and also suggests the most effective anti-biotic. And as such we must relate to the future of clinical pathology and its needs for the remainder of the Twentieth Century and beyond.

These are just but a few of our many probes into the needs of the Health Care Industry and were based upon our view of and ultimate strategies for the 1980's. We are, of course, committed to the industry. But you and we must do this in concert with the direction you and we see as coming in the next decade and beyond. Together we can make it work. The next 20 years will be exciting for all of us in the hospital industry, the users, the providers, and the patients. Exciting with its challenges. Exciting with its changes. Exciting with its frustrations. Preparation for tomorrow, begins today. Our thinking must change. Our approach must change. For tomorrow will be here . . . sooner than we think.

Part Four

Cost Control In Health Care

Chapter Ten

Research and Demonstrations in Prospective Payment

CAROLYNE K. DAVIS and ALFONSO D. ESPOSITO

Introduction

For the past 16 years, hospitals have been paid by Medicare for whatever costs they incurred in providing care to Medicare patients. Hospitals basically file a cost report at the end of the year and allocate their costs according to rules prescribed by the Medicare program in much the same way as corporations file tax returns.

From the inception of the Medicare program in 1965, it was obvious that the method chosen to pay hospitals did not provide any financial incentives to hold costs down. The more the hospital spent, the more it was reimbursed. But there really were no viable alternatives at that time. Medicare could either pay charges as billed by the hospital or pay costs as defined according to Medicare's own "principles of reimbursement."

The result has been a tremendous increase in hospital costs over the past 16 years which cannot be overemphasized. The data show vividly the trends of this inflation:

- In fiscal year 1967, Medicare paid $3.2 billion for hospital services. In FY 1983, we will pay over $37 billion or $3.1 billion a month.
- Medicare expenditures for hospital services have increased 19.2 percent annually from 1979–1982.
- In the first half of fiscal year 1983 when the consumer price index rose 4.1 percent, hospital rates rose 12.6 percent.
- The hospital insurance deductible, which by statute must be increased to correspond with the average cost of one day in a hospital, has risen from $144 in 1978 to $304 this year. Thus, all Medicare beneficiaries who are hospitalized must meet a deductible that has more than doubled over five years.
- While the consumer price index has increased 188 percent since 1967, hospital rates have increased by 460 percent.

But now as a result of a comprehensive program of analyses, evaluation and experimentation, with an investment of over $25 million and the full-time efforts of seven to ten people over ten years, we are on the verge of

135

initiating a new prospective payment system for Medicare. As opposed to the traditional Medicare reimbursement for incurred costs, hospitals will be paid a pre-established rate regardless of actual expenditures.

Early Research Efforts

As early as 1967, Medicare was directed by Congress to experiment with different reimbursement methods and specifically incentive reimbursement on a voluntary basis.

Under this authority, five Medicare incentive reimbursement experiments were conducted. These projects basically offered additional incentive payments to hospitals if they reduced their costs below a target level often established through the use of industrial engineering standards.

The results, however, did *not* support our beliefs that the opportunity to earn the incentive payments would motivate hospitals to contain costs.

Several evaluators cited the voluntary nature of hospital participation as a major drawback to the incentive reimbursement projects. Potential participants were also reluctant to volunteer for experiments that would impose more demanding recordkeeping or reporting requirements. Moreover, hospitals were at liberty to withdraw during any phase of the experiment. In the end, we concluded that the incentive system had little influence on the behavior of providers in containing health care costs.

In 1972, a broader program of experimentation was authorized by Congress. Prospective reimbursement methods were to be devised and tested which would "stimulate providers through positive (or negative) incentives to use their facilities and personnel more efficiently and thereby to reduce the total costs of the health programs involved without adversely affecting the quality of services . . ."

Medicare was also authorized to join rate setting programs which were being operated under state law. In general, our new authority was to test a broad range of methods to determine the rates to be paid to hospitals in advance of the service delivery.

In developing the research strategy, it was necessary to define and resolve the problems that a prospective rate system might be expected to overcome or mitigate in order to become an effective cost containment method. The ultimate goal was to design new schemes where past and present techniques were found lacking or clearly inadequate.

The identification of existing prospective payment systems was made through a national mailing to over 500 health care financing organizations. Each plan was asked whether it had been or was involved in an operating prospective system. This survey effort included the Blue Cross Association and plans, the American Hospital Association, and numerous other health care related organizations.

Our research strategy concentrated on several distinct areas. First, since there were several state and local prospective reimbursement systems operating without Federal involvement, we undertook various efforts to take advantage of this natural learning base.

Contractual arrangements were made with the Harvard Center for Community Health and Medical Care to analyze a selected group of systems. The object was to obtain detailed information on how each plan functioned, how its rates were set, types of problems encountered, and what benefits had been perceived by the sponsors.

Second, we decided to undertake indepth evaluations of six of the more sophisticated programs. These evaluations focused on Western Pennsylvania, upstate New York, downstate New York, New Jersey, Rhode Island, Indiana and Michigan. In general, the results were not statistically significant but suggested that the programs reduced the rate of increase in hospital costs by 1–4 percent per year. However, these evaluations were confronted with major methodological problems. Most importantly, the timeframe evaluated encompassed the Economic Stabilization Program (ESP) (1971 to 1974) and it was not possible to determine how large the differential in inflation rates would have been had ESP not been in effect. Despite the limitation, the studies did indicate that prospective reimbursement programs had sufficient potential to warrant further experimentation and evaluation.

Third, we contracted with numerous individuals for concept papers on each of the research areas we determined would be the focus of our future work and analyzed the incentives and disincentives of various units of payments.

Fourth, by 1975 we had negotiated and engaged in several demonstration efforts and development contracts to explore concepts we believe warranted our support. Demonstrations were initiated in Western Pennsylvania and South Carolina to test budget review systems. In Rhode Island, we initiated a negotiated budget system contained by an overall statewide MAXI-CAP, the aggregate increase in hospital expenditures permitted on a statewide basis. In addition, we initiated our support of the Maryland program to test a public utility approach to hospital rate regulation. By 1975, other developmental contracts were also awarded to Colorado Blue Cross, the California Hospital Association, and Yale University. It is important to note that the 1975 Yale contract involved the development of a hospital payment methodology based on a patient case classification system being developed at the University. By the end of 1975, the contract had resulted in the identification of 317 diagnosis related groups (DRG's) of hospital patients covering the entire acute hospital setting and a corresponding set of 198 DRG's to be used on the Medicare data set. The project had also developed techniques for costing out each of the cases.

In September 1975, we issued a solicitation to encourage a multiplicity of demonstration approaches to prospective payment programs and conducted numerous conferences across the U.S. to encourage submissions.

The basic objectives of our overall demonstration effort were: 1) To improve the state-of-the-art in prospective reimbursement and to demonstrate convincingly that prospective reimbursement is more effective than cost reimbursement; 2) To gain experience on the effects of the operational characteristics of a large variety of program methodologies; and 3) To test the effects of prospective reimbursement programs operating with and without Medicare participation.

Our laboratory consisted primarily of states with the legislative authority to regulate hospital prices or Blue Cross plans and hospital associations with coercive ability to solicit hospital participation in demonstration efforts.

Six new projects resulted from the request. A total budget system was tested in the State of Washington and an improved budget review by exception system was demonstrated in Western Pennsylvania. Developmental contracts were awarded to develop or refine programs in Massachusetts to explore techniques to compare hospital departments; in Connecticut to improve their budget review methods; in New York, with the Blue Cross Association, to develop a regional cap approach to constraining hospital costs; and in New Jersey to operationalize the Yale system to pay hospitals on the basis of diagnosis specific rates.

Several additional demonstrations have resulted from these developmental efforts or by advances in the area precipitated by these projects. Two prospective payment demonstrations were initiated in New York to test an areawide budget concept in which a pool of dollars is split among the hospitals. By 1980, New Jersey was able to initiate its specific payment program and began phasing-in all the hospitals in the state over a three year period. Demonstrations with target rate approaches on a per admission basis were also tried in Georgia and most recently we have approved statewide tests of new programs in New York and Massachusetts.

In addition, in 1978, HCFA contracted with Abt Associates Inc. to conduct a National Hospital Rate Setting Study. This is the most comprehensive evaluation of prospective reimbursement programs undertaken to date. Nine prospective reimbursement programs are being evaluated in detail (Arizona, Connecticut, Maryland, Massachusetts, Minnesota, New Jersey, New York, Washington and Western Pennsylvania) although all programs in existence between 1970 and 1979 will be studied in the hospital cost impact analyses.

Preliminary results from the National Hospital Rate Setting Study were released in the Winter 1981 issue of the *Health Care Financing Review.* The results indicated that mandatory rate setting programs are an effective mechanism for controlling hospital costs. Significant reductions in the annual rate of increase in cost per adjusted admission in the range of 1.9 to 4.6 percent were found for six of the mandatory programs.

The evaluators concluded that the estimated effects are more consistently significant for mandatory programs than for voluntary programs. Based on their analyses, they indicated that mandatory programs appear to have a higher probability of reducing hospital expenditures than voluntary programs without a deterioration of quality. The major findings from the quality of care studies included the following:

> **Fatality Rates** — There was no association between prospective payment programs and fatality rates for hospital patients, either during the hospitalization or from the time of admission to 90 days after discharge.

> **Readmission Rates** — The proportion of patients readmitted to a hospital within 90 days after discharge was no higher as a result of prospective payment.

> **Registered Nurses Per Bed** — The rate of growth of registered nurses in hospitals, the hospital staff most responsible for direct patient care, was unaffected by prospective payment.

Our demonstration experience had led to several other conclusions about prospective payment.

1. *Prospectivity itself seems to be effective in holding down rates of increase of hospital costs.* Mandatory statewide systems are believed to have slowed increases in cost by two to six percentage points.

2. *All systems require consideration of a hospital's case-mix.* Some accomplish this by increasing a hospital's own cost base for inflation ("trending") which implicitly recognizes the uniqueness of the hospital, others group hospitals with similar case mix for the purpose of setting rates, and finally, one state, New Jersey, pays hospitals on a case basis thus explicitly recognizing each hospital's unique case-mix.

3. *When a system does not recognize case-mix adequately an active appeals process has been required.*

4. *Most budget control systems develop a "management by exceptions" process so that every hospital does not go through a complete budget review each year.*

5. *Small rural hospitals require exceptions frequently unless case-mix is explicitly recognized in the payment process.* This is because these hospitals tend to change their case-mix and/or volume rapidly with relatively small shifts in population.

6. *In order to establish payment rates, most systems begin with a*

base year cost report that recognizes Medicare reimbursement principles.

7. *Successful systems require a firm legal basis, strict enforcement and a lack of escape mechanisms* (e.g., control of volume, gaming).

8. *Individual hospital budget review systems are complex to administer and are generally not applicable to single payer systems.*

9. *All systems have inherent undesirable incentives which necessitate that some countermeasures be built into the system.* For example, per diem systems encourage long lengths of stay and per admission systems unadjusted for case mix encourage "skimming" inexpensive cases. However, no prospective payment system contains as many intractable undesirable incentives as do the present cost-based methodologies.

Refinement of the Case Mix Approach

Perhaps the more important developments in the demonstration programs have been in the technical improvements for treating case mix. The prospective payment work initiated in our 1975 contract with Yale University was quickly incorporated into the developmental work by the state of New Jersey.

As part of the New Jersey work the DRG's were refined to 383 patient types by the time the payment phase was initiated in 1980. But by 1979 we had already negotiated a new grant with Yale University to completely redo the DRG definitions to address many criticisms which had been raised as well as to address the problems caused by the completion and adoption of the ninth revision of the International Classification of Diseases. This new version of 467 DRG's was implemented in New Jersey in 1982.

Our other demonstration sites also began to explore the use of DRG's in their systems to account for case mix changes or differences between hospitals.

In Maryland the DRG's were used to limit increases in revenue per admission when problems were encountered with growing use of ancillary services.

In New York a considerable amount of research was conducted to establish standard intensity weights across DRG's for various classes of hospitals. These standards were later used in the New York rate program to more accurately compare hospital costs and disallow excess costs after adjusting for differences in case mix between hospitals.

And finally in Georgia, the DRG's were used as part of their process in grouping hospitals with similar case mixes as well as other characteristics.

But perhaps a more important development at the national level has been our efforts to incorporate case mix considerations in the Medicare reimbursement program.

TEFRA Cost Provisions

The Tax Equity and Fiscal Responsibility Act of 1982 (TEFRA) laid the groundwork for the prospective payment system we embraced. The new authority in Section 101 of TEFRA provided for cost limits to be applied to *total* Medicare inpatient operating costs.

In establishing the limits, each hospital's cost is adjusted using a case-mix index based on Diagnosis Related Groups (DRG's). Previous limits applied only to routine hospital costs and did not include the cost of ancillary services, which account for about half of today's hospital bills.

In addition to the new cost limits, the TEFRA provisions establish target rates which limit the amount by which a hospital's reimbursement can be increased each year. In the first year, hospitals over the target rate lose 75 percent of the cost over the target. Hospitals spending under the target rate will be allowed to keep one half of the savings.

The changes in TEFRA represent important interim improvements in the current system. However, even they do not provide sufficient incentive for hospitals to keep their costs below the limit. Thus, TEFRA does not alter the fundamental nature of retrospective cost-based reimbursement—nor does it eliminate the incentives which reward increased spending by hospitals.

In recognition of the interim nature of the TEFRA provisions, the law included a requirement that the department develop a prospective payment proposal. On December 28, 1982, we presented that report to Congress.

Development of a Prospective Payment System for Medicare

As we worked toward developing a prospective payment system, we established clear objectives. We wanted a system which removes the disincentives of the cost-based system and substituted instead a system which must:

- Be easy to understand and simple to administer.
- Be capable of being implemented in the near future.
- Ensure predictability of government outlays.
- Help hospitals gain predictability of their Medicare revenues.
- Establish the Federal Government as a prudent buyer of services.
- Assure that Medicare expenditures for inpatient hospital services are no greater than the amount that would be spent if the present system of retrospective cost reimbursement with limitations were continued.
- Provide incentives for hospital management flexibility, innovation, planning, control and efficient use of hospital resources.
- Reduce the cost reporting burden on hospitals.
- Continue to assure beneficiary access to appropriate quality of care.

Using these objectives, we began with a rather simple analytical framework based on the two common characteristics of any payment system. Those two characteristics are a *unit of payment* and a *price-setting mechanism.*

We identified the following kinds of units of payment:

- Per diem,
- Per service,
- Per capita,
- Per discharge, and
- Per case (type of discharge).

We identified the following kinds of price-setting mechanisms:

- Cost finding,
- Negotiation,
- Competitive bidding, and
- Formula.

I would like to describe some of the various payment units and various price-setting mechanisms we considered.

A. Unit of Payment

An important consideration here is that whatever the payment unit used, an incentive is created for the provider to maximize the number of units. A basic objective is to establish the government as a prudent buyer of services.

Thus, any per diem system would create an incentive to increase lengths of stay. Similarly, any per service system (e.g., X$ per lab test and Y$ per x-ray) would create incentives to maximize the use of ancillary services.

A per capita system, on the other hand, cannot be implemented quickly on a national basis. In order for such a system to work, it assumes that there is an entity (e.g., a state, an HMO or insurance company), that is willing to go at risk for a certain specified sum of money per enrollee to pay hospitals for whatever medical treatment is needed. Even assuming that such an entity could be found for all areas of the country, it would likely be several years before the system would be in place everywhere. In addition, there are numerous operational obstacles to implementing such a system. Nevertheless, we are interested in capitation as a potential long range solution and are actively exploring this option through our R&D authority.

A single flat rate per discharge is now being used in the new total cost limit system. A flat rate per discharge has one very serious drawback: it does not recognize the different types of cases treated by a given hospital. The need for specific recognition of a hospital's case mix is one of the very clear lessons we have learned over the years from our experimental demonstrations with payment systems. If case mix is ignored, as it is in a flat rate per discharge, a hospital would receive the same amount of money whether it treated a heart attack victim or an influenza patient. Thus, under a flat rate per discharge, a hospital would have a powerful incentive over time to treat less ill patients.

Even if the system were designed in such a manner as to recognize the past case-mix experience of a hospital, it is unlikely that a hospital's case mix will remain static into the future. This outcome has serious, and clearly undesirable, implications for beneficiary access. Alternatively, a retrospective adjustment for case mix would have to be made; however, the principles of simplicity and predictability would then be severely compromised.

Consequently, we believe that payment based on the case (type of discharge) may be the best unit of payment for the prospective payment system. It explicitly recognizes a hospital's case mix because the amount of payment will vary depending on the type of case that was treated.

B. Price-setting Mechanisms

We also considered various price-setting mechanisms.

Cost-finding is the tool now used under the current retrospective cost-based system. It is also the method used by a number of states in their prospective budget reviews of individual hospitals. Reviewing individual hospitals' budgets is highly impractical for a national program with nearly 7000 participating hospitals because it is neither simple nor easy to implement quickly. It is also highly intrusive into the internal management of hospitals, a major flaw of the current system which we wished to correct.

Negotiated Rates have the same problems as do budget review systems. Both are highly intrusive into the internal management of hospitals, and both require a great deal of personnel resources to negotiate rates or review budgets. They are impractical for a national program because each hospital receives a different rate based on the skills of its negotiator.

Competitive Bidding is not an approach that can be implemented quickly on a national basis for hospital reimbursement. It is a price-setting mechanism that remains a long-range possibility. However, it is something that we do want to test through demonstration projects over the next few years.

Consequently, Secretary Schweiker selected a formula-type approach as the best price-setting mechanism. By a formula, we refer to two things: establishing base year costs for all hospitals and then adjusting that base in future years through the use of external proxies such as indexes.

The New Medicare Prospective Payment System

On October 1, 1983, Medicare will begin to implement a new hospital prospective payment system authorized by the Social Security Amendments of 1983. Hospitals will no longer be reimbursed by Medicare for their actual expenditures. Instead, hospital payment levels will be set in advance according to a nation wide schedule of rates for Medicare patients. The new system which will be implemented over a three year period includes the following features:

- Hospitals will be paid on the basis of output. Medicare will establish separate urban and rural national price schedules for each type of patient based on the DRG patient classification system.

- Hospitals in a geographic area will be paid the same rate for the same services. At present, for example, payments for hip replacements can vary from $2100 to $8400, with no difference in quality. Payments under the prospective payment system will recognize existing differences in area wage costs, but all hospitals in an area will receive the same payment for the same service.

- During the three year transition period each hospital will be paid a blended rate developed from three prospectively determined rates which are projected forward based on each hospital's own costs, regional average costs, and national average costs for each DRG. The specific weight given to each component is according to the following table:

Year	Hospital Specific Rate	Regional Rate	National Rate
1	75%	25%	———
2	50%	37.5%	12.5%
3	25%	37.5%	37.5%

In the fourth year rates would be based solely on the urban or rural national rate, although Congress did require a study by the end of 1985 on the feasibility and impact of eliminating or phasing-out the separate urban and rural rates.

- Payment rates will cover all operating costs. Initially, capital and medical education costs would not be included in the prospective rate, but would be paid separately. However, Medicare was required by Congress to study and report on how capital-related costs could be incorporated in the prospective payment system and they specifically legislated that any capital costs obligated after the passage of the new law may be paid according to a different method.

- Teaching institutions will receive a special adjustment to recognize individual hospital differences in indirect costs due to approved teaching activities. The adjustment is based on the ratio of interns and residents per bed.

- Special provisions will be made for outlier cases with extraordinary lengths of stay or cost outlays. The outliers would be defined so that total payments for these cases would be between 5 and 6 percent of total payments.

- The system covers short-term general hospitals. Because of the special populations served by long term care hospitals, psychiatric and children's hospitals, and because the research on DRG's was based on acute care hospitals, these hospitals would not be included in the prospective payment system at this time. They would be paid for services as under current law. Special provision will also be made for sole community providers to assure beneficiaries access to care.

Anticipated Impact of Prospective Payment

For the first time since the inception of the Medicare program, hospitals will be at risk for the cost of the care they provide to Medicare patients. Hospitals will receive a fixed DRG payment rate for each type of patient regardless of their actual cost to provide the care. This change in Medicare payment methods dramatically alters the incentive structure which exists today in our nation's hospitals. In fact, changing hospital behavior is the major reason for the new system. Some of the more apparent changes expected due to these new incentives include the following:

- Hospitals may be expected to first adopt accounting systems to measure their own costs of caring for each type of patient by DRG. Confronted with a fixed price for each DRG, hospitals will need to question not only their cost levels for individual services but also their patterns of care for each DRG. Length-of-stay and ancillary usage by DRG will be the target of considerable attention.

- Hospital administrators will be faced with new challenges as a direct result of the payment system. Because of the risks and rewards inherent in the fixed price system, they will be expected to manage their institution as an efficient business. Fiscal priorities will need to be balanced between the medical, nursing, and administrative staffs. The Board of Trustees will likewise need to be made more aware of the full financial consequences of hospital decisions since each dollar spent on salaries or other operating costs must be balanced against future expansion needs or the purchase of new equipment.

- Nursing cost will be closely examined since it does represent the largest share of a hospital's budget. Hospitals will pay closer attention to the appropriate balance between registered nurses, other levels of the nursing professions, and support personnel. The nursing profession will need to be prepared to demonstrate the importance of nursing positions to a hospital's financial welfare and more research will be conducted on the nursing resources needed for different types of patients. Discharge planning will take on a major role in the new environment and nurses, especially head nurses will be the principal players in developing that function. Nurses will use their clinical abilities to spot complications before they become serious enough to alter a patient's major treatment pattern or length-of-stay.

- Individual hospitals will find that they deliver care in certain DRG's at a profit and others at a loss. Consequently, they may tend to expand in those areas in which they can provide care more efficiently than other hospitals, and to contract in areas where they are relatively less efficient. The more obvious areas to receive attention are highly specialized procedures where costs may be exceptionally high because of low case loads. Further, medical experts believe, and research has shown, that when hospitals and/or individual physicians perform complex medical and surgical procedures infrequently, their proficiency is low and quality of care can suffer. Shared planning for expensive equipment may become more commonplace between hospitals within an area as each hospital will wish to stay within its budget.

- Hospitals will attempt to generate operating efficiencies but this does not necessarily mean that every DRG in the hospital must generate a surplus. Hospitals do have multiple objectives including prestige, research, retention of medical staff and education. Hospitals may subsidize certain DRG cases with surpluses from other clinical areas in order to pursue special areas of interest or to provide a complete range of services. Thus, hospitals would be acting like any other firm which subsidizes one area of operations for another in order to achieve organizational, community, and social obligations. In fact, some hospitals may even decide to diversify into other non-health care related areas in order to subsidize some of their inefficient hospital operations.

- Hospitals will also need to be managed from a clinical cost perspective since individual physician behavior will directly affect the well being of the institution. We expect that hospitals will begin to review physician practice patterns to detect aberrant patterns of care within DRG's in terms of length-of-stays and ancillary usage. In order to effectively use the results, administrative and medical staffs will need to work closely together since peer pressure will be needed to influence any cost ineffective behavior that is detected.

- Hospitals will reassess the need and use of their current facilities, since hospitals with excess capacity will no longer be subsidized for any additional operating capacity associated with the excess.

Conclusion

In conclusion, we believe that prospective payment is a necessary step in our effort to establish appropriate economic incentives in the Medicare program and to establish the Federal Government as a prudent buyer of services.

We believe we have come a long way over the last two decades and now are entering a most challenging era both for the Medicare program and hospitals across the nation.

Chapter Eleven

A Product Approach to Productivity Improvements in Health Care

ROBERT D. FETTER and JEAN L. FREEMAN

I. Introduction

In the last decade national health care expenditures have increased faster than the rate of inflation and now represent almost 10 percent of the Gross National Product. While the largest single component is for hospital care, which has accounted for an increasing share of total health expenditures and has been a major contributor to the relative growth of the health care portion of the GNP [*National Center for Health Statistics: Health, United States*, 1980], ambulatory and long term care expenditures have also grown dramatically. Information on factors influencing health care costs has therefore been essential to the regulatory functions of federal reimbursement programs and state rate setting authorities. It has also been critical to the production and operations management of health care institutions.

Output and cost functions in health care have been theoretically and empirically investigated in a variety of research settings [Lave and Lave, 1970; Ruchlin, 1974]. The major limitation of all these studies is the method used to account for the multiproduct nature of a health care institution. While there is little agreement on the definition of these products, there is concensus that each institution produces an extensive variety of them and that differences in "product-line" play an important role in understanding cost variations among institutions and among patients within an institution.

A system for describing hospital production has been developed and is referred to as Diagnosis Related Groups (DRG's) [Fetter, 1980]. The system has recently undergone extensive revisions to reflect new diagnostic and procedural coding conventions (ICD-9-CM) and suggestions from users based on their experience with the previous group definitions. This paper presents the underlying conceptual framework and operational definitions of the current version of the DRG's. Specific applications for cost control and planning are illustrated plus a description of Ambulatory Visit Groups (AVG's) and Resource Utilization Groups (RUG's) in long term care. The implications of this approach for improved health care management are discussed in the context of these applications. Taken together, these product definitions provide a framework for measuring and comparing productivity in health care at

149

the institutional, regional, national, and international level.

One needs to be able to measure productivity under alternate structural and financial modalities, in order to judge the relative effectiveness of different organizational forms. Further, productivity measures are important for the construction of staffing, budgeting, and control mechanisms in the management of health care organizations. Finally, the measurement of producitivity is important if we are to understand and evaluate the role of various "physician extenders" in health care delivery.

It is often presumed that productivity measurement and control is inherently more difficult in human service enterprises than, for example, in manufacturing. There is, however, nothing intrinsic to such difficulties. Productivity in steel manufacturing is often represented by such measures as tons per worker per year. Interpretation of such aggregate measures is difficult when the product line of the steel companies being compared is vastly different. One particular grade of carbon steel requires rather different inputs than a nickel-molybdenum alloy steel. The skill of the labor and the efficiency of the equipment all serve to confound interpretation of any aggregate measure in a multi-product firm.

Likewise, productivity in health care is most often reported in terms of patients seen or processed per unit time (e.g., visits per hour), average length of stay, patients discharged per year, and the like. It is clear, however, that in such settings as physicians' offices and outpatient clinics, for example, the patient "visit" is not a well defined entity. In hospitals a case of appendicitis is significantly different from a case of acute myocardial infarction.

II. The Products of a Hospital: Conceptual Framework

Defining the Concept of Hospital Product

Chase and Aquilano [1977] define product as "the output from a productive system offered for sale (in the case of a business) or otherwise made available (in the case of a governmental or philanthropic organization) to some consumer." In this context, the outputs of a hospital are the specific goods and services it provides to patients. These include, for example, the x-rays, medication and lab tests ordered by physicians as part of the treatment process as well as nursing care, operating room facilities, and certain hotel and social services. The hospital's inputs are the labor, material and equipment used in the provision of these goods and services. The specific set of outputs provided to each patient is a "product" of the hospital.

The hospital is thus a multiproduct firm with each product consisting of multiple outputs. Its product line is potentially as extensive as the number of patients it serves. Associated with each product is a production function which describes the relationship between input of productive services per unit type and outputs per unit time. Since the product consists of multiple outputs, the relationship is described in terms of a multivariate function: $Y = f(X)$, where Y is the vector of outputs (hours of nursing care, meals, laboratory tests, medication, etc.) and X is the vector of inputs (capital, labor, material).

An Approach to Identifying and Labelling the Products

As with any firm or organization, the particular products a hospital provides may be described in terms of their content (e.g., the specific set of goods and services each patient received) or in terms descriptive of the clients who received them (e.g., women delivering babies). Since matrix organizations are project oriented, it makes sense from a budgeting, cost control, planning, and quality control perspective to identify the products in terms relevant to the project or its objectives. For example, companies in the aerospace industry generally describe their products in the context of the programs that generated the business (e.g., Apollo Project, Mars Project). For hospitals, their "projects" are individual patients. The particular product provided each patient is dependent upon his condition as well as the treatment process he undergoes during his stay.

As noted above, hospitals have a product line that in theory is as extensive as the number of patients each serves. However, while each patient is unique, he has certain diagnostic and therapeutic attributes in common with other patients that determine the type and level of services he receives. Therefore, one method for identifying products is to determine which factors are important in predicting the amount and type of goods and services provided to patients. The different combinations of the levels of these important factors (e.g., age, diagnosis, surgical procedures) describe the classes of patients with similar products.

III. The Products of a Hospital: Operation Definitions According to DRG's

An interactive version of A.I.D. analysis [Sonquist and Morgan, 1964] was applied to a database of information from hospital discharge summaries provided by the Commission for Professional and Hospital Activities (CPHA). The purpose of the analysis was to identify characteristics of patients or "type of cases" with similar patterns of services or resource use. To this end, the A.I.D. approach examines the interrelationships of the variables in the database and determines which ones are related to some specific measure of interest, referred to as the dependent variable. This is accomplished by recursively subdividing observations into subgroups based on values of variables that maximize variance reduction of the dependent variable. Since resource use was the principal measure of interest, length of stay was selected as the dependent variable. At each stage of the analysis a team of physicians reviewed the subgroups recommended by the A.I.D. algorithm and suggested modifications to insure medical interpretability. Their participation in the analysis was particularly critical for the formation of meaningful surgical and diagnostic groups from the ICD-9-CM procedure and diagnostic codes.

The analysis resulted in the formation of 467 distinct patient classes referred to as Diagnosis Related Groups or DRG's. Each DRG is defined in terms of one or more of the following variables: principal diagnosis, operating room procedures, comorbidities and complications (secondary diagnoses), age and in a few cases discharge status. As such, the DRG's represent a multivariable system for classifying hospital discharges from acute care hospitals into patient groups or types of cases with similar expected patterns of resource use. Thus, the DRG's operationally define the products of the hospital in terms of classes of patients with similar sets of services.

The general structure and content of the DRG's and the Ambulatory Visit Groups (AVG's) is described briefly in the following paragraphs. A more extensive discussion may be found elsewhere [The New ICD-9-CM Diagnosis Related Groups Classification Scheme: User Manual, Health Systems Management Group, 1981; Fetter, Averill, Lichtenstein, and Freeman].

Overview of DRG's

In order to insure clinical interpretability, all principal diagnosis codes are condensed into 23 mutually exclusive and exhaustive Major Diagnostic Categories (MDC's). The category to which a particular diagnosis is assigned is a function of the organ system it predominantly affects or the specialist who would typically provide care. Diseases that tend to be diagnosed and treated in similar ways by similar specialists are aggregated in the same MDC regardless of etiology. Under the DRG system of classification, each hospital discharge is assigned to one and only one MDC based on its principal diagnosis code.

With few exceptions, each MDC is then partitioned on the presence or absence of a procedure performed in the operationg room. (All ICD-9-CM procedure codes were intially reviewed by clinicians and a list constructed of those procedures generally requiring an operating room). Discharges with at least one operating room (OR) procedure are referred to as "surgical" hospitalizations and those with no OR procedures as "medical" hospitalizations. In most MDC's, medical hospitalizations are then partitioned into clinically coherent groups of principal diagnoses and surgical hospitalizations into groups of operating room procedures referred to as procedure categories. These procedure categories are hierarchical based on intensity of resource consumption. A discharge with multiple operating room procedures is assigned to the surgical group based on the most resource intensive OR procedure within this hierarchy.

Depending on the MDC, diagnostic groups (corresponding to medical hospitalizations) and procedure categories (corresponding to surgical hospitalizations) may be further partitioned on the basis of age, the existence of comorbidities and complications, and, in a few cases discharge status. Some procedure categories are also partitioned on the basis of principal diagnosis. A compound variable, age 70cc, is used extensively throughout the system. This is a dichotomous (2 level) variable which takes on the value "yes" if age $>= 70$ and/or there are substantial comobidities or complications and "no" otherwise. Substantial complications and comorbidities are defined as those conditions which, in the judgment of the clinicians constructing the system, would be likely to increase the length of stay for 75 percent of the patients by at least one day.

Example: Diseases and Disorders of the Female Reproductive System

As an example of how each MDC is partitioned into DRG's, consider MDC 13: Diseases and Disorders of the Female Reproductive System. The classification of discharges into DRG's or case types within this MDC is summarized in the tree diagram presented in Figure I. Geometric symbols (diamond, circle, hexagon) represent decision points in the division process and contain the variable used in the decision. Lines emanate from the symbol indicating how the groups were split on the basis of that variable. Final groups or DRG's are represented by squares. Inside each square is the sequential DRG number.

Medical hospitalizations in MDC 13 are divided into three diagnostic groups corresponding to diagnoses of malignancy, infection, and menstrual and other diagnoses. Discharges with a malignancy diagnosis are further partitioned on whether or not age is greater than or equal to 70 and/or there are substantial comorbidities or complications. Thus, medical hospitalizations, with a principal diagnosis pertaining to diseases and disorders of the female reproductive system, are divided into four case types of DRG's.

DRG	Description
366	Malignancy of the female reproductive system with age at least 70 years and/or substantial comorbidities or complications
367	Malignancy of the female reproductive system with age less than 70 years and no substantial comorbidities or complications
368	Infections of the female reproductive system
369	Menstrual and other female reproductive system disorders

Surgical hospitalizations in MDC 13 are divided into eight procedure categories: (1) pelvic evisceration, radical hysterectomy, and vulvectomy, (2) other hysterectomy, (3) reconstructive procedures, (4) uterus and adnexa

FIGURE I

MAJOR DIAGNOSTIC CATEGORY 13:

DISEASES AND DISORDERS OF THE FEMALE REPRODUCTIVE SYSTEM

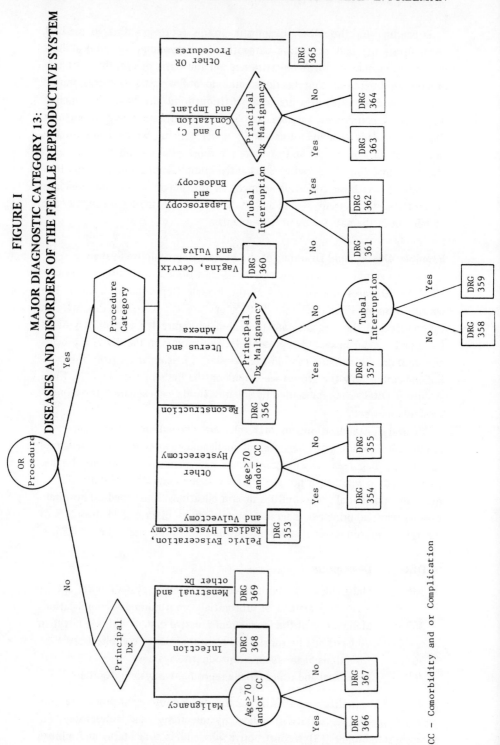

CC – Comorbidity and or Complication

procedures, (5) vagina, cervix and vulva procedures, (6) laparoscopy and endoscopy, (7) D&C, conization, and radio-implant, (8) other OR procedures. The surgical hierarchy of these categories follows in the same order, with pelvic evisceration, radical hysterectomy, and vulvectomy being the most resource intensive and other OR procedures the least. Within this hierarchy, for example, a discharge with both a D&C and a hysterectomy would be assigned to the hysterectomy category. As indicated in the diagram, four of these categories are further partitioned on the basis of age and/or the presence of substantial comorbidities or complications, principal diagnosis of malignancy, and tubal interruption.

In summary, surgical hospitalizations with a principal diagnosis pertaining to diseases and disorders of the female reproductive system are divided into 13 case types, or DRG's:

DRG	Description
353	Pelvic evisceration, radical hysterectomy, and vulvectomy
354	Non-radical hysterectomy with age at least 70 years and/or substantial comorbidities or complications
355	Non-radical hysterectomy with age less than 70 and no substantial comorbidities or complications
356	Female reproductive system reconstructive procedures
357	Uterus and adnexa procedures for malignancy
358	Uterus and adnexa procedures for non-malignancy except tubal interruption
359	Tubal interruption for non-malignancy
360	Vagina, cervix and vulva procedures
361	Laparoscopy and endoscopy (female) except tubal interruption
362	Laparoscopic tubal interruption
363	D&C, conization and radio-implant for malignancy
364	D&C, conization except for malignancy
365	Other female reproductive system OR procedures

Construction of Ambulatory Visit Groups*

Data

The data used to construct the Ambulatory Visit Groups were collected by the National Ambulatory Medical Care Survey (NAMCS) for the years 1975 and 1976. The sample design, data collection, and data processing procedures are documented extensively elsewhere [National Center for

---

*We would like to acknowledge the support of the Health Systems Management Group in this work and especially Robert Elia, Ann Freedman, and Jeanette Ryan.

Health Statistics: National Ambulatory Medical Care Survey, 1967-72 and *Vital and Health Statistics,* 1974].

Data are collected and transcribed to structured abstracts (See Appendix A) by the physician or his staff. Information recorded on the form includes patient demographic characteristics (birth date, sex, race), physician diagnoses (maximum of three), therapeutic services ordered or provided, duration of the patient/provider contact, and general visit information (date, reason for visit, visit status, and patient disposition). The physician's diagnostic information is coded by personnel at the National Center for Health Statistics according to the *Eighth Revision, International Classification of Diseases. Adapted for Use in the United States.* Patients' reported problems were coded using a special classification scheme developed for the NAMCS [May 1974].

A sample of 62,697 visits was collected in the 1975 NAMCS and 51,224 in the 1976 survey. Population totals (e.g., number of visits) may be obtained by inflating the sample counts by their respective sampling weights. However, all analyses reported in subsequent sections of this paper were performed on the *unweighted* data.

Group Formation

In order to insure clinical interpretability and to facilitate the analysis over a wide range of disease conditions, diagnostic codes were condensed into 14 mutually exclusive and exhaustive Major Ambulatory Categories (MAC's). The category to which a particular diagnosis was assigned was a function of the organ system it predominantly affects or the specialist who would typically provide care. Diseases that tend to be diagnosed and treated in similar ways by similar specialists were aggregated in the same MAC, regardless of etiology. A list of the MAC's and their respective codes appears in Appendix B.

The data were initially divided into diagnostic modules corresponding to these MAC's. That is, each visit record was assigned to one and only one MAC based on its principal diagnostic code. For the records within a given MAC, a statistical algorithm was invoked to suggest groupings of observations that maximized explained variance in the value of the dependent variable (provider time) as a function of a set of independent variables (e.g., presenting problem, visit status, age). The particular algorithm employed was an interactive version of the Automated Interaction Detector (AID) method of Sonquist and Morgan [1964, 1980]. The set of independent variables selected as input to the algorithm are described in Appendix C.

General guidelines adhered to whenever possible in creating AVG's were:

- When forming patient groups the use of the variable presenting problem was favored over the use of diagnosis because a primary diagnosis is usually not established until the end of a visit.

- Non-clinical variables such as type of visit or referral were used whenever possible before using clinical variables such as diagnosis or presenting problem.
- Within a MAC attempts were made to be consistent in the way groups were formed. For example, if age is used as a partitioning variable in more than one place in the definition of the AVG's for a particular MAC then the same age categories should be used (e.g., use under and over 65 for all age splits).

In addition, physicians reviewed the partitions formed by the algorithm to insure their content was meaningful from a medical perspective. Thus, at each stage of the process the subgroups were based both on statistical criteria as well as physician judgment.

In summary, the process of constructing the AVG's began with the partitioning of data into 14 mutually exclusive and exhaustive diagnostic categories referred to as MAC's. Each MAC was then examined and divided into subgroups through a recursive process that involved 1) the application of a statistical algorithm to identify clusters of visits that were homogeneous with respect to provider time; and 2) clinical review to modify the partitions in order to insure medical interpretability. The process resulted in the formation of 154 AVG's defined on the basis of one or more of the following variables: age, presenting problem, secondary problem, principal diagnosis, the presence or absence of a secondary diagnosis, visit status, reason for visit, and use of psychotherapy. A description of these groups appears in the Ambulatory Patient Related Groups Report [1980].

TABLE 1

Physician Productivity Report

Physician	Visits/Hours	Visits/Hours Diff.	Diff. Due To Productivity	Diff. Due To Visit Mix	Interact Diff.
NAMCS					
(Std.)	4.47	— —	— —	— —	— —
A	3.82	−.65	−.30	−.25	−.10
B	4.90	.43	.50	−.05	−.02
C	5.50	1.03	.05	1.07	−.09
D	5.35	.88	1.00	−.10	−.02
E	3.50	−.97	−1.10	.20	−.07
F	5.52	1.05	1.02	−.06	.09

Productivity Report

Table 1 contains a sample report presenting hypothetical visit mix related statistics for a set of physicians in a given facility. Of particular interest here is a comparison of their productivity as measured by visits/hour. The precise mathematical formulation of the statistics contained in the report is presented elsewhere [Fetter, Shin, Freeman, Averill and Thompson, 1980], but a brief descriptive summary is presented here in order to demonstrate the application of AVG's in visit mix analyses. In addition, the reader is referred to Hill [1971] and Kitagawa [1955] for a further discussion of the two techniques applied in this context standardization and separation into components.

The first column gives the identity of each subject being compared. In this example, the standard chosen by which to compare individual physicians is the value of the dependent variable given by the National Ambulatory Medical Care Survey for 1975 and 1976, which was 4.47 visits/ hour in these 15 AVG's for all non-federal office based physicians. Then, the set of physicians in a particular group practice is identified and in column 2 is given their productivity rate or visits/hour. The difference between the national rate and the observed value is shown in column 3.

In order to explain this observed difference, it is necessary to break it into components as given in columns 4–6. These show, first, that part of the difference which is due to productivity; that is, the amount of the observed difference due to different performance in treating the same types of visits. Second is shown the amount of the difference due to the fact that each physician sees a different mix of visits. Finally, in column 6 is shown the difference component due to interaction of these two factors.

The separation of the difference into these components is based on the technique described by Kitagawa [1955] and is briefly described here for the reader's convenience. If we let:

a_i = visits/hour for i^{th} physician

a_{ij} = visits/hour for i^{th} physician and j^{th} AVG

p_{ij} = proportion of the ith physician's visits in the jth AVG

and

A = NAMCS visits/hour

A_j = NAMCS visits/hour in j^{th} AVG

P_j = Proportion of NAMCS visits in the jth AVG

then,

$$a_i = \sum_j p_{ij} a_{ij} \qquad\qquad j = 1, \ldots, 154 \,(\text{AVG})$$

$$A = \sum_j P_j A_j \qquad\qquad j = 1, \ldots, 154 \,(\text{AVG})$$

The difference between a_i and A can be expressed as

$$a_i - A = \sum_j P_j (a_{ij} - A_j) + \sum_j A_j (p_{ij} - P_j) + \sum_j (a_{ij} - A_j)(p_{ij} - P_j)$$

| Diff.In Visit/Hour | Diff.Due To Productivity | Diff.Due To Visit Mix | Interact Dif. |

$$j = 1, \ldots, 154 \,(\text{AVG})$$

This may be rewritten as

$$a_i - A = \left(\sum_j P_j a_{ij} - \sum_j P_j A_j\right) + \left(\sum_j A_j P_{ij} - \sum_j A_j P_j\right) + \sum_j (a_{ij} - A_j)(p_{ij} - P_j)$$

$$j = 1, \ldots, 154 \,(\text{AVG})$$

from which we note that the first two differences are computed by subtracting the national rate from the physician rates. The interaction component is the residual or the amount of the difference between the physician and the national average not accounted for by the productivity difference (column 4) or the visit mix difference (column 5).

For example, physician C can be observed to have a visit mix which allows serving 1.07 more visits/hour than is true for the average physician. Conversely, physician D serves one more visit/hour than the national average when we control for visit mix. Thus, while the visits/hour of both are nearly the same, the underlying reason for these rates is quite different.

We may understand even further the productivity of the physicians by looking in detail at their case load. Table 2 shows the breakdown of case types seen by physician F and explains in detail the source of the observed difference in productivity. It can be seen that three-quarters of the difference (column 6, Difference Due to Productivity) is due to his performance with respect to AVG 147. He is treating such patients at a rate almost twice that observed nationally. The remainder of the diffference is due to AVG's 65, 92, 106, and 116. In all other cases his performance is quite close to that observed nationally.

TABLE 2
Comparison of Physician F With Standard

Ambulatory Visit Group	Names of Ambulatory Group	NAMCS Product Dist.	NAMCS Visits Per Hr.	PHYSICIAN F Product Dist.	PHYSICIAN F Visits Per Hr.	Differ Due To Productivity	Differ Due To Visit Mix	Interact Differ
1	Infective, new patient with a venereal disease (e.g., syphilis, gonoccal infections)	.008	3.48	.008	3.76	.002	.000	.000
8	Infective, revisit for a new problem, age 0-12 years, with a childhood disease (e.g., chicken pox, measles)	.006	6.17	.007	6.25	.001	.006	.000
44	Circulatory, new patient, who was referred with a presenting problem of shortness of breath, chest pain, or heart murmur.	.004	1.62	.003	1.60	.000	-.001	.000
55	Circulatory, revisit for a new problem, without periodic exam, who was not referred, without a presenting problem of chest pain, with a diagnosis of hypertension	.021	3.74	.021	3.84	.002	.000	.000
64	Respiratory, new patient who was referred	.015	2.43	.016	2.40	.000	.003	-.001
65	Respiratory, revisit, without a period exam, for medication	.042	12.5	.038	15.00	.105	-.050	-.010
72	Digestive, new patient, with a visit not specified as acute, with a secondary diagnosis	.007	1.94	.011	2.22	.002	.007	.001
82	Digestive, revisit for a new problem, specified as acute, age 0-12 years.	.030	5.15	.032	5.17	.000	.010	.000
87	Genitourinary, new patient, age 40-99, with a presenting problem of breast or gynecologic disorder	.021	2.92	.022	3.05	.003	.003	.000
92	Genitourinary, revisit for a new problem, with a kidney infection or cystitis	.044	4.55	.046	6.55	.088	.009	.004
105	Musculoskeletal, new patient who was referred	.023	2.00	.022	2.15	.003	-.002	.000
106	Musculoskeletal, revisit without a period exam, who was not referred, with arthritis or related diagnosis	.430	3.88	.425	4.20	.142	-.019	-.006
116	Accident, poisoning and violence, revisit for an old problem, with a diagnosis of sprain, laceration, contusion, or eye injury with surgical aftercare	.017	6.60	.018	6.26	-.101	.007	.095
145	Other, receiving a vaccination, immunization, prophylactic inoculation or sensitization	.076	9.35	.072	9.25	-.008	-.038	.001
147	Other, receiving a general medical examination, and not presenting for a gynecological examination	.257	3.08	.259	6.10	.776	.006	.006
	All 15 AVG's listed above	1.00	4.47	1.00	5.52	1.02	-.06	.09

TABLE 3
Casemix Report
Region Average LOS = 6.772

(1)	(2)	(3)	(4)	(5)	(6)	(7)	(8)	(9)	(10)	(11)
	OBS	Avg. LOS	Casemix Adj.LOS	LOS Wgtd. Casemix	LOS Index	Casemix Index	Avg. LOS Diff.	Diff. Due To LOS	Diff.Due To Casemix	Interact Diff.
Hospital 1	12666	7.580	6.850	7.433	1.012	1.098	.808	.079	.661	.068
Hospital 2	24049	6.533	6.591	6.643	.973	.981	-.239	-.180	-.128	.070
Hospital 3	14117	6.798	6.256	6.999	.924	1.034	.026	-.516	.227	.315
Hospital 4	41643	7.479	7.320	6.960	1.081	1.028	.708	.548	.188	-.029
Hospital 5	5499	6.395	6.068	7.072	.896	1.044	-.377	-.704	.300	.027
Hospital 6	8167	6.256	6.585	6.398	.972	.945	-.516	-.187	-.374	.045
Hospital 7	2828	6.493	6.434	7.230	.950	1.068	-.279	-.338	.458	-.399
Hospital 8	20494	4.943	5.457	5.785	.806	.854	-1.828	-1.315	-.986	.473

TABLE 4

Hospital Discharge Casemix Comparison: France, The Netherlands, The United States
(Excluding Discharges with LOS > 100 Days)

Major Diagnostic Category 3: Diseases & Disorders of the Ear, Nose & Throat

DRG Num	Diagnosis Related Group	FRANCE NUM	PCT	MEAN LOS	NETHERLANDS NUM	PCT	MEAN LOS	UNITED STATES NUM	PCT	MEAN LOS
SURGICAL										
49	Major Head & Neck Procedures	140	1.5	17.4	3	0.1	26.0	11459	0.6	22.1
50	Sialoadenectomy	-	-	-	8	0.2	8.8	20247	1.1	4.8
51	Salivary Gland Procedures Except Sialoadenectomy	54	0.6	10.4	8	0.2	10.5	5402	0.3	3.5
52	Cleft Lip & Palate Repair	1	0.0	5.0	10	0.3	18.8	9465	0.5	4.4
53	Sinus & Mastoid Procedures Age > = 18	224	2.4	4.9	127	3.9	8.7	51295	2.9	4.5
54	Sinus & Mastoid Procedures Age 0-17	37	0.4	7.4	32	1.0	8.2	7068	0.4	3.3
55	Miscellaneous Ear, Nose & Throat Procedures	1181	12.8	5.5	550	16.7	6.0	257047	14.4	3.2
56	Rhinoplasty	19	0.2	4.2	189	5.7	6.1	94029	5.3	2.7
57	T & A Proc Except Tonsillectomy &/Or Adenoidectomy Age >=18	18	0.2	5.3	-	-	-	9226	0.5	4.5
58	T & A Proc Except Tonsillectomy &/Or Adenoidectomy Age 0-17	61	0.7	2.8	13	0.4	6.2	113810	6.4	1.8
59	Tonsillectomy &/Or Adenoidectomy Age > = 18	170	1.8	5.3	152	4.6	6.6	112972	6.3	2.3
60	Tonsillectomy &/Or Adenoidectomy Age 0-17	578	6.3	2.6	1747	53.1	2.0	294275	16.5	1.8
61	Myringotomy Age > = 18	12	0.1	4.3	30	0.9	2.9	4734	0.3	2.3
62	Myringotomy Age 0-17	77	0.8	1.9	68	2.1	1.6	61235	3.4	1.2
63	Other Ear, Nose & Throat O.R. Procedures	302	3.3	10.5	14	0.4	9.5	19911	1.1	6.0
MEDICAL										
64	Ear, Nose & Throat Malignancy	416	4.5	15.8	7	0.2	9.3	29778	1.7	9.1
65	Dysequilibrium	440	4.8	10.0	19	0.6	11.6	80939	4.5	5.2
66	Epistaxis	389	4.2	4.5	37	1.1	5.9	14240	0.8	3.6
67	Epiglottitis	2	0.0	0.0	1	0.0	25.0	3043	0.2	4.0
68	Otitis Media & URI Age > = 70 &/Or C.C.	138	1.5	13.7	11	0.3	21.6	87646	4.9	6.5
69	Otitis Media & URI Age 18-69 W/O C.C.	589	6.4	6.4	36	1.1	9.4	122145	6.8	4.2
70	Otitis Media & URI Age 0-17	2865	31.1	5.1	69	2.1	10.3	250257	14.0	3.6
71	Laryngotracheitis	53	0.6	2.5	2	0.1	4.5	36452	2.0	3.2
72	Nasal Trauma & Deformity	505	5.5	4.4	49	1.5	5.2	27301	1.5	2.7
73	Other Ear, Nose & Throat Diagnoses Age > = 18	492	5.3	7.1	67	2.0	8.5	45618	2.6	5.1
74	Other Ear, Nose & Throat Diagnoses Age 0-17	455	4.9	5.3	44	1.3	7.6	17026	1.0	2.8

In Table 3 is shown a similar report for a set of hospitals using length of stay (LOS) as the dependent variable. The difference in average LOS can be seen to be accounted for by differences due to case mix and differences due to productivity. Hospital 4, for example, had a LOS of 7.479 days as contrasted to 6.772 for all the hospitals in the region. Of the difference of about 0.7 days, half a day was due to treating patients differently, that is, using on average half a day more per case when case mix is controlled. The remaining difference was due to treating patients that required on average 0.2 days more than the average requirement for the entire region. In this case we can infer that hospital 4 is significantly less productive than all the other hospitals in its use of bed days. This is even more striking when we consider that the norm used in this case is the average for all the hospitals and hospital 4 contributes significantly to the norm itself.

International Case Mix Analysis

With this approach it is possible to compare hospital case mix and productivity between countries. We have been able to produce a group assignment program using French data by mapping as between ICD-9 and ICD-9-CM for diagnoses and the VESKA procedure codes and ICD-9-CM. At the hospitals of Tilburg University in the Netherlands they have also assigned their records to DRG's. Thus, we are able to present some cross national comparisons for which the measure of performance is average LOS by DRG. Table 4 shows these results for MDC 3, Diseases and Disorders of the Ear, Nose and Throat. The figures for the U.S. are from the Hospital Discharge Survey and the case mix frequency is an estimate of the total for the U.S. in 1980. The French data are from nine hospitals with a total data base consisting of 225,000 records from 1979, 1980, and 1981.

For DRG 53, Sinus and Mastoid Procedures, Age $\geqslant$ 18, it can be seen that the case mix proportion (percent of total cases in the MDC) are 2.4, 3.9, and 2.9 for French data, Netherlands data, and the U.S. The ALOS is 4.9, 8.7 and 4.5 respectively. For DRG's 59 and 60, Tonsillectomy and/or Adenoidectomy, Age $\geqslant$ 18 and Age 0–17, the case mix proportions as well as ALOS can be seen to be remarkably different. Finally, for DRG's 68, 69, and 70, Otitis Media and URI in three age classes, we observe again striking differences in both case mix and ALOS.

Thus, it is possible to examine the sources of observed differences in utilization of hospital resources regionally, nationally, and internationally by this approach. One can, for the first time, compare such utilization and determine the extent to which it is due to the treatment of different kinds of patients, and the extent to which it is due to treating the same patients differently. Insofar as differences are a function of different treatment, then we can legitimately question the relative effectiveness of this differential process. If we spend more of our resources on the same kind of case in one setting than in another, is the patient differently better off?

Hospital Profiles

Individual hospitals can be examined comparatively by DRG to show their relative consumption of hospital resources. Using LOS as the dependent variable, Table 4 shows DRG's 69 and 70, Otitis Media comparing 9 hospitals. For DRG 70, hospital D treated 1164 patients with an average LOS of 3.95 days. Hospital E, on the other hand, treated 508 patients with ALOS of 5.77 days and a median LOS of five days. This two day difference represents over 1,000 bed days consumed by hospital E in treating pediatric otitis media as compared to the performance of hospital D. Hospitals D and E exhibit a similar two day difference for DRG 69, adult otitis media.

The profile for DRG 184, in Figure III, shows hospital D as consuming three days as a median LOS while hospitals E and I use five days. Similarly, for DRG 198, in Figure IV, the comparison is 12 days for hospital D, 14 days for E, and 18.5 days for I. By examination of these profiles, relative productivity can be explored, aand questions raised as to the effectiveness of treatment, given these significant differences in process.

Conclusions

By defining the products of health care institutions, we can for the first time, begin to understand and rationalize the performance of the health sector. As this sector accounts for an increasing share of any nation's resources, it is crucial to be able to monitor and explain the differential behavior and its costs. The product model discussed here is a first step toward this end.

FIGURE II

DRG 69: Otitis Media & URI Age 18–69 w/o C.C.

⇒ Profile DRG 69 Using Hospital Order Median

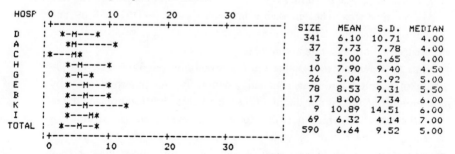

DRG 70: Otitis Media & URI Age 0-17

⇒Profile DRG 70 Using Hospital Order Median

```
HOSP    0        10        20        30
     :+---------+---------+---------+---------: SIZE   MEAN   S.D.   MEDIAN
  H  :  *-M---*                              :   26   3.65   3.14    2.50
  D  :  *M-*                                 : 1164   3.95   3.71    3.00
  B  :  *-M-*                                :   96   3.51   2.68    3.00
  I  :   *-M-*                               :  553   4.75   4.09    4.00
  K  :   *M-*                                :   26   4.58   2.67    4.00
  G  :   *M--*                               :  122   5.22   3.78    4.00
  E  :   *-M-*                               :  508   5.77   4.62    5.00
  A  :    *-M-*                              :  197   6.56   4.43    6.00
  C  :      *---M----*                       :  173  10.86   6.31   10.00
TOTAL:   *-M--*                              : 2865   5.06   4.50    4.00
     :+---------+---------+---------+---------:
       0        10        20        30
```

FIGURE III

DRG 198: Total Cholecystectomy w/o C.D.C. Age < w/o C.C.

⇒ Profile DRG 198 Using Hospital Order Median

```
HOSP    0        10        20        30
     :+---------+---------+---------+---------: SIZE   MEAN   S.D.   MEDIAN
  D  :          *-M---*                      :  437  13.69   8.36   12.00
  G  :          *-M---*                      :   60  14.95   6.38   12.50
  B  :          *--M-*                       :   18  15.61   7.16   13.50
  E  :          *-M--*                       :   29  15.69   7.10   14.00
  A  :          *M------*                    :   97  16.98   8.20   14.00
  H  :          *--M------*                  :   18  18.94   8.19   15.50
  K  :           *M---*                      :   10  20.90  11.20   17.00
  I  :          *---M------*                 :   80  21.27   9.44   18.50
  C  :          *--M-----*                   :   11  30.09  29.95   19.00
TOTAL:          *-M----*                     :  760  15.58   9.40   13.00
     :+---------+---------+---------+---------:
       0        10        20        30
```

FIGURE IV

DRG 184: Esophagitis, Gastroenteritis & Miscellaneous Digestion Disorders Age 0–17

⇒ Profile DRG 184 Using Hospital Order Median

```
HOSP    0        10        20        30
     :+---------+---------+---------+---------: SIZE   MEAN   S.D.   MEDIAN
  K  :  *M*                                  :   92   3.50   2.50    3.00
  D  :  *-M-*                                : 1640   4.23   5.96    3.00
  B  :  *M---*                               :  161   5.52   9.03    3.00
  H  :  *-M---*                              :   36   4.00   3.40    3.00
  G  :  *-M--*                               :  210   5.30   4.90    4.00
  A  :   *-M---*                             :  479   7.18   7.13    5.00
  E  :   *-M--*                              :  581   6.32   5.50    5.00
  I  :   *-M--*                              :  634   6.26   4.85    5.00
  C  :     *---M--*                          :  180  10.67   9.86    8.50
TOTAL:  *-M--*                               : 4013   5.58   6.34    4.00
     :+---------+---------+---------+---------:
       0        10        20        30
```

APPENDIX A

PATIENT RECORD AND PATIENT LOG

B № 881078

B № 881078

PATIENT LOG

ASSURANCE OF CONFIDENTIALITY — All information which would permit identification of an individual, a practice, or an establishment will be held confidential and will be used only by persons engaged in and for the purposes of the survey and will not be disclosed or released to other persons or used for any other purpose

PATIENT RECORD
NATIONAL AMBULATORY MEDICAL CARE SURVEY

As each patient arrives, record name and time of visit on the log below. For the patient entered on line #2, also complete the patient record to the right.

1. DATE OF VISIT Mo / Day / Yr

PATIENT'S NAME	TIME OF VISIT

2. DATE OF BIRTH Mo / Day / Yr

3. SEX
- [ ] FEMALE
- [ ] MALE

4. COLOR OR RACE
- [ ] WHITE
- [ ] NEGRO/ BLACK
- [ ] OTHER
- [ ] UNKNOWN

5. PATIENT'S PRINCIPAL PROBLEM(S) COMPLAINT(S) OR SYMPTOM(S) THIS VISIT (In patient's own words)
a MOST IMPORTANT_____
b OTHER_____

6. SERIOUSNESS OF PROBLEM IN ITEM 5a (Check one)
- [ ] VERY SERIOUS
- [ ] SERIOUS
- [ ] SLIGHTLY SERIOUS
- [ ] NOT SERIOUS

7. HAVE YOU EVER SEEN THIS PATIENT BEFORE?
- [ ] YES • [ ] NO
If YES, for the problem indicated in ITEM 5a?
• [ ] YES • [ ] NO

1

2

Record items 1-12 for this patient

8. MAJOR REASON(S) FOR THIS VISIT (Check all major reasons)
- [ ] ACUTE PROBLEM
- [ ] ACUTE PROBLEM, FOLLOW-UP
- [ ] CHRONIC PROBLEM, ROUTINE
- [ ] CHRONIC PROBLEM, FLARE-UP
- [ ] PRENATAL CARE
- [ ] POSTNATAL CARE
- [ ] POSTOPERATIVE CARE ¬
- [ ] WELL ADULT/CHILD EXAM
- [ ] FAMILY PLANNING
- [ ] COUNSELING/ADVICE
- [ ] IMMUNIZATION
- [ ] REFERRED BY OTHER PHYS/AGENCY
- [ ] ADMINISTRATIVE PURPOSE
- [ ] OTHER (Specify)

(Operative procedure)

9. PHYSICIAN'S PRINCIPAL DIAGNOSIS THIS VISIT
a DIAGNOSIS ASSOCIATED WITH ITEM 5a ENTRY
_____
_____
b OTHER SIGNIFICANT CURRENT DIAGNOSES (In order of importance)
_____
_____

CONTINUE LISTING PATIENTS ON NEXT PAGE

10. DIAGNOSTIC/THERAPEUTIC SERVICES ORDERED/PROVIDED THIS VISIT (Check all that apply)
- [ ] NONE
- [ ] LIMITED HISTORY/EXAM
- [ ] GENERAL HISTORY/EXAM
- [ ] CLINICAL LAB TEST
- [ ] BLOOD PRESSURE CHECK
- [ ] EKG
- [ ] HEARING TEST
- [ ] VISION TEST
- [ ] ENDOSCOPY
- [ ] OFFICE SURGERY
- [ ] DRUG PRESCRIBED OR DISPENSED
- [ ] X RAY
- [ ] INJECTION
- [ ] IMMUNIZATION/DESENSITIZATION
- [ ] PHYSIOTHERAPY
- [ ] MEDICAL COUNSELING
- [ ] PSYCHOTHERAPY/THERAPEUTIC LISTENING
- [ ] OTHER (Specify)_____

11. DISPOSITION THIS VISIT (Check all that apply)
- [ ] NO FOLLOW-UP PLANNED
- [ ] RETURN AT SPECIFIED TIME
- [ ] RETURN IF NEEDED, P.R.N
- [ ] TELEPHONE FOLLOW-UP PLANNED
- [ ] REFERRED TO OTHER PHYSICIAN/AGENCY
- [ ] RETURNED TO REFERRING PHYSICIAN
- [ ] ADMIT TO HOSPITAL
- [ ] OTHER (Specify)_____

12. DURATION OF THIS VISIT (Time actually spent with physician)
_____ MINUTES

HRA 34 3 REV 2/76

DEPARTMENT OF HEALTH, EDUCATION AND WELFARE
PUBLIC HEALTH SERVICE
HEALTH RESOURCES ADMINISTRATION
NATIONAL CENTER FOR HEALTH STATISTICS

OMB 268-R1498

The National Ambulatory Medical Care Survey: 1975 Summary Series 13, Number 33, U.S. Department of Health, Education, and Welfare Public Health Services, National Center for Health Statistics, Hyattsville, Maryland, January, 1978.

APPENDIX B

LIST OF MAJOR AMBULATORY CATEGORIES

Initial Group No.	Initial Group Name	ICDA8 Code	Avg. No.
1	Infective and Parasitic Disorders	017,0171,0179-0189 020-031,0319-0339, 035-0399,050-0619, 067-0689,071-0759, 079-0790,0792-0902, 0904-0929,095-1049, 113-1149,116-1309, 132-1349,136-1369	1-12
2	Endocrine, Nutritional and Metabolic Disorders	193-1949,226-2269, 240-2689,269-2699, 270-2731,2734,2736- 2739,275-2799	13-24

List of Major Ambulatory Categories

Initial Group No.	Initial Group Name	ICDA8 Code	Avg. No.
3	Mental Disorders	290-3159,790-7902, 7930,794-7949	25-36
4	Disorders of the Nervous System	013-0139,0191,040-0469,062-0669,0940-0949,191-1929,225-2259,238,2381-2389, 320-3589,430-4389, 7720-7722,780-7808, 781,7814-7818,791-7919,850-8549	37-39
5	Disorders of the Circulatory System	0930-0939,390-4029 404-4299,440-4459, 451-4519,453-4549, 456,4561-4569,458-4589,782-7826,7829, 795-7959,Y100	40-59
6	Disorders of the Respiratory System	010-0129,0190,034-0341,115-1159,0310, 135-1359,160-1639, 212-2129,231-2319, 450,4509,460-5199, 766-7769,783-7837	60-70
7	Disorders of the Digestive System	000-0099,014-0149, 070-0709,140-1599 210,2119,230-2309, 2690-2691,2732-2733, 2735,452-4529,455-4559,4560,520-5779, 784-7858,Y102	71-84
8	Disorders of the Genitourinary System	016-0169,0192,112, 131-1319,174-1749, 180-1899,217-2239, 233-2379,403-4039, 580-6299,786-7867, 789-7899,792-7929, Y090,Y101	85-94
9	Disorders of the Skin and Subcutaneous Tissue	0170,0791,110-1119, 172-1739,214-2149, 216-2169,232,2322, 680-7099	95-102
10	Disorders of the Musculoskeletal System and Connective Tissue	015-0159,0193-0196, 170-1719,213-2139, 215-2159,2320,2321, 274-1749,446-4479,	105-109

		710-7389,787-7876, Y104	
11	Accidents, Poisonings and Violence	800-8489,860-9999	110-122
12	Disorders of the Eye	0172,076-0789,0903, 190-1909,224-2249, 2380,360-3793,7810- 7812,Y006,Y122	123-132
13	Disorders of the Ear	0173,380-3899,7813	133-143
14	Other		
	Special Conditions and Exam without Sickness	Y00-Y005,Y007-Y089, Y091-Y099,Y103,Y105- Y121,Y123—Y13,Y300- Y302	144-154
	Disorders of the Blood and Blood-Forming Organs	280-2899	
	Complications of Preg. Childbirth and Puerperium	630-6789	
	Congenital Anomalies	740-7599	
	Certain Causes of Peri- natal Morbidity and Mortality	760-7719,7729,773, 774-7759,777-7799	
	Symptoms	7827,7828,788-788-7889 793,7931,7938-7939, 796-7969	
	Miscellaneous	019,0199,195-1999, 200,2099,227-2289, 239-2399,448-4489, 457-4579	

APPENDIX C

Independent Variables*

AGE: The age calculated from date of birth was the age at last birthday on the date of visit.

COLOR OR RACE: On the Patient Record, color or race includes four categories: white, Negro/black, other, and unknown. The physician was instructed to mark the category which in his judgment was most appropriate for the patient based upon observation and/or prior knowledge of the patient. "Other" was restricted to Orientals, American Indians, and other races neither Negro nor white.

PATIENT'S PRINCIPAL PROBLEM(S): COMPLAINT(S), OR SYMPTOM(S) (IN PATIENT'S OWN WORDS): The patient's principal problem, complaint, symptom, reason for the visit as expressed by the patient. Physicians were instructed to record key words or phrases verbatim to the extent possible listing that problem first which in the physician's judgment was most responsible for the patient's visit.

SERIOUSNESS OF PROBLEM IN ITEM 5a: This item includes four categories: very serious, serious, slightly serious, and not serious. The physician was instructed to check one of the four categories according to his own evaluation of the seriousness of the patient's problem causing this visit. Seriousness refers to physician's clinical judgment as to the extent of the patient's impairment that might result if no care were given.

MAJOR REASON(S) FOR THIS VISIT: The patient's major reason(s) for the visit were classified by the physician into one or more of the following categories:

Acute Problem: A condition of illness having a relatively sudden or recent onset (i.e., within three months of the visit).

Acute Problem, Follow-up: A return visit primarily for continued medical care of a previously treated acute problem.

Chronic Problem, Routine: A visit primarily to receive regular care or examination for a preexisting chronic condition or illness (onset of condition was three months or more before this visit).

Chronic Problem, Flare-up: A visit primarily due to a sudden exacerbation of a preexisting chronic condition.

Prenatal Care: Routine obstetrical care provided prior to delivery.

Postnatal Care: Routine obstetrical care or examination provided following delivery or termination of pregnancy.

Postoperative Care: A visit primarily for care required following surgical

---

*The National Ambulatory Medical Care Survey: 1975 Summary Series 13, Number 33, U.S. Department of Health, Education, and Welfare, Public Health Service, National Center for Health Statistics, Hyattsville, Maryland, January 1978.

treatment. Includes changing dressing, removing sutures or case, advising on restriction of activities or routine after surgery checkup.

Well Adult/Child Exam: General health maintenance examinations and routine maintenance examinations and routine periodic examinations of presumably healthy persons, both children and adults. Includes annual physical examinations, well-child checkups, school, camp, and insurance examinations.

Family Planning: Services or advice that enable patients to determine the number and spacing of their children. Includes both contraception and infertility services.

Counseling/Advice: Information of a health nature which would enable the patient to maintain or improve his physical or mental well-being. Included would be advice regarding diet, changing habits or behavior, and general information regarding a specific problem.

Immunization: Administration of any inoculation of specific substances to produce a desired immunity; this includes oral vaccines. (Allergy shots are not included in this category, but are entered in "other").

Referred by Another Physician/Agency: Medical attention prompted by advice or referral for consultation or treatment from another physician, hospital, clinic, health center, school nurse, minister, pharmacist, etc. Does not incude self-referral or referral by family or friends.

Administrative Purpose: Reasons such as completing insurance forms, school forms, work permits, or discussion of patient's bill.

Other: The reason for this visit is not covered in the precedling list.

PRINCIPAL DIAGNOSIS: The physician's diagnosis of the patient's principal problem or complaint. In the event of multiple diagnoses, the physician was instructed to list them in order of decreasing importance; "principal" refers to the first-listed diagnosis. The diagnosis represents the physician's best judgment at the time of the visit and may be tentative, provisional, or definitive.

OTHER SIGNIFICANT CURRENT DIAGNOSIS: The diagnosis of any other condition known to exist for the patient at the time of the visit. Other diagnoses may or may not be related to the reason for that visit.

TREATMENTS AND SERVICES ORDERED OR PROVIDED: These include the following:

Limited History/Exam: History and/or physical examination which is limited to a specific body site or system, or which is concerned primarily with the patient's chief complaint, for example, pelvic exam or eye exam.

General History/Exam: History and/or physical examination of a comprehensive nature, including all or most body systems.

Clinical Lab Test: One or more laboratory procedures or tests including examination of blood, urine, sputum, smears, exudates, transudates, feces, and gastric content, and including chemistry, serology, bacteriology, and pregnancy test.

Blood Pressure Check: Self-explanatory.

EKG: Electrocardiogram.

Hearing Test: Auditory acuity test.

Vision Test: Visual acuity test.

Endoscopy: Examination of the interior of any body cavity, except ear, nose, and throat, by means of an endoscope.

Office Surgery: Any surgical procedure performed in the office this visit, including suture of wounds, reduction of fractures, application/removal of casts, incision and draining of abscesses, application of supportive materials for fractures and sprains, and all irrigations, aspirations, dilations, and excisions.

Drug Prescribed: Drugs, vitamins, hormones, ointments, suppositories, or other medications ordered or provided, except injections and immunizations.

X-Ray: Any single or multiple X-ray examination for diagnostic or screening purposes. Radiation therapy is not included in this category.

Injection: Administration of any substance by syrine and needle subcutaneously, intravenously, or intramuscularly. This category does not include immunizations, enemas, or douches.

Immunization/Desensitization: Administration of any immunizing, vaccinating, or desensitizing agent or substance by any route, for example, syringe, needle, orally, gun, or scarification.

Physiotherapy: Any form of physical therapy ordered or provided, including any treatment using heat, light, sound, or physical pressure or movement, for example, ultrasonic, ultraviolet, infrared, whirlpool, diathermy, cold therapy, and manipulative therapy.

Medical Counseling: Instructions and recommendations regarding any health problem, including advice or counsel about diet, change of habit, or behavior. Physicians are instructed to check this category only if the medical counseling is a significant part of the treatment.

Psychotherapy/Therapeutic Listening: All treatments designed to produce a mental or emotional response through suggested, persuasion, re-education, reassurance, or support, including psychological counseling, hypnosis, psychoanalysis, and transactional therapy.

Other: Treatments or services rendered which are not listed in the preceding categories.

DISPOSITION: Eight categories are provided to describe the physician's disposition of the case as follows:

No Follow-up Planned: No return visit or telephone contact was scheduled for the patient's problem on the visit.

Return at Specified Time: The apteint was told to schedule an appointment or was instructed to return at a particular time.

Return if Needed, P.R.N.: No future appointment was made, but the patient was instructed to make an appointment with the physician if the patient considers it necessary.

Telephone Follow-up Planned: The patient was instructed to telephone the physician on a particular day to report on his progress, or if the need arises.

Referred to Other Physician/Agency: The patient was instructed to consult or seek care from another physician or agency. The patient may or may not return to this physician at a later date.

Returned to Referring Physician: Patient was referred to this physician and was not instructed to consult again with the physician or agency which referred him.

Admit to Hospital: Patient was instructed that further care or treatment will be provided in a hospital. No further office visits were expected prior to that admission.

Other: Any other disposition of the case not included in the above categories.

DURATION OF VISIT: Time the physician spent with the patient, but does not include the time patient spent waiting to see the physician, time patient spent receiving care from someone other than the doctor without the presence of the physician, and time spent reviewing records, test results, and so forth. In the event a patient was provided care by a member of physician's staff but did not see the physician during the visit, "duration of visit" was recorded as zero minutes.

REFERENCES

Ambulatory Patient Related Group, Health Systems Management Group, Yale School of Organization and Management, April 1980.

R. E. Berry, "Cost and Efficiency in the Production of Hospital Services," *Milbank Memorial Fund Quarterly*, Vol. 52, pp. 291-313, 1974.

————, "Product Heterogeneity and Hospital Cost Analysis,"*Inquiry*, Vol. 7, pp. 67-75, 1970.

R. B. Chase and N. J. Aquilano, *Production and Operations Management*, Richard D. Irwin, Inc., 1977.

Diagnosis Related Group Reports for PSRO Databases, Center for Health Studies, Yale University Institution for Social and Policy Studies, April 1978.

M. S. Feldstein, "Hospital Cost Variation and Case-Mix Differences," *Medical Care*, Vol. 3, pp. 95-103, 1965.

R. B. Fetter, Y. Shin, and J. L. Freeman, *et al.,* "Case-Mix Definition by Diagnosis-Related Groups," *Medical Care*, Vol. 18 (supplement), February 1980.

R. B. Fetter, R. F. Averill, J. L. Lichtenstein, and J. L. Freeman, Ambulatory Visit Groups: A Framework for Measuring Productivity in Ambulatory Care, Health Systems Management Group, Yale School of Organization and Management (To Be Published in *Health Services Research*.)

R. B. Fetter, Y. Shin, J. L. Freeman, R. F. Averill, and J. D. Thompson, "Case Mix Definition by Diagnosis Related Groups," *Medical Care,* 1980, 18 (supplement).

B. A. Hill, *Principles of Medical Statistics,* New York, Oxford University Press, 1971.

E. M. Kitagawa, "Components of a Difference Between Two Rates," *Journal of the American Statistical Association,* 1955; 50: p. 296.

J. R. Lave and L. B. Lave, "Estimated Cost Functions for Pennsylvania Hospitals," *Inquiry,* Vol. 7, pp. 3-14, 1970.

J. R. Lave, "A Review of the Methods Used to Study Hospital Costs," *Inquiry,* Vol. 3, pp. 57-81, 1966.

J. R. Lave and L. B. Lave, "The Extent of Role Differentiation Among Hospitals," *Health Services Research,* Vol. 6, pp. 15-38, 1971.

J. R. Lave and L. B. Lave, "Hospital Cost Functions," *American Economic Review,* Vol. 60, pp. 379-95, 1970.

M. L. Lee and R. L. Wallace, "Problems in Estimating Multiproduct Cost Functions: An Application to Hospitals," *Western Economic Journal,* Vol. 11, pp. 350-63, 1973.

National Center for Health Statistics: National Ambulatory Medical Care Survey: Background and Methodology, United States, 1967-72, *Vital and Health Statistics,* Series 2, No. 61, DHEW Publication No. (HRA) 74-1335. Health Resources Administration, Washington, U.S. Government Printing Office, April 1974.

National Center for Health Statistics: Health, United States, 1980, DHEW Pub. No., (PHS) 81-1232, Public Health Service, Washington, U.S. Government Printing Office, 1980.

National Center for Health Statistics: The National Ambulatory Medical Care Survey: Symptom Classification, *Vital and Health Statistics,* Series 2, No. 63, DHEW Publication No. (HRA) 74-1337, Health Resources Administration, Washington, U.S. Government Printing Office, May 1974.

New ICD-9-CM Diagnosis Related Groups Classification Scheme: User Manual, Health Systems Management Group, Yale School of Organization and Management Group, Yale School of Organization and Management, 1981.

H. S. Ruchlin and I. Levenson, "Measuring Hospital Productivity," *Health Services Research,* Vol. 9, pp. 308-23, 1974.

J. A. Sonquist and J. N. Morgan, *The Detection of Interaction Effects,* Institute for Social Research, University of Michigan, 1964.

Part Five

New Productivity Techniques

Chapter Twelve

Productivity in Health Care

CHARLES T. WOOD

Health care expenditures are a source of increasing concern the world over —not only to hospitals and other health care institutions, but to governments, government agencies and the consumer as well. While it is not accurate to pinpoint unrealistic accounting and budgeting methods as the cause of all of the current problems, they do compound misrepresentations as well as inefficiencies within the delivery system.

When institutionalized health care was primarily limited to custodial care for the dying indigent consisting of room, board, and minimal therapeutic, palliative services, the cost for such care was determined by an all-inclusive average rate per patient, per day or per occupied bed day. This early measure was a fairly accurate cost allocation. Early health care institutions were dealing with a medically homogenous population with nearly identical service needs. As medical care became more sophisticated and the patient population became more diverse, accounting and budgeting methods did not reflect these changes. Cost finding techniques continued to be based on division of total operating cost by total patient days or occupied bed days, thereby neglecting the differences in service intensity by diagnosis and point-in-progress toward recovery among patients.

Historically, the nebulous definition of the components of per diem costs which should be included in the calculation of productivity statistics has resulted in varying services per unit of cost between institutions as well as within a single institution. In some hospitals the routine per diem cost currently includes a per occupied bed per diem fraction of the expected annual cost of providing all services including the specialized services (such as anesthesiology, radiology, operating room, pathology laboratory, etc.) whether a particular patient receives the service or not.

I believe we health care managers have had our mind set far too long on averaging everything into a per diem rate, and in order to change to productivity management in health care we not only have to build management systems, but we have to build management systems that are meaningful.

To challenge your current thinking, I want to tell you a story that was published in an article of mine in the *Harvard Business Review* [Wood, pp.

177

97-104]. Once upon a time there was a vehicle rental agency called Hurtz. Mr. Hurtz rented out fourteen-wheelers, ten-wheelers, heavy trucks, light trucks, small cars, and luxury cars. Mr. Hurtz had rental divisions all over the world. Let's imagine now that he approached cost-finding the way we do in health care. With his average per diem mind set, he took the direct cost of all of these vehicles plus his overhead and divided it by the sum of the days each vehicle was used and he came up with a figure that he called "cost per vehicle day." Now, I ask you, if you were Mr. Hurtz, could you manage an operation like that? Could you really manage an operation where you take all of your expenses and divide that figure by the number of days your vehicles were rented and come up with a cost per vehicle day and expect to use that figure to measure productivity? You would say, "That guy is crazy. How can he do that? Why doesn't he cost out his heavy trucks and his light trucks all separately so that he will know what the different costs are?"

But in health care, we have been managing our businesses just like Mr. Hurtz for many years—that is, averaging our heavy trucks and our lighter cars. It didn't make any difference years ago because all we were doing as institutions was giving care consisting of room, board, and minimal therapeutic services. However, as technology increased and treatment methods changed in the health care field, somehow or another we neglected to change our method of determining cost.

I have another story. This one concerns a shoe manufacturer. In one year the shoe manufacturer produced 17.5 million pairs of shoes at a total cost of $160 million. The manufacturing cost per shoe was $9.14. Does this sound familiar? What kind of a productivity statistic is that? Whether that company makes sneakers or boots, whether the company uses expensive materials on some shoes and inexpensive materials on others, we are expecting the company to divide all the expenses by the number of pairs it produces and identify a cost per shoe.

If a shoe company did its costing in this way, any one of us could drive it out of business by manufacturing only the less expensive items in the product line. We could undercut the shoe company's price and still make a profit because we would have properly identified specific product cost and would not use this item to subsidize more expensive ones.

What we are doing in health care is averaging too many things, and because we average too many things we don't really know what our costs are for them individually. We can't be sensitive to productivity if we don't know the resources that go into our operations.

I could go on with this little shoe fantasy. I could tell you that this particular shoe manufacturer has different plants all over the country, some in the South and some in the North, East and West. The company is frustrated because it is afraid someone is going to get into competition with it and therefore it wants to keep costs down. Remember, it is costing just like hospitals—so many dollars per shoe, regardless of the actual cost elements. How is it going to keep its costs down? The CEO gets his management team together and says, "The only way we can keep our costs down is to put some ceilings on the budgets of those guys out in the plants. We must measure cost-of-living indexes, inflation factors, and then we will send out a memorandum from the home office which says, 'Next year when you do your budgets, we are not allowing you to raise your cost per average shoe more than 8 percent. Do anything you want to, just don't produce shoes in your plant which average more than the ceiling,'"

One of its plants is in New England where the weather is more severe; the cold winds are blowing and snow is falling. Its market for boots is growing rapidly. Most likely the plant manager is going to write to the home office and say, "I can't tolerate your ceilings. My product mix is changing towards more boots and you at the home office are trying to limit me to 8 percent increase as a ceiling per average shoe. Besides, someone nearby has opened a factory producing sneakers and I am not selling as many sneakers as I used to. How am I going to keep my cost per shoe at $9.14 plus 8 percent? With fewer sneakers and more boots, my cost will be at least 15 percent higher next year."

Another plant in Georgia is making lighter shoes. Business is increasing in sneakers. Yet the manager is allowed to raise his cost per average shoe by the 8 percent although his cost per average shoe will actually drop as he reduces boot manufacture.

The point I'm making here is that we can't be competitive with each other and efficient in terms of productivity unless we use reliable data for measuring costs. If we want to be productivity conscious, we have to have a data base that is meaningful in terms of identifying true costs. All of which brings us back to the title of this presentation—"Changing Productivity Measurements and Managerial Techniques."

Our approach to health care management should be cost accounting, budgeting, and identifying cost of production units measured by resource output (Table 1). We should have management audits to measure and control productivity efficiency of the individual service units. In other words, productivity management measurable in resource output. What does it cost us for a fourteen-wheeler? What does it cost us for a luxury car? We can cost out the heavy load or the small load or the light load; at the very least we will know the cost of the heavy load or the light load even if our pricing decisions do not always follow the cost.

We should measure resource output by unit. Cost out the sneakers, cost out the boots, cost out the high fashion designs in a unit that is measurable

TABLE 1

Productivity Management

---

1. Cost Accounting and Budgeting by Productivity Units Measurable in Resource Output.
2. Management Audits to Measure and Control Productivity Efficiency by Units of Service.
3. Monitor Resource Utilization by Diagnosis by Physician by Units within a Hospital and between Patients.

---

so that we know what the true cost is. If we in health care don't do that, somebody is going to open up a sneaker plant next to us and guess what will happen? He's going to make sneakers for $2. He doesn't even have to practice productivity management to beat our price. He can undersell us without even trying because we are still averaging our costs, boosting the price of the sneakers to subsidize the boots. He can even run the most inefficient plant in the world and sell sneakers at $3 and still beat our $9.14 because we averaged our entire product line.

The problems of productivity measurements are not unique to the United States. Dr. Barry Catchlove of Melbourne, Australia feels that the present method of measurement is at best "a method of financial accounting. Certainly not a lot of management." [Catchlove and Hall, 1978]. He also says in his paper "the need for output measures to assess hospital performance and costs, length of stay, average daily census, number of admissions, occupancy, daily bed cost, and cost by inpatients treated—the common parameters used to compare performances—are all dependent on case mix and do not indicate a hospital's real performance. A short length of stay may indicate efficiency but more likely indicates a predominance of minor surgery and relative absence of more serious cases such as cancer and spinal injuries. Average daily admissions and occupancy are really only a measure of the hospital's ability to keep beds full and a decrease in length of stay for legitimate reasons will eventually decrease occupancy. Daily bed cost, i.e., cost of inpatients treated, still ignores the case mix and assumes all patients, all diseases use the same services."

After a hospital organizes for costing by units, what are the benefits? You would measure and control efficiency of these production units. In other words, you would know the efficiency of your institution. Mr. Hurtz would know what his ten-wheelers cost to operate. That is productivity management. Wouldn't you like to know if the cost for the same products is different at different institutions? You should know. And you should also know why. That is Number 2 of Table 1—Management Audits to Measure and Control Productivity Efficiency by Units of Service.

Statement Number 3 on Table 1 is what we can give free of charge to the consumer to save his health care dollars. You see, once we have a productivity system which identifies cost by units measured by resource output, and management audits to measure efficiency, we can start monitoring resource utilization by diagnosis, by physician and by units within a hospital or between hospitals. We can open up a whole new world of information. I suspect that while we are talking about the hard decisions we will have to make because our monetary well is drying up, we will find a lot of health care dollars can be saved before we come close to denying people excellent health care. But we can do this only by having good data, a productivity audit system and a system to measure resource utilization by institution, by diagnosis, and by physician. We can use these data in an educational process. Once we know the cost of our units, we can decide how many of these units we need to use to move this load from New York to California as in the Hurtz story. No more and no less, only what's needed to do a good job.

An example in our own health care system is the operating room. Remember back in the days when we used to cost our O.R.'s by surgical procedure? We did a very good job of it. We measured the number of hours by procedure, the O.R. team by procedure, the supplies by procedure. We developed a laundry list of costs and prices. That was good for about the first week the list was in operation. But the first person who changed a procedure rendered the list inaccurate. When we went to do our budgets for the O.R., how did we do it? If you did yours like I did mine, you negotiated with the operating room supervisor and she said, "I need more people." You said, "You don't need more people." She said, "I do need more people." You said, "Why do you need more people?" She said, "Because I have more work." And then the surgeons joined in on the side of the O.R. supervisor. None of you had productivity statistics but you negotiated. You said, "Well, we will have a 10 percent increase in the O.R. costs next year over this year, so we'll go down our laundry list and add 10 percent to all of those procedures. And that is our budget." Everybody here probably sets budgets this way. I did, and a lot of people in the United States are still doing it. But, to have productivity statistics you need an accurate accounting of personnel time in the O.R. and supplies by surgical procedure. Most of us are familiar now with productivity measurements in the O.R.

Nursing services, on the other hand, have traditionally been costed for and accounted for in the average per diem basis. Until recently, this created little incentive on the part of the Nursing Department to collect personnel hours by diagnosis statistics which would reflect true involvement by diagnosis and acuity. In other cases, this information has been available but since it was not tied to cost-finding and/or reimbursement methodologies, nursing budgets continued to be a function of patient days or occupied bed days.

At the same time the phenomenon of a shortened length of stay is being applauded as a quality-enhancer and cost-saver. It has a punitive effect on labor-intensive nursing departments. Yet as the length of stay decreases, the intensity of care per day usually increases. The prime target for cutbacks is the single largest line item of the hospital's operational budget—salaries and wages—and that means nursing. Thus, nurse staffing becomes a function of total patient days rather than workload. The result is two-fold: decreased availability of care during hospital stay and/or inappropriate early discharge of a patient to an alternative institutional setting or home, in which case the probability of repeat hospitalization is increased further increasing care.

The patient day or occupied bed day has prevailed as a unit of measurement although it's incompatible with the dual goals of high quality patient care and aggregate cost effectiveness and efficiency throughout the health care system.

The fallacy of the average per diem statistic became evident immediately when it was suggested for the producers of goods or services of industries other than health care. Should all cars be sold at the same average cost per car? It is like building a Cadillac and a Chevelle and selling them as a unit called Cadelle [Weaver, June 1977, p. 32].

Costing nursing care by output measures leaves us a little breathless. We are almost afraid to look at it. But as early as 1970 PETO developed an acuity measurement system at the Eugene Talmadge Hospital of the University of Georgia [Poland et al, July 1970, pp. 1479-482]. The Nursing Department was assessing and meeting the patient care needs by work load measurement. PETO was one of the earliest groups to work on acuity measurement. The Janna Plus system is a grandchild of PETO. The system at our hospital, the Massachusetts Eye and Ear Infirmary, is also a grandchild of PETO. PETO was originally and still is an acuity measurement system for developing nursing staffing patterns by nursing management.

Why were nurse managers the first to try productivity management? Why did the nurses feel they had to set up an elaborate management system for staffing their departments? I am guessing that they did it because too many times they walked in to see the administrator and said, "We need more nursing staff," and he said, "You can't have that because the 3.5 nursing hours per patient per day is what we have been using as a basis for the last 20 years and our hospital is getting reimbursed this way and I can't afford to give you any more nurses."

As you can see in Figure I, as the length of stay decreased, nursing work-

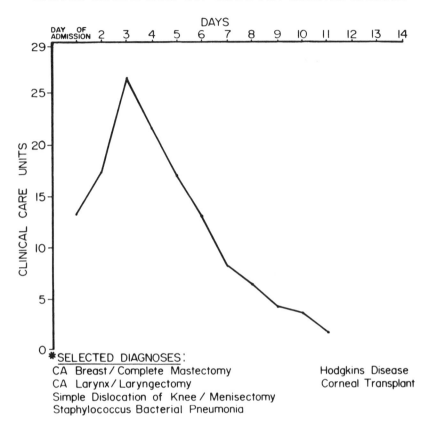

FIGURE I

AVERAGE CLINICAL CARE UNIT CURVE PER SELECTED DIAGNOSIS*

*SELECTED DIAGNOSES:
CA Breast / Complete Mastectomy
CA Larynx / Laryngectomy
Simple Dislocation of Knee / Menisectomy
Staphylococcus Bacterial Pneumonia

Hodgkins Disease
Corneal Transplant

load went up if a hospital was measuring nursing hours per patient day or by occupied bed day. Yet there was no way to measure this as long as the only measurement we used was patient days.

You don't think the nurse managers would have gone to all the trouble to set up sophisticated systems if every time they walked into the hospital administrator's office he said, "Oh, sure, take all of the nurses you want. Just tell me what you need and we will put it in the budget for next year." They had to prove that a need existed. That was probably the first real productivity management system in nursing care.

Staffing by acuity measurements was developed in the 1970's, long before health care administrators figured out that the system would change into competitive markets and productivity management. A good productivity system should identify the areas of direct patient care (such as the categories I have illustrated in Table 2) and give them a relative value according to work

TABLE 2

Categories

Diet	Suction
Toileting	Bath
Vital Signs	Activity
Respiratory Needs	Treatments

time necessary to complete the task. I am not particularly concerned that you worry about what system or whose system. If a hospital has statistics on nursing hours for diagnosis by day of hospitalization, that hospital has all of the data necessary for a relative value system. Even if such complete information is nonexistent, you can still build a relative value system. However, there is a system, Janna Plus, that bridges the gap between acuity measurements for staffing and systems for budgeting and cost accounting.

Earlier than most health care facilities, my hospital, the Massachusetts Eye and Ear Infirmary in Boston, was beset by problems related to a shortened length of stay due to improved surgical techniques and advances in Otolaryngology and Ophthalmology. By the 1960's, management, trustees, and medical staff saw the need for separating out the true costs involved in the intense, short length of stay characteristic of the specialized treatment delivered at the Massachusetts Eye and Ear Infirmary. The result of this concern was our approach to costing and budgeting. Our system closely parallels the Janna Plus system.

In 1975, we implemented a new system that measures more accurately the true cost of the care being delivered to patients. This system is both an effective and broad management tool. What was formerly the patient day, or occupied bed day category, has been split into three parts, each covering a range of services which are essential elements of a hospital stay: cost per patient (hospitalization cost), cost per (patient) day, and cost of clinical care.

I. Cost Per Patient (Hospitalization Cost). This is the measurable cost of being a hospital patient. It is each patient's equitable share of the costs involved in being scheduled for admission, the admission process, a set of medical records, the billing procedures, and cashier operations. It also includes a per patient apportionment of plant and administrative overhead—in effect, the cost of the hospital's availability and readiness. It is a one-time cost, or charge regardless of length of stay or illness. The cost centers covered by this are admitting, scheduling, medical records, and cashier, etc.

$$\frac{\text{Direct Cost + Apportioned Overhead}}{\text{Number of Patients}} = \text{Cost Per Patient}$$

In Fiscal Year 1982, the Massachusetts Eye and Ear Infirmary's direct cost and apportioned overhead totaled $3,201,048 with 12,450 discharges, resulting in a one-time fee of $270.30 for every patient admitted.

II. Cost Per (Patient) Day. This category encompasses the routine daily costs for room, meals, laundry, routine pharmaceuticals, medical and surgical supplies and incidentals.

$$\frac{\text{Direct Cost + Apportioned Overhead}}{\text{Expected Number of Patient Days}} = \text{Daily Room Cost}$$

During Fiscal Year 1982, the daily room rate was $69.80.

Traditional comparisions of per diem rates are meaningless because the routine services category is used as a catch-all for many cost factors; when the true costs of providing a hospital room are isolated, acute care hospitals' daily rates can be competitive with each other as well as with other lower level institutional settings.

III. Cost of Clinical Care. This is the cost of direct patient care in accordance with diagnosis, surgical procedure and the patient's point-in-progress toward recovery.

The unit of measurement for clinical care is a clinical care unit (CCU). A CCU is the value assigned to the amount of time it takes to provide a direct patient care service.

$$\frac{\substack{\text{Inpatient Nursing Department Cost} \\ + \\ \text{Inpatient Physician Cost} \\ + \\ \text{Additional Overhead}}}{\text{Expected Number of CCU's}} = \text{Cost per CCU}$$

The cost per CCU at the Massachusetts Eye and Ear Infirmary was $7.40 in Fiscal Year 1982. The CCU's used at the Massachusetts Eye and Ear Infirmary are based on the PETO System developed at Eugene Talmadge Hospital. It identifies areas of direct patient care and assigns points or units of time to the treatment modality. The modalities are: diet, toileting, vital signs, respiratory needs, suction, bath, activity, and treatments.

In this system, a CCU equals approximately seven and one-half minutes of staff time.

TABLE 3

Category	Description	Clinical Care Unit Value
Treatments	Once in 8 Hours	1
	Twice in 8 Hours	2
	Three Times in 8 Hours	4
	Four Times in 8 Hours	8
	More than Every 2 Hours	12

TABLE 4

Category	Description	Clinical Care Unit Value
Vital Signs	Routine-Daily Temperature, Pulse, and Respiration	1
	Vital Signs Every 4 Hours	2
	Vital Signs Monitored, or Vital Signs Every 2 Hours	4
	Vital Signs and Observation Every Hour, or Vital Signs Monitored, Plus Neuro Check.	8
	Blood Pressure, Pulse, Respiration and Neuro Check Every 30 Minutes	12

TABLE 5

Category	Description	Clinical Care Unit Value
Toileting	Toilets Independently	0
	Toilets with Minimal Assistance	1
	Toilets with Supervision, or Specimen Collection, or uses Bedpan. Hemovac Output	2
	Up to Toilet with Standby Supervision or Output Measurement Every Hour. Initial Hemovac Setup	4

The unit value is an indicator of the relative difficulty and staff involvement for each task.

Samples of three modality assignments may be seen in Tables 3, 4 and 5.

Prerequisite to the development of CCU assignments, is a comprehensive patient data base of average daily clinical care requirements from the day of admission to the day of discharge by diagnosis. The existence of these data obviates the need to continue routine measurement of the actual clinical care workload effort expended per patient per day. Rather, the fixed statistic of average number of CCU's by diagnosis by point-in-progress toward recovery, can be used as a productivity measure.

This total Eye and Ear Infirmary system has made information available which can be used appropriately for internal management as well as societal decision making. The statistics generated by this system will help health care institutions, government, and the public to have a better understanding of the intensity of care provided to individual patients or types of cases. Since the system accounts for the true cost of services provided and measures cost effectiveness and produciticity, meaningful comparisons can be made between hospitals which can be used in the regulatory arena in attaining its goal of cost control.

One of the societal implications of this system is the opportunity it affords for the integration of multilevels of care within one institution. In the United States, in an effort to contain national expenditures for acute hospital care, patients requiring lesser degrees of skill and technological support have been placed in specifically designed institutions. This introduction of separate facilities has been, in my opinion, the single most important factor in increasing total health care expenditures. In other words, instead of attacking the disease we responded to the symptoms. The disease was retrospective cost reimbursement on a per diem basis which went out of control. The symptom was the apparently less expensive service of the skilled nursing facility down the street.

The addition of new non-acute hospital based beds, while acute care hospital beds go unfilled, is a vivid illustration of the unnecessary duplication of resources. A multilevel care facility integrating and providing the services each patient requires, and calculating the cost of that care accordingly, provides the greatest potential for maximum occupancy at minimum cost and efficiency.

It could readily achieve cost-effective, continuous, high-quality care appropriate to each patient's condition, i.e., economies of scale.

You've heard a great deal lately about vertical integration; one corporation owning and operating several facilities, each giving different levels of care. That's not what I am talking about. From a management standpoint, the multilevel facility makes more sense because providing mixed levels of care within one institution, and even on the same nursing station, would ensure:

- Avoidance of duplication of construction cost;
- Greater efficiency from continuity in paperwork;
- Greater flexibility and utilization of facility through a more diverse patient mix.

In the multilevel facility, equally important medical and social advantages would accrue to patients, such as:

One-time Placement — By entering and remaining in one institution throughout a course of illness, patients would be spared disruptive moves, the hazards of transfer of personal belongings and medical records, and the expense of ambulance transportation.

Continuity of Nursing Care — Uninterrupted hospitalization also encourages important familiarity with clinical staff members and consistency in treatment.

Continuity of Physician Responsibility — A patient's physician would be better able to follow through in supervision of care. His continued availability to the patient is assured in the single facility, mixed, multilevel care setting. Under present arrangements, the attending physician in an acute care facility is unlikely to be mobile enough to even attend the patient at the skilled nursing facility to which the patient is transferred. Instead, should complications develop, the patient is transferred back to the acute care facility.

Adaptability to Change — When the spectrum of acute care to skilled nursing care is available within a single institution, there is also more receptiveness to new concepts of patient care as they evolve.

Length-of-stay Monitoring — Presently, there exists a multitude of patients in acute care facilities because no beds are available in skilled nursing facilities. This backlog is expensively inefficient as long as we are dealing with per diem cost accounting. Under a multilevel care facility concept with proper cost identification, patients would be billed only for the amount of care their condition required on each hospital day.

Beyond the cost of transferring patients back and forth, the vertical integration system conceals extensive and expensive duplication of:

- Admitting costs
- Administration and management support operations
- Record keeping
- Social services
- Rehabilitation guidance
- Plant and utilities costs.

We feel that a new cost accounting system allows us to accurately identify the cost of patient care in our hospital even as clinical care needs change. At our hospital, once a patient has paid the one-time hospitalization charge of $270.30, ongoing charges consist only of the $69.80 rate per patient day and the charges for the required CCU's. If, for example, a long-stay patient needed six CCU's every day, at the Infirmary's 1982 rates the bill would come to $69.80 plus $44.40 or a total of $114.20 a day. This figure compares favorably with the daily charge in many skilled nursing facilities in our area, and duplications, inefficiency and inconvenience would be reduced to a minimum.

On a more internal management level, this productivity-based cost accounting system is a valuable tool for budget forecasting, staffing, placement of patients, scheduling of patients, and determining cost and charge per unit of care.

This system gives accurate historical patient data based on diagnosis, which can be used to project CCU requirements for future admissions. The one-time charge that has no relationship to length of stay or nursing care would be an excellent candidate for co-pay.

The first step in budgeting at our hospital is agreement by all concerned parties on volume and case mix statistics for the upcoming year. Once this step is completed, appropriate expense and staffing budgets can be developed throughout the hospital. Rather than making most cost centers a function of patient days, they work with statistics appropriate to their cost and productivity statistics. For example, the Admissions and Medical Records Departments work with discharges while Nursing works with clinical care units.

In conclusion, let me repeat what I said at the onset. First, it doesn't matter what payment, reimbursement, or delivery system we have or are likely to have. None of them will work unless we have cost data that are specific to resource input—in other words, relative to work effort. We need to find a more meaningful tool than patient days or occupied bed days.

Secondly, we need to organize a system for management audits between hospital cost centers and between hospitals.

And thirdly, we need to have a utilization review system that encompasses not just length of stay monitoring. We need to monitor all resources going into caring for a specific disease, by doctor and by hospital.

REFERENCES

R. B. Catchlove and J. Hall, "The Need for Output Measure to Assess Hospital Performance and Costs," The Royal North Shore Hospital of Sydney, Speech presented 1978.

M. Poland, et al, "PETO—A System for Assessing and Meeting Patient Care Needs," American Journal of Nursing, 70:7, July 1970, pp. 1479-482.

P. G. Weaver, "Cost Analysis by Patient Diagnosis," *Dimensions in Health Service,* Vol. 54, June 1977, p. 32.

C. T. Wood, "Relate Charges to Use of Services," *Harvard Business Review,* March/ April 1982; also in "Saving Our Health Care System, *Harvard Business Review,* 1982, pp. 97-104.

Chapter Thirteen

Improving Productivity in Health Care Through Quality Circles

JOHN E. BAIRD

Administrators in health care—particularly those having direct responsibility for the institution's employee relations function—find themselves today facing three areas of rapid change:

A. Economic Realities

Reductions in government funding, combined with decreased patient census attributable in part to high unemployment, have caused hospitals to give more attention to their costs, incomes, and employee productivity. The need to compete effectively with other health care institutions has caused administrators to seek ways of reducing patient care costs, and an increased emphasis upon employee productivity and cost-effective human resources management has been the result.

B. Management Theories

Scholars writing about the "best" ways to manage people are emphasizing worker participation in organizational decision making. In his widely-acclaimed text *Theory Z: How American Business Can Meet the Japanese Challenge,* William Ouchi stresses the importance of trust between employees and their managers and suggests that the development of such trust can occur only when employees and management participate together in organizational decision making and problem solving. In turn, this trust has been shown to bring about increased productivity, improved worker morale, reduced turnover and absenteeism, improved quality of work, and enhanced organizational success.

C. Employee Values

Employees today have a set of expectations concerning how they are to be treated and what role they are to play in the organizations that employ them, and when their expectations are not met they often become disenchanted and nonproductive. Increasingly, those expectations are centering upon decision making and communications. In her article "Winds of Change Sweep Nursing Profession," for example, Barbara Ellis points out that one of

191

the major reasons nurses are leaving their profession is that "nurses want some control over their professional practice . . . whether it is in defining what is their role within the work setting or whether it is in time commitment versus their personal lives." [Ellis, 1980, p. 95]. Similarly, Gail Hallas [1980, p. 17] in "Why Nurses Are Giving It Up," indicates that 25 percent of all nurses are dissatisfied with hospital-wide communications and with their own inability to shape their work environment.

This changing value system has been illustrated by our own research, conducted in hospitals over the past four years. Nearly 250,000 health care employees working 423 hospitals have completed an employee opinion survey administered by Positive Personnel Practices, Inc., a Chicago-based employee relations consulting firm. As a part of those surveys, employees were asked to complete the "faces" scale measure of general satisfaction and to answer 140 questions about all aspects of their work environment (Figure I illustrates the "faces" scale general satisfaction measure). When a multiple regression analysis was used to calculate the impact of each portion of the survey upon the general satisfaction measure, the factors found to have significant impact were, in order from most to least impact:

FIGURE I

INSTRUCTIONS: Consider all aspects of your job. Circle the number between the faces which best expresses how you feel about *your job in general.*

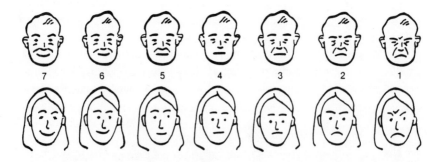

1. Work itself, or the extent to which employees found their jobs interesting, challenging, leading to personal growth, etc.
2. Communications, or the extent to which employees perceive themselves to be involved in decision making and problem solving in their workplace.

3. Supervisors' Communication Skills, or the effectiveness with which employees perceive their supervisiors and managers to communicate with them.
4. Management Concern, or the extent to which employees perceive hospital administration to care about their happiness and well-being.
5. Coworker Relations, or the degree to which employees have and enjoy contact with their fellow employees.

Since the "faces" scale has been found to predict accurately such factors as turnover, absenteeism and productivity by health care employees, the impact these survey factors have upon general satisfaction becomes even more important. In effect, those hospital employees who perceive themselves to be challenged, involved, communicated with, cared about, and part of a real work team show lower absenteeism and turnover and higher productivity than do hospital employees who perceive their work environment to be lacking in those things. Such, then, is the nature of today's health care employees' value system.

Significantly, and perhaps happily, all three areas of change are leading in the same direction. The need for increased productivity suggests that all health care employees become actively involved in cutting costs, reducing waste, and improving the quality and efficiency of their own work. The evolution of management theory similarly suggests that worker involvement is the cornerstone to increased organizational strength. And the new employee value system indicates that employees themselves want to be involved in making the decisions that affect their work lives, and that they become frustrated and disillusioned when such involvement is not forthcoming.

One method for achieving that involvement is "Quality Circles." Briefly, Quality Circles are groups of employees from the same work unit who meet together regularly to identify, analyze and solve quality and efficiency problems in their area. As such, then, Quality Circles are not particularly new or mysterious; they simply are common sense. However, because they are "fashionable" and because they incorporate elements which ought to be in every system of upward communication, they now are proving highly successful in increasing hospital productivity and economic strength. The purpose of this paper is to discuss the Quality Circles concept as it applies to health care, and to outline the procedures through which they are implemented successfully in the hospital setting.

History of Quality Circles

Twenty years ago, products labeled "made in Japan" were regarded as cheap, often shoddy merchandise. Today, Japanese products are considered to be among the best made and most reliable available. Although a variety of factors contributed to this rise in Japanese production quality and efficiency, one of the most important was the involvement of Japanese workers in improving quality through Quality Circles. Thus, it was in Japan that Quality Circles first were implemented and proven on a nationwide scale.

Following WW II, General Douglas MacArthur, who was commander of the United States forces occupying Japan, decided to do all he could to revive the Japanese economy as quickly as possible. He saw that Japan's island economy would make it necessary to trade with other nations rather than relying upon natural resources, but he also saw that Japan's poor reputation for quality would seriously damage their trade efforts. Thus, he asked Dr. W. Edward Deming to come from the United States to work with Japanese industrial leaders in improving their levels of quality.

Dr. Deming introduced the Japanese to the concept of statistical quality control—a concept which immediately was adopted by the Union of Japanese Scientists and Engineers (JUSE) as the cornerstone of their program. In 1952, at a conference in Syracuse, New York, Dr. Deming introduced the founder of JUSE, Mr. Koyanagi, to another American, Dr. Joseph Juran, an expert on quality control. During the next few years, Dr. Juran visited Japan several times, teaching the Japanese his approach to quality improvement—an approach which stressed participative decision making. This approach was to serve as the basis for the Quality Circles program which followed several years later.

Through the 1950's and 1960's, the Japanese conducted a nationwide drive to improve quality. Radio programs stressing quality were broadcast each week, and in 1960 a weekly television program on quality was initiated. Awards were given to individuals and corporations achieving unusual improvements in quality, and the Japanese government developed their "JIS" symbol to be put on only those products which had exceptionally high quality. November was named "national quality month" in 1960, and during that month it was common to see quality posters, "Q" flags, and quality-oriented seminars and conferences.

In 1961 the editors of the Japanese magazine, *Quality Control,* decided to involve first-level foremen in the quality improvement process. They established a discussion session for foremen called "The Duties of the Shop Foreman in Quaity Maintenance" as a part of the Annual Quality Control Conference, and invited shop foremen to join the discussion panel. They also developed a new magazine for shop supervisors called *The Foreman and QC,* and published the first issue in July, 1962. This magazine was intended to educate first line supervisors in quality control methods, and through the magazine the editors sponsored the organization of "QC Circles," to be led by foremen who could serve as the central points for quality control activities within an organization. The Quality Circles concept thus was born.

Quality Circles (also called "QC Circles") spread rapidly in Japan, first in manufacturing and later in finance and merchandising. Today, nearly ten million workers are involved in Quality Circles throughout Japan.

The Quality Circles concept spread to the United States in the early 1970's, when a visiting team of JUSE Quality Circle leaders were invited by the American Society for Quality Control to present their programs to a conference at Stanford University. This conference sparked the interest of several representatives from the Lockheed Corporation, who studied the concept at length and ultimately installed a Quality Circles program at Lockheed. This program proved highly successful, and similar programs were put into place in such organizations as J.C. Penny Co., Uniroyal, Chrysler, General Motors, Ampex, Firestone, R. J. Reynolds, Bendix, Michigan Bell Telephone, and many others. At present, thousands of American workers in all types of organizations are participating in Quality Circle groups, contributing to the improvement of their organization's operations and their own working lives.

The impact of Quality Circles upon the organizations which have implemented them has been dramatic. For example, Lockheed reported documented savings in the first two years of the program of $2.8 million (achieved by only 15 operating Quality Circle groups) [Zemke, 1980, p. 18]. Honeywell, Inc. reported a 40 percent increase in machine and equipment utilization in one division, and a 6 to 1 return on investment in operating savings from Circle activities in another. At the Tarrytown, New York, General Motors assembly plant, the introduction of Quality Circles brought about a decrease in outstanding grievances from 2,000 in 1972 to 30 in 1980, a decrease in average absence rate from 7 percent to 2.5 percent, and a reduction in percentage of bad body welds from 35 percent to 1.5 percent within a few months of installation of a Quality Circle in the area responsible for body welds [*Industry Week,* 1979, p. 17]. The Westinghouse Defense and Electronic Systems Center near Baltimore, Maryland reported a cost savings of over $800,000, brought about within 16 months of Quality Circles implementation [Burck, 1981, p. 68]. Many other similar success stories have been reported elsewhere [Baird and Rittof, 1983]. What is clear is that Quality Circles have proven successful in the United States in increasing productivity and employee job satisfaction among employees in virtually every industry.

Quality Circles in Health Care

The history of Quality Circles in health care organizations is much more brief. Two hospitals—Mount Sinai Medical Center in Miami, Florida, and Barnes Hospital in St. Louis, Missouri, each claim to have been the first American hospital to implement the Quality Circles concept. Both began their Circles in 1980. Shortly thereafter, Henry Ford Hosptial in Detroit, Michigan began a limited Quality Circles program, and many other hospitals subsequently followed. Although it is impossible to gain an exact count on the number of American hospitals currently conducting Quality Circles programs, the author is aware of nearly 100 who have implemented Quality Circles in one or more departments [Baird and Rittof, 1983].

Quantifiable results from Quality Circles programs are only now beginning to emerge. Norma Ederer, Director of Human Resources at Mount Sinai, reports measurable improvements "not only in cost savings but also in time savings, reduction in errors, increased efficiency, reduced absenteeism, reduced turnover and the number of grievances, improved employee morale and attitude and greater cooperation." [Johnson, 1981, p. 69] Similarly, Rusti Moore, who coordinated implementation of Quality Circles at Barnes Hospital, reported that "There's been a definite increase in employee morale and communication. People are talking to each other a good deal more openly, according to the supervisors. Absenteeism appears to have dropped and productivity has grown in most of the departments that have circles."[1]

Some specific improvements brought about by Quality Circle groups include:

1. A dietary Quality Circle which solved the problem of giving the wrong food to patients who order items not on the hospital's menus [Johnson, 1981, p. 68].
2. A transportation Quality Circle which brought about an increase in the number of wheelchairs returned to the transportation area [Johnson, 1981].
3. A nursing Quality Circle developed an improved system for transporting and storing patient valuables, with a resultant time savings of three hours per employee per month.[2]
4. A pharmacy Quality Circle developed an improved poison control system.[3]
5. A biomedical engineering Quality Circle developed an improved maintenance request and tracking system.[4]

---

[1] Personal interview with Ms. Rusti L. Moore, Director, Department of Education and Training, Barnes Hospital, St. Louis.

[2] Results of Quality Circle measurements taken six months after program implementation by large hospital in Illinois.

[3] Results of Quality Circle measurements taken six months after program implementation by large hospital in California.

[4] Results of Quality Circle measurements taken two months after program implementation by medium-sized hospital in Texas.

These are but a few of many examples of improvements directly attributable to Quality Circles in health care institutions. Quantifying productivity and quality in a hospital is more difficult than quantifying those factors in a manufacturing environment; nevertheless, the evidence is clear that all elements of a health care institution can benefit from implementing Quality Circles. Alvin Goldberg, Executive Vice President and Chief Executive Officer of Mount Sinai Medical Center, summarized his observations in this way: "Within a short period of time, our investment started to pay dividends in a swelling enthusiasm where we previously had seen lackluster behavior. What kind of price tag do you put on behavioral changes? How do you calculate dollars when a group of employees who were previously disinterested or criticizing, become actively involved in identifying, researching and developing solutions to the nagging day-to-day problems they fight." [Johnson, 1981, p. 69] Quality Circles therefore seem certain to play a major role in the management of many hospitals during the coming years.

The Quality Circles Structure

There are six basic elements in an organization's Quality Circles program (illustrated by Figure II). These include:

1. Circle participants
2. Circle leaders
3. The Program Facilitator
4. The Steering/Advisory Committee
5. Non-circle management
6. Non-circle employees

At the top of the structure is the Advisory Board or Steering Committee consisting of top-level managers or administrators. Formed to oversee and guide the program, this board may also serve as a source of expertise for the Circles and it may provide a base of power that assists the Circles in accomplishing their tasks. Often members of the Steering/Advisory Committee include the hospital Administrator, the Director of Finance, the Director of Nursing, the Director of Ancillary Services, the Director of Human Resources or Personnel, and the Director of Public Relations, among others. Indeed, every major area of the hospital should be represented on the Steering/ Advisory Committee.

The Quality Circles Program Facilitator also is a member of the Steering/ Advisory Committee. This individual (or in larger hospitals these individuals) has responsibility for monitoring the entire system, meeting regularly with Circles and other employees in the hospital, scheduling meetings between a Circle and top level management, assisting the implementation of Circle recommendations, and teaching problem solving and communication skills

FIGURE II

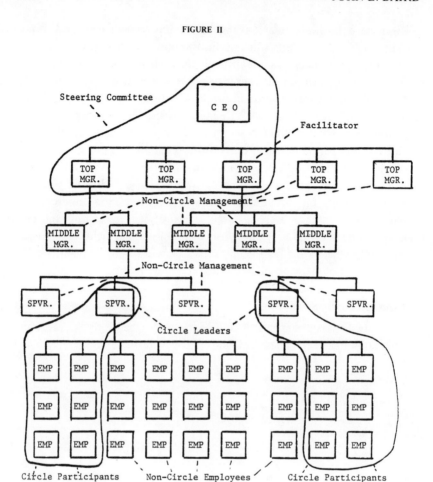

to Circle leaders and participants. Typically, the Program Facilitator is a member of upper management or administration who is particularly supportive of the Quality Circles concept, is skilled as a communicator and instructor, and is viewed as credible by other administrators and employees throughout the hospital. This person acts as the "driving force" behind the entire program, and therefore must be carefully chosen if the process is to succeed.

Circle leaders generally are first-line supervisors or department heads trained to facilitate meetings without dominating them. Clearly, Circle leaders must be chosen carefully. They must be skilled in preventing their supervisory role from inhibiting employee interaction and contributions, and they must have good relations with their employees. The Circle leader's function is to lead the group by scheduling meetings, developing agendas, keeping minutes, encouraging everyone to contribute, controlling the participants who are over-talkative, inviting visiting participants, resolving conflict, and so on. However, the leader must not make decisions or in any way discourage discussion among the participants. Usually, Circle leaders need formal training in these techniques for conducting group meetings.

The Circle participants are, of course, the basic components of the entire system. These are employees who volunteer to participate in the program, who work in the same general department or area, and who number from three to 15. It is important to note, however, that these are the permanent Circle participants; during a particular meeting, temporary or visiting participants may be invited to take part. If, for example, a Circle has identified as one of its major problems the quality of raw materials they receive from Purchasing, they may invite someone from the Purchasing Department to meet with them and discuss purchasing procedures, alternate suppliers, and so on. Similarly, if the group needs information from an engineer, an accountant, or any other specialist in the organization, they may invite that person as a visiting participant.

Non-circle management consists of those supervisors and managers who are not directly involved in the Quality Circles system. It is important to the success of the program, however, that these people be taken into account whenever possible. They should be invited to attend Circle meetings whenever they like; they should be kept informed by the Circle leaders of the things which the Circles are considering; they should be consulted whenever appropriate for their input in developing solutions to work-related problems. Each manager should meet regularly with all Quality Circle leaders (along with non-Circle supervisors) in his or her department to review the Circles' progress. In addition, if a department manager encounters a problem which ought to be considered by the Circle members, he or she should refer that problem to the group. Typically, the Circle participants feel honored when their manager makes such a request, and they will attack the problem immediately and energetically. Above all, non-circle managers should be kept informed about the program, and they should be invited to contribute to the program in any way they wish. They must not feel that the program undermines their authority in the organization, or that they have no role to play in the program's success.

Non-circle employees are impacted by Quality Circles, for any suggestions made by a Circle which administration implements has some influence over the work done by all employees in the organization. Again, it is important that non-circle employees be encouraged to contribute their ideas or problems to Circle participants, and that they be informed of the things which Circles are achieving. Moreover, when the Quality Circles sytem is expanded beyond its original pilot basis, many of these employees are likely to become Quality Circle members. Their participation in the program will be encouraged if they are kept informed, and the transition occurring when they are added to the program will be much smoother if they know what the Circles have been doing.

All of this should make it clear that Quality Circles fit within normal organizational operations. Circle communications follow established lines of communication, and Circle members have no more authority or access to organization staff than do non-circle members. In most organizations, the first line supervisor carries information from employees to management; in Quality Circles, the supervisor/Circle leader plays that same role. In most organizations, people having new ideas need to send them to top management, who then decides whether the ideas have merit and whether they can practically be implemented. So it is with Quality Circles. In effect, Quality Circles provide a formal structure for things which probably are already happening on an informal basis in the organization, or which may not be happening, but should happen.

Two important changes do occur when Quality Circles are implemented, however. First, the skills of the participants, leaders and facilitator(s) are improved. Through the training these individuals receive when Quality Circles are implemented, their abilities as communicators, problem solvers and leaders are strengthened, making them more effective not only as participants in Quality Circles but as members of the organization. Second, the relationship between employees, supervision and management often changes. Quality Circles stress, and in fact demand, participative decision making. Employees are given a greater voice than ever before in determining their own work environment, and an atmosphere of mutual respect and trust between employees and management is encouraged. Thus, Quality Circles often change attitudes as well as changing work. But in both instances, the changes are for the betterment of the organization.

Implementing Quality Circles

No two organizations implement Quality Circles in exactly the same way. Every organization is unique, and therefore every organization must go through a relatively unique process to implement its Quality Circles system. However, there are some basic stages through which most organizations proceed, and these are outlined below.

A. Discovering Quality Circles

The first step usually is for someone in the organization to discover the Quality Circles concept. Upon hearing of it, he or she may search for literature providing additional information, and may talk to other people about the idea. Information also may be obtained from the International Association of Quality Circles (IAQC). Gradually, people in the organization come to know about the system.

B. Developing Initial Support

At some point, someone having a reasonably high office in the organization must endorse the idea. Often, this person is the individual who "discovered" the concept originally. Just as often, however, this person is told of Quality Circles by a subordinate, finds the concept interesting, and asks for more information. Eventually, this person may decide that "we should do this here." He or she may talk to other managerial personnel, and they may also support the idea. Eventually, these people provide the initial impetus for the program.

C. Setting Preliminary Objectives

Early in the process, the support group must define what the objectives of the Quality Circle program will be. This set of objectives could be stated as simply as: "Enhance the quality of service and working life;" on the other hand, the objectives could be stated in much more detail:

1. Reduce errors and enhance quality.
2. Inspire more effective teamwork.
3. Provide job enrichment.
4. Increase employee motivation.
5. Create problem solving capabilities.
6. Build an attitude of "problem prevention."
7. Improve house-wide communication.
8. Develop harmonious employee-management relations.
9. Promote personal and leadership development.
10. Develop a greater safety awareness.
11. Improve employee morale.
12. Improve public relations efforts.
13. Provide opportunities for recognition.
14. Improve patient relations.

Naturally, the list they develop may not include all of the items listed above. However, it is important that the support group have an opportunity to participate in developing objectives that are important to them. Later, it is these objectives which may encourage all members of management to support the system, and which will guide the activities in which Quality Circles become involved.

D. Building Management Support

Three important principles are involved in developing support for the program among hospital management. First, support must be provided from the top of the organization. Managers at lower levels often have expressed the concern, "I support the concept, but I am afraid to stick my neck out until I find out whether it has support at higher levels. I have been burned too many times in the past." This concern is set to rest only when the Chief Executive Officer of the organization has endorsed the concept.

Second, the management groups having responsibility for the areas in which Quality Circles are begun must support the concept. Indeed, the areas selected for implementation of Quality Circles often are those in which management has been most openly supportive.

Third, depth of management support is important: as many people in the management structure as possible should be supporters of the program. Such support can be built over time by the initial support group, who takes every opportunity to talk to other managers about Quality Circles, to supply them with information, etc. It is important that the initial group make this effort, for non-supportive managers occasionally attempt to undermine the Quality Circles effort, or their lack of enthusiasm may in turn dampen the enthusiasm of their employees.

E. Deciding to Start

Finally, the decision to start will be made. Again, this should occur at the highest level of the organization. This decision must not take the form of: "All right. Go ahead and do it." Rather, it must be: "We are eager to move forward and will provide the kind of support necessary to make this an organizational commitment."

F. Engaging a Consultant

Often, hospitals at this point contract with a consultant experienced in Quality Circles in health care. This individual works with the hospital to structure the program, to train the facilitators, leaders and participants, and to guide the hospital through the initial phases of implementation. This individual must have a background not only in Quality Circles, but in training and education, personnel management, and health care. Since Quality Circles impacts the entire hospital, this individual must have a broad enough background to understand and control that impact.

G. Organizing the Steering Committee

As we already have seen, the Steering Committee is the group which provides direction and guidance for the Quality Circles system. Members are management level personnel who have an interest in the program and who represent each of the major functions in the organization. In many unionized organizations, union leadership is invited to participate on the Steering Committee as well.

H. Selecting the Facilitator(s)

One of the key initial steps taken by the Steering Committee is the selection of the person or persons who will act as facilitator(s). This person or group will have primary responsibility for implementing the coordinating of the Quality Circles system.

I. Finalizing the Objectives

The preliminary objectives already have been established, but these need to be refined into a final set of system goals. All members of the Steering Committee should have input into these objectives and should support them enthusiastically.

J. Developing the Implementation Plan

This plan is a combination of two documents. One is the Quality Circle policy and procedure which defines the goals, rules, practices, and responsibilities involved in the Quality Circles system, and which defines the way Quality Circles will mesh with the entire organization. This policy and procedure statement may also define those issues which cannot be addressed by Quality Circle groups. Second is the implementation time table, which indicates all of the activities which must occur to implement the system and when those activities should happen.

K. Collecting Pre-implementation Data

Ultimately, the administrative group will need to measure the impact Quality Circles are having. Such measures require base line information against which later measures can be compared. Thus, pre-implementation data should be collected in such areas as quality, cost, absenteeism, turnover, employee attitudes, safety performance, schedule adherence, patient and physician relations, and so on. Certainly, these measures should reflect the objectives established earlier in the process.

L. Conducting Briefings for Management and Union

There may at this point be many people in management who have not been directly involved in Quality Circle activities. These people need information about current Quality Circle activities and about future plans, for their support later on will be crucial. Their fears that Quality Circles will represent some kind of threat to their own position and power also need to be addressed. Typically, a briefing meeting convened by the Chief Executive Officer and featuring the Quality Circles consultant will be the best forum in which these matters can be considered.

Union officials also should be briefed about what is occurring so they can respond to questions from their membership. Normally, union officials are among the most ardent supporters of Quality Circles, so that providing them with information about current activities and future plans serves to advance the program. In addition, on rare occasion one or more union officials have perceived Quality Circles as a potential threat to their position and power in the organization, and again administration needs to let them know that such is not the intent of the program.

M. Selection Pilot Program Circle Leaders

When all supervisors and managers have been briefed about the nature and intent of the program, volunteers to act as Quality Circle leaders should then be requested. Initially, only six to ten Circles should be started in the pilot program; thus, this is the number of leaders to be selected initially. Generally, there are more volunteers than there are available Circles. The Steering Committee and/or the facilitator should interview each of the applicants, and select those which seem best qualified.

N. Developing Leader Performance Goals

The facilitator next should meet with each individual leader to discuss the performance objectives they will strive to achieve through Circle activities. Measurable objectives should be agreed upon by the facilitator, leader and leader's immediate superior, and provision should be made for regular feedback so both the leader and his/her manager will know how successfully each goal is being met. These goals become a part of the leader's own regular performance review.

O. Issuing Pre-publicity to All Employees

Naturally, there will be curiosity about what is going on. If administration does not act to provide information, the grapevine will. However, the kind of information given is important. If Quality Circles are made to sound too enticing, there will be a deluge of requests by employees wanting to become involved in Quality Circles. Those not selected may be disappointed and disillusioned, and those chosen may find that Quality Circles do not live up to their inflated expectations. On the other hand, if the information is too uninteresting, no one may volunteer.

At this point, then, what is needed is complete but simple information about the Quality Circles system: the nature and objectives of the program, the fact that it is being initiated on a pilot basis only but that gradual expansion is anticipated, the fact that it involves work on the part of employees involved, and so on. This information should be transmitted through letters to employees' homes, employee newsletters or magazines, large group meetings, smaller departmental or unit meetings, individual conversations between supervisors and employees, bulletin board announcements, or pay envelope "stuffers." The greater the number of communication channels used, the more likely it is that complete and accurate information will reach everyone.

P. Conducting Training Classes

The facilitator is trained first, either by the consultant or by sending the facilitator to an outside training seminar. The Circle leaders receive training next, with the facilitator and consultant working in concert to provide that training. Typically, these leader training classes are attended by other members of management who have an interest in Quality Circles, but who may not be involved actively in the pilot program. If members of the Steering Committee are available, they too should attend the leader training sessions.

Q. Initiating Circles

The Circle leaders, freshly trained in Quality Circle techniques, select the membership for their own Circles. This in itself may not be an easy task: in the Medical Records department of one large hospital, 29 of 32 employees working in that department asked to participate. The Circle leader solved the problem, after considering a variety of options, by putting all 29 names in a hat and pulling out eight of them. Other Circle leaders have simply chosen those employees who they feel would perform best in the Circle activities, while still others have used seniority as a selection criterion.

R. Participant Training

Brief training classes are used to teach Circle participants basic communication and group decision making skills. Then during the first several weeks of meetings, the participants learn problem solving techniques by attacking a real problem of their own choosing. Thus the facilitator provides the initial classroom instruction, while the Circle leader teaches problem solving skills during actual meetings. The facilitator should attend each Circle's initial meetings to assist the instructional process where necessary, but the bulk of the instruction must be provided by the leader.

S. Periodic Review by Steering Committee

Like any other activity, Quality Circles requires managing. Goals must be established, and measurable milestones must be identified to allow evaluation of the system's progress. The Steering Committee's success in measuring the impact of the Quality Circles system depends, in part, on the care with which the original implementation plan was constructed. Assuming that measurable check points were established in that plan, the Steering Committee should conduct regular (probably every two months) reviews of Circle progress and should transmit the results of their reviews to all members of management and of the Quality Circles system. This periodic review also provides information necessary for making modifications and corrections in Circle activities, thus laying the groundwork for expansion of the system (and indeed, allowing the system to be adjusted to enhance its chances for success).

T. Expanding the Program

Ultimately (typically within about six months), the program will be expanded to include new departments and groups. Managers who initially were non-committal about (or even opposed to) the program now may be enthusiastic about it due to the successes which have occurred in other areas, and they may be eager to have their own people become involved. Employees who volunteered initially but were not chosen still may want to participate. Thus, using the lessons learned by the pilot project, the next stage is to expand the program to new areas, teaching new Circle leaders and Circle participants the skills they will need, and then implementing new Circles in their areas.

U. Ending Group Involvement

Eventually, Quality Circle groups will cease to be effective and should be phased out or replaced. Perhaps the group has run out of problems or ideas; perhaps they have become interested in other things; perhaps they simply have participated long enough and need to step aside to allow others an opportunity. In any event, this group must receive some recognition for its contribution before it is disbanded.

Again, the actual sequence of events occuring in a specific hospital may vary somewhat from the sequence outlined above. For example, an employee opinion survey may occur before any of these steps (rather than as a part of collecting the baseline data), or it might reveal that Quality Circles should be started in some departments but not others. The facilitator might be chosen (or self-selected) before the Steering Committee is constructed, or pre-publicity to all employees may occur before Circle leaders are selected. In any event, the sequence is less important than the functions: at some point in the process, each of the stages outlined above must occur if the Quality Circles system is to have maximum effectiveness.

Quality Circle Procedures

When the Quality Circles structure has been established and training of the leaders and participants completed, the Circle meetings begin. These meetings usually occur weekly, with each meeting lasting approximately one hour. Meetings take place during the employees' normal work schedule, or if they must be held before or after working hours, the employees are compensated at overtime rates.

During the meetings, the participants first identify specific problems which prevent them and their peers from achieving maximum productivity and quality. These are listed during "brainstorming" sessions, and then the priority problems are selected from that list. Using various means of decision making, the single most important problem finally is selected for analysis.

When the problem has been identified, participants next go about analyzing causes of that problem. Often, this step requires additional investigation by the Circle members beyond their weekly meeting; however, these efforts must be completed on the employees' own time. The facilitator works with the Circle leader to provide the circle with any resources they need, including financial data, purchasing information, engineering data, and so on. The facilitator may arrange for in-house experts to meet with a Circle, or for Circle members to visit another part of the organization. The information collected by the Circle members is analyzed through such information display tools as Pareto Charts, histograms, pie charts, line graphs, scatter diagrams, pictographs, and work flow process charts. Ultimately, the group must settle upon the major factors which seem to have caused the problem they identified.

Suggesting possible solutions via brainstorming occurs next, with the group then narrowing the list of possible solutions to four or five which seem particularly viable. Each of these potential solutions is investigated, again often requiring outside work or assistance, and the best solution is chosen.

Finally, the group develops a specific action plan whereby the selected solution can be implemented. This action plan must take into account all aspects of the solution, including time frames, responsibilities, costs involved, availability or generation of funding, coordination among all work units involved, and so on. Indeed, more time usually is spent developing this action plan than is spent on any of the preceding activities.

When a Circle has developed an action plan for solving a problem, the members make a formal presentation to their department head (or to any member of middle management having responsibility for their work area), who reviews and, if necessary, revises the plan. Then it is presented by the members to the Steering Committee, who again review and perhaps revise. Finally, the same presentation is made to all members of the administrative team, who make a final determination about the advisability and practicality of the plan.

Certainly, it is important that these presentations proceed smoothly. Much of the employees' reward for participating in Quality Circles is their opportunity to present their ideas directly to top management. If the presentation goes poorly, the experience is punishing rather than rewarding, and their subsequent participation may be reluctant. Some training in making formal presentations therefore may be given the Circle members prior to their presenting their action plan to management.

After hearing a Circle's recommendations, administration must respond, preferably by implementing the employees' idea. A major source of satisfaction derived by Circle members stems from seeing their ideas put into action and from the recognition they are given publicly for their contributions.

However, if management decides it cannot or chooses not to implement the Circle's plan, it must meet again with the Circle to explain the decision and the reasons behind it. At the same time, management should encourage the Circle to continue its efforts to improve operations in the organization. Happily, experience indicates that 94 percent of all Circle recommendations are implemented without modification, while only slightly more than one percent are rejected outright.

Making Quality Circles Work

While employees usually are eager to participate in Quality Circles, there are some conditions which must be met before Quality Circles can succeed. These include:

1. Some value placed on innovation. Managers or supervisors (or particularly hospital administrators) who feel "We've always done things this way, so we should continue to do so" will not be receptive to Quality Circles action plans and suggestions, and a Quality Circle in their area of responsibility probably would have little chance for success. Quality Circles are designed specifically to bring about creative, improvement-oriented change, and such change must be valued by the organization before Quality Circles can be of benefit.

2. Some expertise among employees and supervisors. If everyone in the organization is relatively new, or if employees and supervisors do not know their jobs very well, then asking them to participate in Quality Circles probably would be unproductive. Participants must have had a chance to get to know their job-related problems reasonably well before they are asked to participate, and they should have some knowledge of how their problems might be attacked. As a general rule, persons having less than six months experience in their present position are excluded from participation in Quality Circles.

3. Reasonable clarity in the organization's structure. People must have a clear idea of who reports to whom in the organization; otherwise, the Quality Circle system will be difficult and confusing to administer, and the Circle members are likely to become frustrated at management's inability to respond to them.

4. General employee satisfaction with compensation. While no one believes he or she is paid enough, employees must be reasonably satisfied with their compensation before they are asked to volunteer to participate in Quality Circles. If the workers believe strongly that they are not paid fairly or competitively, they will not be enthusiastic when asked to devote their time and effort to identifying and solving the organization's problems.

5. General employee satisfaction with supervision. The immediate supervisor acts as Circle leader. Thus, if the group is to function well, the Circle participants must be reasonably favorable in their feelings toward that individual. If Circle meetings are conducted by a supervisor who is strongly disliked by his or her employees, they are likely not to be enthusiastic about participating.

6. Reasonable levels of job security. Employees who are concerned about their jobs due to impending layoffs, reductions in force, potential firings, and so on generally are too preoccupied with these fears and are unable to concentrate fully on Quality Circle activities.

7. A desire to participate. Not every employee will find Quality Circles appealing. Some simply want to do their jobs and be left alone. For that reason, participation in Quality Circles must be on a voluntary basis; people should not be forced to participate if they have no desire to do so.

8. Some value placed on people. A few managers believe that "employees should be seen and not heard." Often they are autocratic in their style of management because they believe employees have nothing to offer. They tell employees what to do and how to do it. Although such managers could gain most by having Quality Circles in their departments, they also are least likely to support the program or to be interested in the proposals which employees offer. For that reason, Quality Circles should not be started in their work areas. Once the pilot program is started and successes are being publicized, these managers may decide that a more participative approach to supervision may be appropriate in their own departments as well. But initially, extremely autocratic supervisors and managers should not be involved in Quality Circles, and a hospital administered very autocratically should not attempt the program at all.

These conditions for success apply to organizations of all types. Hospitals, however, also have some unique characteristics which similarly must be taken into account when Quality Circles are implemented.

In every hospital, infection control committees, patient care committees, policy and procedure committees, and so on already are in place and dealing with many of the problems which would be attacked by one of more Quality Circle groups. To have these committees functioning independently of the Quality Circles system is to have duplication of effort, and thus less efficiency rather than more. In addition, standing committees may resent the creation of Quality Circles that overlap their authority, and these individuals may work actively to undermine the Quality Circles system.

Standing committees should be incorporated into the Quality Circles program. They may act as adjuncts to the Steering Committee; they may take the role of facilitators; they may have representatives sit in on each Quality Circle meeting. In any event, they must play an active part in contributing to and reviewing the recommendations made by each Quality Circles group.

The medical staff also must be taken into consideration. Obviously, many of the decisions and recommendations made by Quality Circles will affect the medical staff. If the physicians are not included in the decision making process, they may resist the changes recommended by the Quality Circles, thereby frustrating the Circle members and perhaps destroying the process.

Moreover, nurses are particularly anxious to be viewed as physicians' teammates and to have a voice in designing patient care systems. By having Quality Circle groups comprised of nurses and medical staff members, this desire among nurses may be met, and better quality recommendations may be developed. In any event, the medical staff must be represented on the Steering Committee, and they must be kept informed of each Circle's progress.

Quality Circle experts often argue that Quality Circle discussions should focus strictly on work-related issues, not personal or emotional problems. Circle leaders are trained to get the discussion "back on track" when such problems arise, and to view social-emotional topics as non-productive. In hospitals, however, there often exists a need for precisely that sort of discussion, particularly among nurses. The recent development of Staff Support Circles which provide nurses with social and emotional support in dealing with the pressures and stresses of nursing illustrates the need for such interaction. Circle leaders must therefore be trained in techniques for facilitating, not discouraging, this sort of discussion. Many of the problems faced by employees in health care are social or emotional in nature, and resolution of those problems is just as beneficial to the hospital as is resolution of work flow blockages.

Successful implementation of Quality Circles in health care thus involves two important factors. First, the organization must be sure that the eight conditions listed above are present, either throughout the organization or in those areas of the hospital where Circles are to be started.

Second, the Quality Circles concept must not be implemented in the same manner that it has been used in industry. The health care environment is unique, and unique procedures must be followed if the system is to have maximum success.

Conclusion

The potential for Quality Circles in health care clearly is enormous. By allowing them to analyze and solve their work-related problems, Quality

Circles give health care employees the voice in hospital decision making which they are demanding. By enabling them to develop their own scheduling and patient care systems, Quality Circles enable employees to contribute to the reduction of stress and pressure on the job. By letting them share their fears and concerns with one another, Quality Circles help health care employees to provide one another with social support and reassurance. And by bringing about improved work methods, reduced costs and waste, improved morale, recruitment and retention, and improved supervisory and management development, Quality Circles help hospital administrators to achieve long-lasting improvements throughout their organizations.

For all of these reasons, then, it seems clear that Quality Circles will continue to spread throughout health care world wide, and to contribute to the productivity improvements which today are so desparately needed.

REFERENCES

John E. Baird, Jr. and David J. Rittof, *Quality Circles Facilitator's Manual,* Prospect Heights, Illinois: Waveland Press, 1983.

Charles G. Burck, "Working Smarter," *Fortune,* June 15, 1981, p. 17.

Barbara Ellis, "Winds of Change Sweep Nursing Profession," *Hospitals,* January 1, 1980, p. 95.

Gail G. Hallas, "Why Nurses Are Giving It Up," *RN,* July 1980, p. 17.

Donald E. L. Johnson, "Quality Circles Put Workers In Charge of Their Productivity," *Modern Healthcare,* September, 1981, p. 69.

"Quality Control Circles Pay Off Big," *Industry Week,* October 29, 1979, p. 17.

Ron Zemke, "Quality Circles: Can They Work in the United States?" *Journal of Applied Management,* September/October, 1980, p. 18.

Part Six

The Changing Role of Nurses

Chapter Fourteen

Delivery Systems and Nursing in the 21st Century

GLORIA S. HOPE

Introduction

Predicting future trends in any profession cautions one to carefully review the present and past trends. In the past two decades, the health care industry in the United States has undergone major changes due to the impact of knowledge and science explosion. Advances in health and life expectancy alone have created dramatic changes. The gain in life expectancy for adults has surpassed that made between 1940 and 1964 with the advent of antibiotics. In fact, the recent rate of gain exceeds that of any other time in this century. The life expectancy proposed for the rest of this century may turn out to be even more significant. The rights of the elderly become another dimension of concern along with the "rights" of women and minority groups, physically handicapped, patients and human rights. These rights accompanied shifts in new values and social changes in families, groups and work ethics. These social changes have shaken the basic roots of the family and one often feels that churches, community life and schools have also lost much of their influence. Drug abuse, alcoholism, mental illness, teenage pregnancy, venereal disease, child and aged abuse, are all on the rise. Suddenly one begins to realize that social changes are compounding the crisis in health care. Two major aspects seem to be involved in the crisis.

First, most citizens and much of the policymaking apparatus of our nation have come to view health care as a "right." The consumer demands access to quality care. Second, the institutions which pay for health services (notably government and insurance companies) are extremely sensitive to any proposal designed to increase active demand for services. In something approaching panic, the third party payors are placing cost containment as high as they can on the public agenda [Kale, 1974, pp. 25-32].

Reforms addressed to several aspects are proposed almost daily. Some reforms are directed at small parts of the problem, and some propose to wrestle the whole system to the ground singlehandedly. I suspect some of my comments may appear to be at both extremes; however, I admit my bias is toward nursing.

215

Perspective of the Last Two Decades

The decade of the 1960's became an era of growth, social change, productivity and investment in the health care system. In general, more citizens received better medical care than ever before. Medicare and Medicaid assured persons who were aged or indigent that they would no longer face financial barriers to health services. For the first time, positive action was being taken to provide health services to populations with limited access. Investment in basic and applied research was increased. Regional medical programs were created to disseminate and make use of the research and oversee the dissemination of funds. Community mental health centers, drug and alcohol treatment centers were introduced and comprehensive Health Planning Committees were organized. As more individuals took advantage of these health services, there was a dramatic need for increased numbers of health professionals. Federal funds were allocated for increasing health professionals and allied health care workers. Shortages of health manpower became the "catch phrase" of the industry.

Along with these increases, the rate of scientific and technological advances skyrocketed. There was an emergence of sophisticated, highly technical procedures and treatments in every health care delivery system. These investments in technology gave rise to spiraling health care costs. During this decade, it has been noted that very little was not done to build up the capacity of the health care delivery system to meet the expected increase in demand.

As we entered the 1970's, there was a cutback in federal investments in health care. Medicare was amended; monies for hospitals and schools for health professionals dried up; support grants for health profession education and research were also cut back. The cost of illness provoked a need for regulation and control. Health Maintenance Organizations (HMO's) were introduced, hospital rates reviewed and changed, cost sharing was increased, certificates of need arrived and, by the end of 1979, revenue caps in hospitals were proposed. These reactions were primarily governmental in origin.

It is generally thought the rising cost of health care is due in part to technological change and a health insurance system that provided change for hospital care. This hospital care, being the more lucrative, has resulted in increased utilization of physicians, hospital nursing homes, and other related services. Medicare and Medicaid amendments brought more with them to health care industry than financing. There was, too, the burden of complicated regulations.

The 1970's brought the movement of multi-hospital systems. According to Ludam and Christensen [1981], the movement was motivated by regulatory and economic pressures:

In the National Health Planning and Resources Development Act of 1974

(PL 93-641), for example, Congress identified three national priorities: the development of "multi-institutional systems for the coordination or con-solidation of institutional health services"; the creation of "multi-institu-tional arrangement for the sharing of (hospital) support services"; and the capacity to provide health care "on a geographically integrated basis." These priorities seek to facilitate the rational allocation of services and facilities and to help contain costs by eliminating duplication and excess capacity.

The number of hospital beds represented by multi-hospital systems has grown to at least one third of all U.S. hospital beds. Some projections esti-mate that by 1985, half of the nation's hospitals will belong to the system [Bisbee, 1981].

Impact on Nursing

During the past two decades, there was a general sense that nursing was in turmoil and that professional nursing may become extinct. Even nurse leaders often reinforced these feelings, that the registered nurse, as a nursing practi-tioner, was fast becoming extinct. Alfano wrote that within the next 10 years, a registered professional nurse may well become a luxury which society may decide it is unwilling to support [Alfano, 1970]. Fortunately, there has been a renewed sense of being able to cope with the social and technological changes. Proudly, I state, the nursing profession has demonstrated that it can cope and have data accumulated indicating the importance of nursing and how nursing care is affecting patient outcome in and out of hospitals [Georgopoulus, 1962].

The introduction of the Clinical Specialist and the Nurse Practitioner role has changed the clinical practice of nursing. These roles were in response to the problems of maldistribution of both geography and speciality of the existing health professions, plus the escalating costs. As a result, the public had improved access and reduced cost. There is a great deal of evidence to show successful outcomes of care as measured by standards of cost and quality with regard to the nurse in primary care [Sox, 1979]. Data from re-search indicate that nurse practitioners make a difference in continuing care of patients with selected chronic disease [Runyon, 1975; Haurie and Kline, 1979].

While clinical nurse specialists and nurse practitioners practice in a variety of settings, there were also changing demands in the nature of care in tradi-tional settings; the hospital. Highly skilled nurses were making a difference in acute care settings as well as caring for the long-term patient and the elderly. In essence, nursing responded well to the forces of change of health care in the last two decades and remains the single largest category of professional health care providers.

Paradoxically, being the largest does not signify the most potent force in setting direction. Growth in the number of nurses and increased demands for nursing services have not heightened our profession's sense of direction within the health care arena [Aydelotte, 1982A] . One of the major obstacles pointed out by Aydelotte, [1982B] in our path toward professional autonomy, has been nursing's failure to achieve autonomy in practice. Perhaps the greatest obstacle to achieving power and autonomy has been the Bureaucratic organization of the hospital industry. Hospitals have been the primary employers of nurses since the mid-1930's and today, approximately 60 percent of all registered nurses are employed by hospitals. Institutional nursing has been characterized by regimentation, rigid division of labor, and intense supervision. Unfortunately, in the majority of settings, nursing services are billed as "room and board."

Until recently, nurses were rarely assigned to specific patients, and nurses served as agents of the hospital who also carry out physicians' orders. In these settings, nurses are obscured by the fragmentation of their roles by competition for patient attention of a variety of hospital employees. Consumers, health organizations and other health professionals tend to overlook nursing's contribution in these settings. Documentation of nurses' dissatisfaction with this type of employment is evidenced by union contracts, high turnover rates and more recently, by studies [Wandelt, 1982] and reports that conditions in the structure of hospital organizations actually inhibit professional nursing. Conflict arises as one perceives ourselves as professionals engaging in nursing practice while administration views nurses as employees carrying out the job of nursing. This inability to exericse control over clinical practice has produced feelings of career stagnation and has caused members to leave the profession.

In another study of nurses' job satisfaction, Hurka [1974] found that nurses working in public health and education were more satisfied with their jobs than nurses working in the hospital. He identified lack of clarity with respect to limits of authority as one of the reasons for job dissatisfaction within the hospital. Fortunately, in the last few years, hospital management began to listen and hear what was being said in regard to nurses' need to control their practice. Hospital administrators heard when they were forced to close beds because of a lack of nurses. The American Hospital Association National Commission on Nursing held hearings across the country and the message was clear that professional nurses today seek autonomy; the ability to perform the work for which they have been educated, without requiring authorization by members of another profession and, ability to exercise control over the clinical practice of nursing.

Graduates of baccalaureate, graduate and doctoral programs in nursing in this decade are united and self-determined regarding their control over nursing practice rather than being controlled by the institutional environment in which the nurse practices.

Health Care in the 21st Century

As we have discussed thus far, health care delivery in the United States is a power struggle between diverse vested interests with shifting alliances, depending on the issue and the disparate interests therein [McEwan, 1980]. In a democratic society, we have come to realize that group efforts and participation of many people are seen as useful approaches to the solution of common problems. Today, more and more people are questioning health care programs and expenditures as they never did before. Health care workers, including professionals, are prepared to provide input into the nature and shape of the health care system. Such input, from varied sources, if sound, will contribute to optimization of human and physical resources in the pursuit of improved health care of a nation.

Adversely, no one can be precise in foreseeing and forecasting the events as we prepare for the 21st century, but I would like to identify some of the key ingredients that will continue to interact and will shape and guide the directions of delivery sytems in health care.

● The principles and relationships of an Integrated Governance and Management Process (IGMP) developed by a multi-hospital system ideally supports a system of participation in governance in health care delivery. The document clearly articulates three basic principles: collegiality, subsidiarity and accountability [National Commisson on Nursing, Public Hearing, 1981].

Collegiality deals with the quality of relationships among those involved in governance and management within the multihospital system. Collegiality demands a spirit of collaboration, consensus seeking, and cooperation, all of which stem from a basic respect for the dignity and worth of each individual. In a collegial environment, opinions are openly sought and valued irrespective of position or status. Open dialogue, effective communication, mutual trust, recognition of the limitations as well as the gifts of all persons, the presence of true listening to the views of others, all are indicators of collegiality.

Subsidiarity calls for vesting decision-making authority and responsibility as close as possible to the point in the organization where the impact of the decision will be felt and vesting that authority in those most competent to make the decision. The principle is based on the belief that persons should retain as much influence as possible over decisions that affect their working environment, their job tasks, their professional and personal development, and their fulfillment as individuals and groups.

Accountability requires that individuals and groups be answerable for how authority has been exercised and responsibilities discharged. Accountability is viewed as a constructive and positive principle because it gives individuals and groups the opportunity to demonstrate the extent to which goals and objectives are fulfilled.

• Improved automation of patient support services in hospitals, computerized robots for delivery of materials; individual computerized medication banks in patients' rooms that dispense the medications, tells the patient what he's getting and when to take the next one: many other areas of technology can be applied that would free nurses to engage in the clinical practice of nursing and reduce costs and numbers of personnel. Nurses must reassess the true practice of nursing and be concerned with the caring functions rather than in numerous patient support activities. Hospitals have a well-documented problem of the inadequacies of middle management in many professional and support departments. Lacking appropriate standards and accountabilities for performance of these services results in poor service. Nursing is particularly vulnerable to systems failure because of the primacy of their accountability. Therefore, they must assume the responsibilities not adequately fulfilled by other services. This results in a sense of futility and negativism.

More advanced automation and computerization could remedy a good deal of inadequate patient support services.

As I prepared for retirement after 30 years in one organization, I was asked to reflect on the past and make some predictions for the future. One very startling factor surfaced: in nursing practice today, one is still expected to do all I was doing 30 years ago and a hundredfold more activities. Probably no one profession has done that—nursing has not let go of certain areas, while taking on new activities, as a result of specialization and scientific advances. I do not believe an individual nurse can continue in the 21st century to carry out all the caring functions from the simple to the most complex. There must be shifting organization patterns and role delineations for the various levels of workers in nursing. I foresee professional nurses going to a patient unit when nursing services are necessary; they will not be part of the bed and board. Just as community public health nurses have done for years; go to the client when there is a need. This will accelerate the "costing" of nursing care and third-party reimbursement, a more accurate understanding of the costs and benefits of specific nursing care.

• There will be increased ambulatory programs which will eliminate the barriers which prevent direct access to nurses for health services. Nurse-managed clinics for children and teenagers, pre- and post-natal care, nursing-determined home care, and care of the elderly will be available as nursing plans for an increasing variety of delivery mechanisms. One which is embryonic, but bound to grow, is the independent nurse practitioner functioning in private, group practice with other nurses or with other health professionals.

- Health Maintenance and self-help programs will be readily available. The consumer will assume greater responsibility and accountability for maintaining health. Nurses will participate in the preparation of materials and teaching health maintenance.

- Free market competition will be the dominant issue in health care delivery. Services which can be provided effectively with more cost efficiency will be sought by consumers and this era of competition and free enterprise will provide opportunities for the public to have access to more economical and appropriate care.

- By the year 2000, one out of every eight people in the United States will be 65 or older, thus triggering the emergence of a four-generation society. The dramatic aging of the American population and its impact on health care delivery systems will bring about major changes of ways in which health and social services will be delivered and financed [Abdellah, 1979]. Home care will become an essential component of the health care delivery system. Proprietary and private, non-profit entities will be seeking opportunities to enter the home care field. Some agencies have already begun such programs which provide a full spectrum of services; health and social services.

In these instances, it will be the nurse fulfilling a multi-factored role of assessor, planner, care giver, coordinator and supervisor of care provided by others. The major objective will be to keep the elderly out of long-term care institutions and to add not only "years to life," but "life to years" by enabling the elderly to live more independently. Nurses can capitalize on their years of experience in community health by surging ahead with new models of community health planning.

- Ethical problems, resulting from the explosion of medical and science technology which provides heroic methods for maintaining "life" will increase and special attention will be required to the basic question of ethical theory and to real life, day-to-day problems of ethical decision making.

- Patients' rights will take on new directions and health professionals will be accountable for their practice. Health professionals hold expectations that a working environment will be provided them to permit them to provide humane care and to be involved in ethical decisions that affect their practice and lives. As patient advocates, nurses see themselves upholding patients' rights to be involved in decisions about their care.

Conclusion

This paper has discussed a spectrum of issues dealing with the social, economic and technological changes in health care during the past two decades. The impact on the nursing profession has been discussed and it has been shown that when nursing has been successful in regulating its practice and in meeting the health care needs of society, there remains no question—that the profession of nursing will continue to exist. Nursing's task, as it moves to meet the demands of a more sophisticated consumer in a society characterized by moral pluralism, is to adjust roles so that professionals and patients will work together to promote the well being of individuals.

Now that we are on the threshold of the 21st century and bombarded by technology, let us determine its usage so that we may plan our contributions at higher and more humane levels of participation in health care.

I remain optimistic about the future. I believe that it is brighter for nursing than a decade ago because nursing has finally begun to speak out with a clear sense of professional identity and self determination to change today's health care delivery systems. Nursing has demonstrated its commitment to the issues of reducing health care costs, increasing primary care and demonstrating that nursing interventions have low cost/high benefit results.

Nursing is ready to become actively involved in setting and designing programs of health care, promotion and prevention in the 21st century. As a philosopher once said, "We might feel some sympathy for the one who tried and failed, but only pity for the one who never even tried."

I say to you today, "Nursing has tried!"

REFERENCES

Gearase Alfano, "Nursing in the Decade Ahead," *American Journal of Nursing,* 70, (10), p. 2117, 1970.

Faye B. Atdellah, Ed.D, "Preparing for the Health Care Issues of the 1980's," NLN Monograph, *Health Care in the 1980's, Who Provides? Who Plans? Who Pays?* pp. 1-11, 1979.

Myrtle K. Aydelotte, "The Path Toward Professional Autonomy," *Military Medicine,* Vol. 147, pp. 1048-50, December 1982.

Gerald E. Bisbee, *Multi-hospital Systems: Policy Issue of the Future,* Chicago, 1981.

B. S. Georgopoulos and F. C. Mann, *The Community General Hospital,* New York, McMillian, 1962.

C. M. Haurie and C. Kline, "Cost Effective Primary Care," *Nurse Practitioner,* 4:5, p. 54, 1979.

Slanek J. Hurka, "Organizational Environment and Work Satisfaction," *Dimensions in Health Service,* 51, p. 43, January 1974.

Joseph C. Kale, "The Role of Comprehensive Health Planning in the Development of a Health System," NLN Monograph, *The Future is Now,* New York, 1979.

James E. Lumlam, Esq. and Jay D. Christensen, Esq. *et al.* "Multi-hospital Arrangements and the Federal Anit-trust Laws," *Multi-hospital Systems: Policy Issues for the Future,* The Hospital Research and Educational Trust, Edited by George E. Bisbee, Jr., Chicago, Illinois, p. 25, 1981.

David Mechanic, "Rationing Health Care: Public and the Medical Market Place," *The Hastings Center Report,* Vol. 6, No. 1, pp. 34-7, 1976.

Duncan E. McEwan, "The Realities of Medicare," *Health Management Forum,* Vol. 1, No. 1. pp. 27-38, Spring 1980.

J. W. Runyon, "The Memphis Chronic Disease Program: Comparisons and Outcome and the Nurse's Extended Role," *Journal of the American Medical Association,* pp.241-44, January 20, 1975.

H. C. Sox, "Quality of Patient Care by Nurse Practitioners and Physicians Assistants: A Ten Year Perspective," *Annals of Internal Medicine,* 91, pp. 459-68, 1979.

Mabel Wandelt, P. N. Pierce, and R. R. Meddnissan, "Why Nurses Leave Nursing and What Can Be Done About It," *American Journal of Nursing,* 81:76, 1981.

Chapter Fifteen

Strategic Planning for Nursing Administration

LYNDSEY STONE

"Strategic planning" is the latest fashion in management. It is often "sold" to managers as the panacea for survival in unstable economies in relatively prosperous countries, countries in which enterprises can afford the leisure and resource expenditure that the formal strategic planning process requires. Fashions are related to realities, however, and despite its pitfalls, comprehensive strategic planning, management and implementation do address some of the main dilemmas of the 1980's. Strategic planning accepts as a premise the variability of internal organizational circumstances and external environmental conditions. Alternative future scenarios can be "played out" theoretically and alternated in reality as circumstances change. There are criteria for making day-to-day managerial decisions. When things go wrong, as they inevitably do, there is a structure for analyzing the error sequence and for choosing different alternative future actions. This process, formal strategic planning, is public, presumably rational, data-based and expressed in a written document which is available to the manager of the organization.

What is meant by strategic planning; what is this mystical process for looking into a crystal ball (or a series of crystal balls) in order to have better future options? Actually, the strategic planning process is quite mundane and easy to define. The complexity comes in the creation of a plan and its implementation in an actual organization. A strategy is "a unified, comprehensive, and integrated plan designed to assure that the basic objectives of the enterprise are achieved . . . Strategic planning is that set of decisions and actions which leads to the development of an effective strategy . . . Strategy is the means used to achieve the ends (objectives). A strategy is a plan that is unified—it ties all the parts of the enterprise together. A strategy is comprehensive—it covers all major aspects of the enterprise. A strategy is integrated—all parts of the plan are compatible with each other and fit together well" [Glueck, 1976, p. 3].

Why should nursing be involved in strategic planning? Nurses are frequently vice presidents of the health care organizations in which they work. They are full members of the executive management group. As such, nurse administrators are increasingly required to develop strategic plans which fit within the overall strategy of the entire organization. Nurses are the largest single group of human resources in health services institutions. The goals of nursing and methods may be crucial for the success of the hospital as a whole.

Strategic planning can revolutionize the work of nursing administrators. Traditionally, nursing has followed medicine in functioning via the crisis model, which is a reactive, emotionally exhausting and inefficient means of providing care or organizing health services. Strategic planning is actually a means of organizing the delivery of services so that short- and long-term objectives are served. Future oriented thinking must occur. Philosophical issues must be reflected upon, for philosophy guides strategy development.

Issues to consider: Who will give care — Licensed Professional Nurses?; Licensed Practical Nurses?; Aides? To whom will care be given and under what circumstances? Will unit managers make real administrative decisions under a decentralized system or will nursing be centrally directed? Philosophically, a hospital staff utilizes highly educated nurses with advanced degrees as much as possible. It has been postulated that it is less expensive to have one highly competent nurse than several technicians. Technicians are not licensed to perform many essential tasks. Their efforts must always be directed by a Licensed Professional Nurse, and much time-consuming follow-up and documentation must occur. For every hour a technician works, an hour of supervisory time is spent, time when the Licensed Professional Nurse could be providing patient care. Furthermore, aides and technicians have high turnover (about 150 percent per year) due to low salaries and an absence of professional commitment. A decision to use the Licensed Professional Nurse is a multi-faceted one—economic, since costs are weighed; and philosophical, since a commitment to highly skilled nursing care guided the evaluation of alternative nurse staffing patterns.

The use of a business context in strategic planning dictates that marketing strategies be discussed and developed. Physicians are defined as the primary consumers of nursing care. Patients do not admit themselves, nor do administrators admit patients. In a given geographic area, physicians retain admitting privileges at a number of hospitals and can choose where they place their patients. When a hospital has a reputation for providing superior nursing care, physicians are attracted to that hospital and they remain content with the affiliation. One could assume that patients cannot evaluate the quality of medical care, but they can and do evaluate the "hotel services"—whether the nurses are kind and friendly; whether the nurses respond to bells and lights rapidly; whether food and medication are brought on time. Sometimes patients do request hospitals as a consequence of hearsay or previous experience. It is a known fact that patients do sometimes influence a physician's choice of hospitals, especially when physicians have multiple admitting privileges and utilize several hospitals with regularity.

When a hospital adopts a marketing approach to its mission, then nursing is challenged in its ability to remain flexible and in its attitudes toward physicians, as these attitudes are expressed in nurse/physician interaction. For example, flexible operating room schedules are important to physicians. In the past nurses have often said, "You can have 2:00 on Thursday. Take it or leave it." Nurse socialization has often been anti-physician; in part because physicians and nurses frequently compete for direction and management of patients. There is not always a clear demarcation line between physicians and nurses in their knowledge base and skill level and there may be disagreement about the needs of patients. A market-oriented nursing department devises policies which describe how complaints about physicians can be diplomatically handled.

There are many side benefits when a marketing-oriented strategy is adopted. In one situation a consequence was that the decision was made to phase out technicians (aides) and assistants through attrition, using junior and senior nursing students as assistants. These student assistants were drawn from new clinical affiliation programs and each worked two or three days per week. The students were highly motivated and competent, and recruitment strategy, designed to attract new Licensed Professional Nurses, was greatly enhanced.

By providing opportunities for students, the interest of faculty members was attracted. Now, some of those faculty members work part- or full-time at that hospital. Master's prepared nurses are attracted to the environment and nurse externs (baccalaureate students) are almost all available upon graduation. In a period where there is a shortage of highly educated nurses, the marketing orientation of this hospital's strategic plan was notably successful.

Costs are held down and multiple agendas served. Without a comprehensive strategic planning effort, it is unlikely that staffing patterns would be re-examined for nursing. The philosophical, economic and marketing considerations dovetailed. One consequence was a competitive edge over other hospitals in the area, an area where there is a surplus of tertiary care hospital beds.

The importance of the philosophical premises of an institution for economic effects should not be underestimated. It is believed that people will remain at work if they are happy, and that the applicant pool of nurses will be of higher quality as the hospital becomes known as a place where "nurses want to nurse." If nurses are hired who are well prepared to make clinical decisions and judgments on their own, then professional autonomy can be granted. Decentralization of nursing administration, with downward delegation of authority and responsibility and upward accountability is possible. The strategic planning process met the needs of all audiences—physicians, nurses, patients, administrators, students and faculty.

At this point it should be evident that a business administration context for strategic planning does not make nursing "less humane" or less patient oriented. In fact, it clarified and harmonized the interests of patients with a variety of audiences, and with the economic needs of the survival of the hospital. It also seems clear that nurses do not need complete autonomy or client or organizational control to plan and implement strategic goals. Further, strategy and operations can be organically fused.

How this fusion is accomplished is dependent upon the way in which strategic planning is approached by the nursing administrator. It is essential to realize that the strategic planning of today is very different from the long-range planning of yesterday. The long-range planning so popular in the past assumed high internal and external stability and usually relied on future scenario, that of present conditions. A static entity, long-range planning was based on assumptions which are unworkable in the 1980's. Long-range planning customarily did not deal explicitly or in depth with premises, philosophy or short- and long-term tradeoffs made under shifting definitions of the purpose of the institution.

Modern strategic planning centrally assumes that there will be directional choices (and roads not taken); that there must be an orientation around which strategy is developed; that the strategic plan must be congruent with operational capability; and that strategy must be responsive to changing internal organizational and external market conditions, many of which are not completely predictable at any point in time.

The foregoing suggests that in these days of intense competition hospitals would benefit from a marketing orientation. Other orientations within the conceptual model include product, technology and production orientations [Tregoe, 1980]. Once an orientation is selected, it narrows the perspectives of the planners so that depth is achieved in one area, such as marketing, and activities in the other areas, such as products, production and technology are weighed in relation to the basic area of orientation. For example, whether to order computer consoles for patient monitoring (technology), whether to offer a visiting nurse service (a new product offered) and whether to hire a greater number of nurses with advanced degrees (greater production capability) are evaluated in terms of market needs.

A description of each orientation should clarify the choices available to nurse administrators engaged in strategic planning. A market needs orientation focuses upon development of a means of filling the current or anticipated needs of specific market segments such as physicians, administrators and patients, or customer groups such as the elderly, parents, children, etc., in order to accomplish broader organization goals. The planners of the organization will constantly explore new or emerging needs of relevant market segments in order to remain competitive. This approach is compatible with

Drucker's description of the essence of marketing. According to Drucker,

> There is only one valid definition of business purpose—*to create a customer* ... The want a business satisfies may have been felt by the customer before he was offered a means of satisfying it ... it remained a potential want until the action of businessmen converted it into effective demand ... [marketing is] the whole business seen from the point of view of its final result, that is, from the customer's point of view ... True marketing ... says, 'These are the satisfactions the customer looks for, values and needs.' [Drucker, 1974, pp. 61, 63, 64]

A marketing perspective forces planners to externalize their notions of nursing service. For example, most patients do not think nursing quality is high if three different nursing staff members must identify, verify and adjust an IV which has infiltrated or when it ran out of fluid. From the patient's perspective, the first individual to reach the IV should have been able to reset it immediately, and in any event, IV checks should have been more frequent to avoid patient discomfort from infiltration into the skin. A marketing orientation directed toward patients would require re-examination of the time spans between IV checks and of the disadvantages of using technicians and aides rather than Licensed Professional Nurses who can "do the whole job once." Team nursing might be re-examined with a view toward implementing primary nursing, where specific patient responsibility rests with a single nurse.

A product orientation, in contrast, emphasizes the offering of a wide variety of nursing services individually or as a group based on their common characteristics or common appeal, in order to accomplish broader organization goals. With a product orientation, new products will be evaluated in part due to their similarity to old products and their ability to serve familiar markets. Organization efforts will be directed toward selling the product mix and toward improving the mix. This strategic approach for nursing would be apparent when a health care institution expands its services to the elderly, a well developed market for them, by adding on direct phone hookups to a special elderly care unit for emergency consultation by home-bound patients and by hiring visiting nurses specializing in geriatrics. One constraint on the marketing orientation would be the need for stability of market position. One opportunity would be that the ease of adding other services could enhance patient/customer loyalty, thus protecting the market share of the institution and enhancing its comparative advantage *vis-à-vis* competing institutions.

The technology orientation would result in a search to improve the technological capability of nursing service and/or the skills and knowledge of nurses to accomplish broader organization goals. A technological orientation would lead nurses to identify and incorporate systems, equipment and support facilities to increase the sophistication of the nursing services available. For example, a technologically oriented nursing service would constantly scan its environment for innovative methods and techniques which could be incorporated into the services provided for its clientele. The expenses of technology would be a constraint, but the excitement of new knowledge and equipment would be an enjoyable challenge.

A production capability orientation would seek to expand the quantity and depth of services offered by nursing in order to accomplish broader organization goals. For example, a visiting nurse service might adopt a production capability orientation so that a sufficient number of visits per day are made by nurses, allowing the organization to survive and potentially to expand. This model is driven by the need for efficiency and is coming into vogue in the 1980's due to economic retrenchment. A nursing service could also act as a job shop with a production capability orientation, contracting to utilize its staff and programs for the benefit of other organizations lacking the necessary production capability. For example, a larger tertiary care center provides in-service nursing education for rural hospitals in surrounding areas and earns additional income by using the staff of its nursing resource department fully and profitably. One advantage of a production orientation is the potential ease of increasing revenue. One constraint is the resistance of nurses to "being production line workers."

Some basic premises are implicit in this analysis. First, it is possible to examine a situation and decide upon the most appropriate focus at a specific point in time. As examples, a hospital nursing department in a highly competitive environment where many hospitals have excess bed capacity might choose a marketing orientation. A hospital nursing department in a stable environment with a well satisfied clientele might choose a product orientation. A nursing department in a sophisticated tertiary care center might reflect a technology orientation. A nursing department in a hospital which is financially marginal might look carefully at a production orientation.

Questions such as these help the organization decide upon a new strategic orientation—What are the comparative advantages of the organization in its market area? What does the internal and external environment appraisal say about the market segment and market share? What internal capabilities affect the potential for success with different strategic orientations? What alternative strategies fit the financial base, management thrust and market picture? How would the selected strategy be implemented and evaluated? Basic orientation of a strategic plan for nursing may change over time, but it should be congruent with the overall plan of the hospital if there is one. As new opportunities and constraints arise, or as an organization moves through the life cycle, changes in strategic orientation are inevitable [Kimberly, 1980]. The need to change a plan is problematic only for those who regard the plan as a "bible" rather than a working document subject to periodic revision.

The notion of strategic planning may be difficult to sell to the naive administrator who asks, "Why plan if the internal and external environments are constantly changing?" It may be equally difficult to convince the cynical administrator who asks, "Why plan when politics are so influential in organization decision making?" The former can be answered that one can be manipulated by change, or one can direct it, based on the extent of one's willingness to accept shifting realities which can be described, evaluated and rationally influenced. To the latter, it can be said that political variables can be built into the alternative scenarios developed to operationalize strategic goals, and that politics are frequently predictable as are most classes of events.

Evaluation is the area where most strategic plans fail in both specification and precision. Success targets should be carefully and realistically described in the initial plan and on an annual basis. Some brief and partial examples are illustrated here. "Home health care nurses shall make at least an average of 4.5 visits per day during each work day per year" (production capability). "In this fiscal year the nursing department shall expand the number of distinct and separate services offered to the elderly by at least 20 percent" (product). "In this fiscal year the nursing department shall add ten patient monitors to the cardiac care unit" (technology). Or "In this fiscal year the nursing staff shall include at least 80 percent Licensed Professional Nurses, of whom 40 percent have at least a baccalaureate education and 10 percent have at least a master's degree." It is evident that a strategic plan has important quantitative anchors so that the objective criterion of success is described in the formal document.

What makes a nurse executive a successful strategic planner? First, the nurse executive must be well matched with the institution in personal goals, philosophy and competencies. The management style of the nurse executive must complement those of the chief executive officer. Ideally, both should be entrepreneurial and view internal and external changes as challenges rather than headaches. Second, the nurse executive must be careful to acknowledge the limits of a "blank check" as a top level decision maker. The limits are set by the history of the hospital, current chief executive, financial and staff resources and strategic goals. Third, the nurse executive must have the ability to sit in the corporate boardroom and make contributions to discussions on a wide range of topics as an experienced team player. This is essential for credibility. Fourth, the nurse executive must present proposals based on facts not value judgements, refining quantitative information for appropriateness to the needs and capabilities of the hospital. Investments must be projected for accuracy and completeness.

Fifth, the nurse executive should be willing to make sacrifices beyond those asked for when the hospital is in difficulty. Rather than "nickel and diming" the chief administrative officer, the nurse executive should fully support that individual, even at short-run costs to the nurse executive's own turf. Overproduction earns "idiosyncracy credits," resulting in chief executive support and greater future resources and credibility.

Strategic planning is really a balancing act between the past and the future. It is a process by which an organization invents its own future as part of the drive toward success. The process is both abstract and concrete. It requires both creativity and dull, routine monitoring of ongoing events. The strategic planning process challenges the ability of organization members to function as goal-directed team members striving to meet measurable outcomes. Strategic planning assumes that there will be conflict and negotiation over goals, capabilities and resources, but that the end result will be working cooperatively for the common interest.

For the nurse administrator, strategic planning requires executive level skill, and the ability to work with the variety of business areas of hospital management, including budgeting and finance, marketing, management information systems and organization behavior. Because nursing is the core of ongoing health service in hospitals, nurse executives are increasingly called to the boardroom to engage in strategic planning. It is truly an opportunity to influence hospital policy and to advance the nurse executive's interest in professional nursing and improved patient care.

At this point one might wonder how strategic planning and its applications for nursing would apply to countries other than the United States; countries whose administrative patterns differ as a consequence of tradition and culture. The strategic planning process is theoretically applicable anywhere. There are some assumptions which one makes here. The first is that explicit and deliberate decision making occurs, with an identifiable group of people involved in an ongoing process in a relatively permanent organization with stability and continuity. Without stability and continuity, there cannot be any tracking of the successes and failures of a plan.

A second assumption is that authority explicitly resides with a group of people who have considerable freedom in directing the efforts of the enterprise. Thirdly, strategic planning can work only if this freedom allows the executive group to adapt managerial action to external circumstances. A fourth assumption is that management is competency-based, so that mere political decisions do not overwhelm the rational planning process. A fifth assumption is that the organization has a well-defined mission within which the business purpose can be framed after sufficient debate.

For nursing, a sixth assumption is crucial. Nursing must be regarded as an executive area of managerial expertise. The chief nurse administrator must be a full participant in the strategic planning process of the hospital, with considerable latitude for departmental planning and control. In some countries, nursing has not received this level of recognition and nurses are still viewed as the handmaidens of physicians.

Cultural context also affects strategic planning. The American assumption of rationality is often looked upon as quaint by nationals of other countries. Nevertheless, high quality strategic planning in any country requires systematic collection of information from many levels of employees and from the broader economic, political, social and geographic environments. The success of strategic planning depends heavily on the "fit" of the organization with its environment and on a mutuality of needs.

In some countries, an elite with a right to rule make strategic decisions without the participation of lower management; caste, rather than ability or knowledge, can skew the plan. The possibilities for success are reduced by authoritarian, elitist strategic planning systems. There are also a number of areas which must be explored when the strategic planner is from one country and is consulting in another country [Holt, Spring 1982, p. 8]. Different organization customs must be accounted for. As an **example,** "cradle to grave" employee security, differences in vocations, safety and health requirements, unemployment costs and comprehensive benefits are evaluated.

In many countries, there is a stronger political component to decision making than in the United States. Strategic choices may be heavily constrained by alliances and factions within and outside the organization. Managerial prerogatives may be limited by complex legal requirements. In some countries there are legal protections against layoffs, staffing patterns may not be negotiable, and representation on committees of significance may be fixed by law. The habits and customs indigenous to any country set the subtle but real outer limits upon changes in organization life. For example, automated equipment which is technologically sophisticated may be difficult to introduce due to a cultural bias toward low unemployment and job security.

The strategic planning effort in health care is further impacted by national priorities. Hospitals must often plan to deliver those services which the government has decided are most important at a particular period of time. Within these boundaries, the strategic planner must be creative in defining the plan and describing its means of implementation.

For strategic planning to exist, a formal, deliberate, explicit and ongoing commitment is necessary by the chief executive of the organization. This individual's support and participation often determines whether the plan actually guides action. For nursing to be fully included, the chief executive officer must understand the importance of the profession to patient care, and the significance of nursing services to physicians and hospital administrators.

We will see further development of alternative structures for the strategic planning process which are specific to institution mission, cultural content, and economic and personnel resource levels. When this occurs and strategic planning matures as a management specialty area, health administrators and nurse executives will have greater ease in establishing plans that work. For nurse executives, complete membership on the executive team may still be a future expectation. Nursing, the "sleeping giant" of the health care system, must become knowledgeable about strategic planning. When necessary, such knowledge can enhance the nurse executive's influence upon the hospital and acceptance as a key decision maker.

REFERENCES

William F. Glueck, *Business Policy: Strategy Formation and Management Action,* New York: McGraw-Hill Book Co., 1976, p. 3.

Benjamin B. Tregoe and John W. Zimmerman, *Top Management Strategy,* New York: Simon and Schuster, 1980.

Peter F. Drucker, *Management: Tasks, Responsibilities Practices,* New York: Harper and Row, 1974, pp. 61, 63, 64.

John R. Kimberly, Robert H. Miles and Associates, *The Organizational Life Cycle,* San Francisco: Jossey-Bass, 1980.

David H. Holt, "Changing Planning Roles, Strategy Formulation and Host-Country Manager," *The Collegiate Forum,* Spring 1982, p. 8.

Chapter Sixteen

Why Strategic Planning for Nursing?

**DOROTHY H. FOX and
RICHARD T. FOX**

Increased attention is being paid to institutional strategic planning; that is, planning at the top administrative level which affects the institution as a whole. Everyone will agree that some degree of sophisticated forethought is essential for the continued, successful operation of a health care facility. The institution must look ahead—plan for its future. Tomorrow's activities must be a reflection of today's sound decisions. And so it is with the department of nursing —the most labor intensive component of the entire institutional system.

Why strategic planning for nursing? To answer this question, it is helpful first to define strategic planning in somewhat simple terms and then review the main points of the planning process as they apply to nursing before discussing benefits specific to the department.

What Is Strategic Planning

Planning can be simply defined as "devising a detailed scheme which is aimed toward accomplishing some goal." Strategic planning is more specific in that it refers to "using tools or techniques designed to conserve scarce resources—capital and human resources—while working toward the achievement of a goal." Peter Drucker makes three important points as he describes strategic planning [Drucker, 1974, p. 125]. He says that strategic planning is:

- A continuous, systematic process of making risk-taking decisions today with the greatest possible knowledge about their effects on the future;
- Organizing efforts needed to carry out these decisions; and
- Evaluating results of these decisions against expected outcomes through reliable feedback mechanisms.

In short, the formal planning approach (1) determines what is desired, (2) maps out the overall action phase, and (3) measures the degree of success in reaching the desired goal.

A strategic plan for nursing might be thought of as a systematic approach to decisionmaking in the present for the future well being of its patient clientele, the department, and the institution. Critical thinking about the organization's mission and the department's philosophy preceed the actual development, implementation, and evaluation of the strategic plan to be used by nursing.

How Are the Phases of the Planning Cycle Linked

Answer to this question not only complements the definition of strategic planning, but it helps us to better understand the rationale behind why this type of planning is a must for nursing. Figure I shows the linkage of the five critical phases of the planning cycle which involves:

- Identifying institution values and mission;
- Collecting data and processing;
- Determining department goals and objectives;
- Implementing operations; and
- Evaluating results (outcomes).

Using this linkage as a guide, nursing should examine the values or basic beliefs that underlie decisions made by policymakers of the institution. These values are fundamental to the process of planning; therefore, they are used in defining the mission or basic purpose of the whole organization. Nursing's understanding of the philosophy and intent of the policymaking body is a good starting point in putting together a strategic plan for nursing.

We see that the progressive linkage—values to mission to goals to objectives —is directly related to the hierarchy of the organizational structure. This means that the "mission statement" initiated by the policymaking board functions as a general directive to top administration which, in turn, compiles "official goals" to be used throughout the institution. Nursing now enters the picture as its department, after reviewing pertinent data, makes these goals more explicit and operational. That is, institution goals are broken down into department goals which are further broken down into objectives. Objectives are the specific end points or targets which, when reached, bring about the reality of the goals. Precision in operationalizing these objectives in clear, concise, measurable (quantitative) terms is required because they direct the concentration or usage of resources. In the end we see that the values inferred in the mission statement become actualized as nursing's goals and objectives openly address the dynamic state of nursing practice.

However, before a final decision is made as to its goals and objectives, nursing first must gather baseline information about the present status of nursing practice. This involves identifying key factors and trends which could ultimately affect the department and its patient clientele. For instance, alternate modes of nursing care delivery and utilization rates/case-mix data of individual nursing divisions should be analyzed. Specifically, nursing is urged to carefully examine some of the recent information concerning:

- Political issues and legal requirements affecting nursing practice;
- Marketing capabilities and innovations;
- Physical and social work environments of nursing personnel;
- Technological advances; and

- Nursing productivity measures.

Again, a clear understanding—both quantitative and qualitative—of the nursing department's internal and external environment is strongly recommended prior to establishing standards in the form of goals and objectives.

Operations is the next action phase of the planning process when nursing personnel as a group actively work together to achieve the department goals and objectives. It is important to note that the transition of plans into policy and practice is the main reason for the whole planning process. Second, this operational phase is directly connected to all other management functions, such as organizing, directing, and controlling. It is during this phase that we see the strategic plan come to life.

Evaluation is often thought of as the final action signifying closure of the planning process. However, this is not always the case. In fact, evaluation—the comparison of actual outcome against desired outcome—takes place not only at the end of the planning cycle, but at each of its preceeding critical phases. For example, before a program requiring expanded physical space and/or additional manpower is implemented, economic feasibility of the project must be projected and evaluated. The more comprehensive type of evaluation is due at the end of the operation period. Its purpose is to measure final outcomes against the desired, goal-oriented objectives by making qualitative and quantitative comparisons. Use of quantitative comparison techniques is highly recommended because of the greater degree of objectivity.

In summary, the linkage of values and mission to data to goals and objectives to operations to evaluation make up the planning cycle. We see that (1) output from one phase acts as input to the next, and (2) periodic and final evaluations are essential to round out the planning process. It is of utmost importance that the nurse administrator and others who participate come to acquire the sense of sequence and interrelationship demonstrated in Figure I before attempting the outline of a plan.

Why Strategic Planning for Nursing?

Strategic planning in the long run is a good investment. Authorities on the subject, such as George Steiner and Henrick Blum, tell us that we can expect a significant improvement in overall department performance when systematic planning is substituted for a day-to-day "gut feeling" approach now used by many nurse administrators [Steiner, 1979, p. 44; Blum, 1974, p. 43]. It makes sense that decisions affecting the short run can be made with more certainty if some long run point has already been investigated and established. Planning offers a benefit package to nursing that should not be overlooked:

- Planning provides a sense of direction to the department over time.

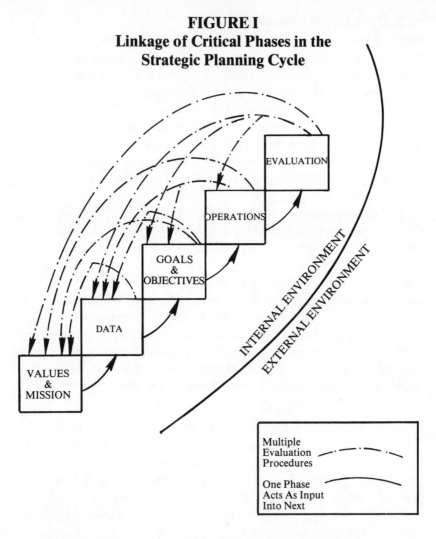

FIGURE I
Linkage of Critical Phases in the
Strategic Planning Cycle

- Planning functions as a control mechanism by setting limits and monitoring variance from the intended course of action.
- Planning helps to conserve both capital and human resources.
- Planning deals concretely with complex projects/programs in multiple stage, time sequences.
- Planning is a source of professional satisfaction for those who are involved in the process.

Since strategic planning methodology necessitates the outlining of ways and means believed useful to reach some defined destination, a direction course of action evolves. Unlike courses of action may be chosen by nurse planners in different facilities for various reasons: One wants to work toward maintaining the status quo while another works to rapidly progress toward newly identified goals. Regardless of which path is followed, active involvement in a strategic planning program coordinates and guides present and future department activities.

Use of control mechanisms, such as monitoring with patient classification data and manpower budget reports, gives a good indication as to whether the department (1) is proceeding on course as anticipated, or (2) is off course to a significant degree. Patient classification determines the total hours *needed* for nursing care delivery whereas manhour budget reports summarize the total hours *used* for nursing care delivery. A quantitative comparison between the two data sources—hours needed versus hours used—can be done on a daily, a monthly, and a yearly basis. (Projected figures of nursing hours needed for each of the nursing divisions function as standards, and are noted in the written plan.) During this past year we have seen nursing departments alter their courses when timely adjustments of decreases in manhours were made in response to lowered rates of occupancy in hospitals.

Conservation of scarce resources is a primary objective of strategic planning. March and Simon emphasize the fact: Any degree of activity on the part of the oganization absorbs scarce resources [March and Simon, 1958, pp.199-210]. Therefore, nursing must choose between two options:

OPTION 1   □   Persist in making short sighted decisions with no well defined objectives in mind.

OPTION 2   □   Think critically about where the department is going, why, and by what means.

Outcome of Option 1 is misdirected activity which, more often than not, inapprorpriately absorbs costly resources. Outcome of Option 2 is deliberate, directed activity which lessens the chances of wasting these same resources. Simply stated, both material and human resources can be saved when nurse administrators select the latter option and put systematic planning into practice. This second approach is rated as being especially helpful when undertaking a multiple stage project or program. Advanced specifications are used to show how and when complex parts of a project fit together, and what are the expected results.

Finally, actual involvement in strategic planning can be both personally and professionally rewarding in terms of the satisfaction perceived as management and staff work together to develop, implement, and evaluate a comprehensive planning program.

We should remember that it is impossible for a nurse administrator to initiate or follow through on a systematic plan for the nursing department without receiving backing and encouragement from the chief executive officer.

Together, they must agree that applying the five principles basic to the strategic planning process will be beneficial to both the institution and the community which they serve. These principles include:

- Thinking critically about past, present, and future states of affairs aids in the development, implementation, and evaluation of a well formulated plan.

- Sensitivity to the needs of the institution and its personnel, as well as to the clientele it serves, is fundamental to strategic planning.

- A structured plan is both flexible and adaptive to environmental changes.

- Accuracy is increased when goal/objective related outcomes are measured in quantitative terms as compared to qualitative terms.

- Advanced planning is positively related to the making of sound decisions in the present.

REFERENCES

Henrik L. Blum, *Planning for Health,* New York: Human Sciences Press, 1974, p. 43.

Peter Drucker, *Management: Tasks, Responsibilities, Policies,* New York: Harper and Row, Publishers, 1974, p. 125.

James G. March and Herbert A. Simon, *Organizations,* New York: John Wiley and Sons, 1958, pp. 199-210.

George A. Steiner, *Strategic Planning,* New York: The Free Press, 1979, p. 44.

Chapter Seventeen

Economic and Employment Issues in Health Care: The Nursing Perspective

RICHARD C. McKIBBEN

I. Introduction and General Considerations

Nursing faces many challenges. As individuals, the nation's 1,800,000 registered nurses confront a variety of choices regarding their careers. These include differing work patterns, alternative employment opportunities, specialization, and additional education. As a profession, nursing continues to struggle with attainment of equitable compensation, advancement of professional recognition and status, agreement about the role of the professional association, resolution of the educational base for nursing practice, and extension of nursing's influence in health care organization, delivery, and policy.

These challenges, and many others faced by nurses[1] and their profession, involve economic and employment considerations. Both the development of an individual's career and the progress of a profession are intimately influenced by economic and employment issues. These range from obvious factors—salary levels and scheduling patterns, for example—to more subtle ones, such as the effects of changes in reimbursement levels for various health services on utilization rates, and thereby on nursing employment. Whether they are obvious or subtle, the economic and employment issues that affect nurses and nursing are often inadequately understood. These issues may also be more powerful and influential than is generally believed.

An understanding of the role of economic and employment issues is essential to nursing in the 1980's, because most of the challenges nursing faces are related to these issues. As the 1980's progress, it appears that many of the choices and challenges that nurses and nursing face in the United States are

---

*Adapted with permission from the author's "Nursing in the 80's: Key Economic and Employment Issues," the first of ten monographs in *Economic and Employment Issues for Registered Nurses,* published by the American Nurses' Association (copyright, 1982).

[1] The term "nurses" in this analysis refers only to registered nurses, not to other categories of nursing personnel (licensed practical nurses, nurses' aides, attendants, and so forth).

significantly different from those of a decade earlier. Some concerns are entirely new, such as emerging speculation that the shortage of nurses may end,
to be replaced by an era of nursing manpower surpluses. This development,
if it occurs, would have far-reaching effects on nursing employment and related economic factors. The impact of the recent prolonged recession, the
effects of major federal budget cuts for Medicare and Medicaid and other
health programs, and the consequences of new Medicare payment mechanisms
on hospitals and other employers of nurses are other developments of immediate concern.

Some choices and challenges faced by nurses and nursing, however, have
been remarkably persistent over time. Adequate income, improved fringe
benefits and pensions, third-party reimbursement for nursing services, the
establishment of the baccalaureate as the educational base for professional
nursing practice, and improved professional standing and autonomy have
all been sought for many years. The American Nurses' Association's economic and general welfare program was established in 1946, 28 years before
amendments to federal labor laws that facilitated the more rapid development
of unionization among registered nurses. The nurse shortage has been a mainstay of discussion, debate, and policy attention since the end of World War
II. Many other economic and employment issues have also persisted over
time.

Some way of understanding, responding to, or acting upon these issues,
new or old, must be developed or acquired. Some may believe that nurses
are underpaid without ever having examined salary schedules or other related
information for nurses or other professionals; others may reach the same
conclusion (or a different conclusion) only after extensive study of the
situation. On any particular issue, individual opinions, knowledge, or beliefs
may be highly varied, vague or explicit, correct or inaccurate. Relatively few
health care professionals have had formal education or training in economics,
business administration, accounting, finance, or related fields that would enable them to better assess the impact of economic and employment issues
on them and their profession. As a result, too many health professionals—not
just nurses but also members of all categories of health professionals—may
have difficulty in confidently developing appropriate understandings of,
responses to, and actions upon those economic and employment issues.

For example, consider the following questions:

- What facilitates salary increases?
- Why do salaries increase at different rates among different professions
  or within the same profession in different locations, different specialties,
  or different employment settings?
- What effects has unionization had on nurses' salaries?

- How do wages paid to registered nurses relative to those of licensed practical nurses affect the employment levels of those two groups?
- How much does the predominance of women in nursing affect their salaries, working conditions, and professional status?
- How has the opening of new employment opportunities for women affected the relative attractiveness of nursing as a career?
- What factors influence the willingness of nurses to work full-time, part-time, or not al all?
- How can the adequacy of alternative pension and retirement arrangements be evaluated?
- How are nurses affected by changes in hospital costs, reimbursement levels, utilization rates, and related factors?
- If the nurse shortage disappears and a surplus emerges, how will this impact nurses' salaries and employment patterns?
- How much will federal cutbacks in support for Medicare, Medicaid, and other health programs reduce nursing employment?
- How would reimbursement for nursing services affect nurses' incomes?
- What effects do the continued existence of educational programs of significantly different setting, focus, and length have on salaries, career advancement, and professional status?
- How can the concepts of "pay equity" and "comparable worth" be defined, measured, achieved, and enforced? What actual impact would they have on nurses?
- What effects do temporary employment agencies for nurses have on staffing, nursing costs, and work patterns?
- What effect does the growth in multihospital systems, for-profit hospitals, HMO's, and other organizational and ownership arrangements have on nurses?
- How will new and proposed federal policies such as prospective, DRG-based Medicare payment mechanisms, the "new federalism" and pro-competitive health care systems affect nurses and nursing?
- How are the foregoing concerns interrelated?

This list, which could continue with many other related questions, serves to illustrate two points: first, a large number of economic and employment issues are of concern to registered nurses, and second, few if any of these concerns have responses that are either simple or obvious. The discussion that follows provides summary descriptions of key economic and employment issues organized around these topical areas:

- The impact of the general economic situation on nurses and nursing
- Changes in the health delivery system
- Salaries of registered nurses

- Fringe benefits for nursing employment
- Economic and general welfare efforts
- The demand for nurses: shortage or surplus?
- Economic issues in nursing education
- The work setting: scheduling, career ladders, and alternative mechanisms for the provision of nursing services
- Nurses' political-economic role
- Reimbursement for nursing services
- Other economic and employment issues

II. The Impact of the General Economic Situation on Nurses and Nursing

General economic trends have a profound effect on everyone; nurses are no exception. Economics has been casually defined as "everybody's business," a phrase suggestive of this general impact. Formally, economics relates to choices and exchange transactions that determine how scarce resources (land, capital goods, and labor services) are allocated among competing uses, how the production of goods and services is organized, and what methods are utilized to distribute those goods and services. The pervasive influence of the general economic situation is evident when some recent economic trends are considered:

1. Rapid escalation in health costs;
2. Increased labor force participation by females;
3. High interest rates, particularly in real (inflation-adjusted) terms;
4. The recent recession and the highest unemployment rate in more than 40 years; and
5. Federal budgetary problems, including massive deficits and fundamental philosophical disagreement over budget priorities and programs.

All people are affected in one way or another by these general economic trends. Rapid increases in health costs have led to a focus on cost control and efforts by the federal government to reduce its commitments to pay for health services. Increased labor force participation by women is restructuring both work and family patterns. High real interest rates reduce investment expenditures of various kinds; for example, they have devastated the housing industry and made employees very reluctant to transfer from one location to another. The impact of the recent recession and the accompanying unemployment of more than 10 million people is felt throughout the economy. Federal budget cutbacks are affecting the funding of a variety of health programs, the employment of nurses, and the ability of citizens to gain access to needed health services.

Nurses and nursing are affected by these general economic trends in various ways. Individual nurses feel the effects of recession and high interest rates. Nurses may be more reluctant than ever before to terminate their employment because of reduced alternative employment opportunities and the increased uncertainty and loss of confidence in the economy associated with the recession. These major economic trends all affect both individual nurses and the nursing profession.

III. Changes in the Health Delivery System

The nation's needs for health delivery change over time. These needs reflect changes in a variety of factors, including health status, age distribution, the specific incidence of health disorders, lifestyle and environmental factors that affect health, medical technology, the availability of financing to support the utilization of health services, and organizational arrangements for the delivery of health services.

The delivery of health services in the United States has undergone profound change, and the pace of change continues to be rapid. Many of these changes have been fostered by changes in the payment system, such as the shift toward government financing of health services, which began with Medicare and Medicaid, and the increased reliance on other third-party payments. A variety of other factors also contribute to the rapid pace of change in health delivery.

On the surface at least, the health services delivery system of today resembles the system 25 years ago or more. For example, hospitals remain the "keystone" of the system. They provide the most complex services, expend more than 40 percent of the total costs of health delivery, provide a research and teaching base for the entire delivery system, and employ some 4 million people (approximately three-fourths of all health workers), including more than 800,000 registered nurses.

The resemblance of a hospital today to its counterpart of 25 years ago may be only "skin deep," however: the substance of the hospital and its activities have changed remarkably. Dramatic technical advances, the development of many new categories of health workers with specific responsibilities in particular areas of expertise, increasing bureaucratization brought about by the dictates of organizational complexity, new procedures, and the enhanced survivability of patients who would have died in earlier years are all part of this transformation to what we now identify as a "modern" hospital. Changing ownership and organizational patterns are also widespread. The numbers of for-profit, investor-owned hospitals have increased, especially in "sunbelt" locations, and multihospital systems are proliferating. All of these developments affect nurses and nursing.

Changes outside the hospital are even more dramatic. It would be impossible to explore here all of the major developments that have affected health care delivery. The rapid rate of technological change in health services delivery is one factor that has profoundly affected both the health care system's ability to sustain people's lives and the way in which health care professionals practice. Group practice, HMO's, the extension of widespread third-party coverage for health care, health promotion activities, the rapid growth of nursing home care and extended care facilities, ambulatory service alternatives to hospitalization, "deinstitutionalization" of the mentally impaired, and dialysis centers and at-home care for those with end stage kidney disease are but a few other developments. Overall, these changes have a profound impact on where and how nurses practice, and on what they do in the course of their practice.

IV. Salaries of Registered Nurses

Nurses rightly believe that they were significantly underpaid for many years. This situation was the result of a combination of factors, including (1) the relative lack of professional status accorded nursing; (2) the possible abuse of monopsony power, arising from the fact that only one or a few hospitals are the major employers of nurses in certain local areas, allowing hospitals to hold nurses' wages down; (3) the presence of discrimination against women in the labor market, coupled with the fact that nursing is a predominantly female occupation; (4) the traditional view that hospital and other health care work involves an element of "voluntarism," or service that need not be compensated at market rates; and (5) the effective prohibition of significant union activity and collective bargaining among nurses prior to legislative changes in 1974. In combination, these factors were responsible for fundamental inadequacies in nurses' salaries. These factors also provided, and continue to provide, the impetus for nurses to organize to exert more influence over their economic and general welfare concerns.

Nurses' salaries have increased dramatically in recent years. Average salaries for nurses are approaching $20,000 per year, although there are widespread variations in salary levels as a result of location, employment setting, position, education, experience, and other factors. Much of the increase in nurses' salaries, however, merely offsets similarly dramatic inflation and its corresponding erosion of real earnings. Still, nurses' salaries have improved relative to those of a number of other employee groups with whom nurses' salaries are frequently compared—female professional and technical workers, teachers, and other health care workers.

Special problems also exist for nurses' salaries that merit increased attention. For example, most employers of nurses recognize only a few levels or steps within their salary system. As a consequence, unlike most other professions, nursing has a relatively flat lifecycle earnings pattern. Nurses with many years of experience may earn little more than newly hired staff members, a fact that can lead to frustration and career dissatisfaction. Thus, strong general arguments can still be made that nurses' salaries are inadequate and need further improvement to make them comparable with those of other employees in comparable work settings.

V. Fringe Benefits for Nursing Employment

While nurses' salaries have shown some improvement relative to other groups, fringe benefits for nursing employment are an area in which significant inequities exist and to which increased attention is warranted.

Fringe benefits take a variety of forms. They include employer contributions for health insurance; vacation time; sick leave; allowances for educational, uniform, and other expenses; overtime premiums; shift differentials; and contributions for social security and/or private pension plans. For U.S. industry overall, employer expenses for fringe benefits currently approximate 37 percent of wages and salaries. Of all industry groups, hospitals and retailers devote the smallest proportion of salaries to employee fringe benefits, according to Audrey Freedman, senior labor economist for the Conference Board [Freedman, 1981]. This is confirmed by the U.S. Chamber of Commerce which has reported that, for 1981, hospitals were next to the lowest of 20 industry groups surveyed in terms of employee benefits as a percent of payroll. The figure was 31.0 percent for hospitals compared to a 37.3 percent average for all industries [U.S. Chamber of Commerce, 1982, p. 9]. While this percent has been increasing over time, it still represents a level below that for nearly all other industry classifications.

One type of fringe benefit for nurses merits particular scrutiny—retirement income programs. A broad variety of retirement income programs are now available to individual employees, including public programs (social security and state and local government retirement plans) and private programs (employer pension plans, Keogh plans for the self-employed, and Individual Retirement Accounts–IRA's).

Women are disadvantaged under many retirement income programs. Traditional pension plans reward long years of service and high earnings. Typically, women employees have interrupted work patterns due to childbearing and rearing, other home responsibilities, and, in the case of nurses, relatively frequent job changes. Because full vesting (entitlement to a pension benefit) may not occur for up to 10 years or more in a private pension plan, these factors restrict the ability of women to attain adequate retirement income security.

Still other factors point to the significance of retirement income for women. Because women live longer than men, on average, aged women are more dependent on retirement income programs than are men. Moreover, employed women tend to be concentrated in fields of employment least likely to offer pension plans. In the private sector, pension coverage is least frequent in the service and trade industries; 61 percent of all employed women, as opposed to 31 percent of all employed men, work in these industries [Dittmar, 1983, p. 4]. According to the President's Commision on Pension Policy, "the most serious problem facing our retirement system today is the lack of pension coverage among private sector workers" ["Wealthy Beware . . .," *National Journal,* 1982, p. 1165]. This problem of lack of coverage is particularly acute among women workers, including nurses, for whom earning levels, as well as employment discontinuity, are significant inhibiting factors.

Serious questions can also be raised regarding the adequacy of various private pension plans, on which long-term workers depend in large part for retirement income. Many private plans provide for a relatively low "replacement rate," the percentage of pre-retirement annual earnings paid by the pension. Private pension plans may also provide no inflation adjustment in pension benefits so that retirees find the real values of their pension benefits declining year after year. There are other problems with many private pension plans which limit their adequacy as a source of income for retirement.

Until the law was changed in April 1983, a considerable number of hospitals and other employers of nurses had filed notice of their intention to withdraw from the social security program. The Research and Policy Analysis Department at the American Nurses' Association estimated in 1982 that the group of hospitals that had formally indicated their intention to withdraw from social security would remove coverage for social security from more than 40,000 registered nurses. This development would have had a profound impact on the access to and adequacy of retirement income programs as a fringe benefit for nursing employment. Fortunately, however, changes in the Social Security Reform Act of 1983 eliminated this particular problem, although some more general concerns about the financial stability of the Social Security program in future years remain.

As a relatively mobile work force, the majority of whom are married, nurses have traditionally not placed great emphasis on retirement planning; the view among married women may have been that their husbands' coverage would be sufficient for retirement. Increasingly, women and nurses specifically recognize the importance of retirement planning, and this recognition needs to be turned into action to improve the ability of nurses to attain a secure income for retirement.

VI. Economic and General Welfare Efforts

The American Nurses' Association instituted its economic and general welfare program in 1946. Since that time, the association and its state members have played an active role in advancing the economic and general welfare concerns of registered nurses.

Programs for economic and general welfare involve primarily organized union activity, as well as certain other efforts. Unionization is concentrated in the Mid-Atlantic, East North Central, New England, and the Pacific regions [Hoffman, 1982, p. 66]. More than 100,000 registered nurses are represented for collective bargaining by the state nurses' associations that are the members of ANA; they represent approximately 78 percent of all registered nurses who are unionized [Becker, 1982, p. 7].

While the state nurses' associations represent the largest proportion of registered nurses who are unionized, there has been a growing interest among other labor unions in organizing service workers and women employees, including nurses, in recent years. Part of the impetus for this development has been the relative employment growth in the service industries, including health care, in comparison to stagnant employment levels in manufacturing enterprises, the traditional base of most unions. Increased interest by other unions in organizing health care workers and nurses has important implications for ANA and its member state nurses' associations.

The growth of union activity among nurses has occurred primarily since the National Labor Relations Act was amended in 1974 to cover employees of private, nonprofit hospitals. A number of studies have examined the impact of hospital unionism on nurses' salaries; virtually all find that union activity raises wages, but there is no agreement about the exact extent to which it does so [Feldman, 1982; Link, 1976; Sloan, 1979, 1980]. A new study of the effects of collective bargaining on wages and fringe benefits for nurses indicates that four generalizations can be made from the available evidence [Becker, 1982, pp. 10-11]:

> First, a statistically significant positive collective bargaining effect has almost always been obtained from studies in hospital and other areas. Typically, unions have had a smaller effect on professional nurses' and other professionals' wages than for nonprofessional occupations. . . Second, collective bargaining affects a hospital employee's pay even when he or she is not a union member. These spillover effects may be either internal or external. . . Third, strikes and other work stoppages have important consequences for wages; the effects of collective bargaining in hospitals having work stoppages is substantially higher than collective bargaining effects without work stoppages. . . Fourth, there is some evidence that the union effect on wages is higher when the union has been in place for a number of years.

Unionism in hospitals is, therefore, a potent force for raising nurses' wages. About one-half of the state nurses' associations do not engage in active union organizing or collective bargaining activities. In those associations, economic and general welfare programming is more limited. Educational materials and programming may be provided. It is not possible to systematically assess the effectiveness of such efforts because of a lack of data and an inability to identify cause and effect relationships in this situation.

VII. The Demand for Nurses: Shortage or Surplus?

If the literature on nursing manpower in this country has one primary theme, it is that there is a shortage of nurses. A shortage of registered nurses has been discussed since the late 1940's; federal programming to help alleviate the shortage was initiated in the Nurse Training Act of 1964. Vacancy rates, the number of budgeted but unfilled positions in hospitals, are the most frequently cited measure of the nurse shortage. According to data assembled by Donald Yett, vacancy rates for general duty nurses in hospitals ranged between 11.2 percent and 23.2 percent between 1953 and 1969, for those years for which data are available [Yett, 1975, p. 138]. The AHA hospital personnel survey for September 1980 found a 9.5 percent vacancy rate for staff nurses, representing nearly 62,000 vacant positions [American Hospital Association, 1981]. This vacancy rate was the highest of all categories of hospital personnel in the survey. One year later, however, vacancies had declined by 13 to 21 percent, nationwide, and 41.5 percent of hospitals reported no registered nurse positions vacant at the time of the 1981 survey, compared to 27.6 percent in 1980 [Mullner, 1983, p. 547].

However, another recent study casts doubt on the usefulness of using "budgeted but unfilled" positions as an indicator of the nurse shortage, primarily because the meaning of the term is ambiguous [Hixson, 1981, pp. 13-16]. That report suggests that the shortage is not a truly general one, but is limited primarily to hospitals, and most specifically to evening and night shifts and to the more intense or demanding specialties, such as ICU/CCU units. Moreover, vacancies occur more frequently in rural and inner-city hospitals in smaller institutions, and where the ratios of patients to registered nurses are relatively high and ratios of registered nurses to licensed practical nurses are relatively low [Hixson, 1981, p. 16].

The existence of an overall shortage of nurses has been challenged. Paul Feldstein, a noted health economist, has argued thus [Feldstein, 1979, p. 374]:

> An analysis of the market for registered nurses appears to indicate that it is currently performing well. That is, as demand for nurses increases, the wage of registered nurses rises so that there is no economic shortage or surplus of nurses.

For a number of years, funding for nursing education has been drastically reduced, and even more drastic reductions have been advocated by Presidents Nixon, Ford, Carter, and now Reagan. These proposals are also based on arguments that the nurse shortage, if it exists, is not as chronic or severe as it once had been.

Does a shortage of nurses exist? Reasonable people may reach different conclusions based on the available evidence. Differing interpretations may be attached to (1) the importance and meaning of an "unfilled budgeted position," (2) the concept of a shortage itself—whether it is based on perceived *need* for nurse personnel or on *demand,* actual employer willingness to pay for nurses' services, and (3) the presumed effectiveness and efficiency of the nurse labor market in terms of its responsiveness to changing wage rates and other factors.

In an effort to assist with evaluation of the continued existence and extent of a shortage of nurses, ANA has developed a national index of help-wanted advertising for registered nurses. This index provides information analogous to that available monthly for all help-wanted advertising from the Conference Board, an independent, nonprofit, economic research institute [Preston, 1977; "Help Wanted Ad Index . . .," *The Wall Street Journal,* August 26, 1982, p. 42]. Changes in the volume of help-wanted advertising provide current evidence regarding changes in the relative availability of jobs for registered nurses. Initial data from this project indicate that the volume of help-wanted advertising for registered nurses has fallen significantly in 1982 in comparison to 1981, indicating a reduction in the nurse shortage. Also, for the U.S. as a whole, the volume of help-wanted advertising for registered nurses declined 31 percent in the first quarter of 1983 from the comparable period in 1982, indicating further reductions in available employment opportunities. This effect is as expected during a period of recession, when fewer new jobs are created, nurses are more reluctant to change jobs, and some nurses who would not otherwise be working have taken jobs to supplement spouses' incomes. Information on the volume of help-wanted advertising for registered nurses is now being published on a monthly basis by the *American Journal of Nursing.*

Some authors and studies project significant manpower surpluses among physicians and certain other categories of health care workers by 1990 [Graduate Medical Education, 1981]. As a result, some speculative discussion has begun regarding future "turf battles," intensified professional jealousies, and other related factors in an era of manpower surpluses [McTernan, 1982]. Whether or not a surplus of nurses will emerge in the future is an empirical question that cannot be answered without a crystal ball. Prevailing views, based on manpower forecasting models such as that developed by the Western Interstate Commission on Higher Education (WICHE), indicate that nursing will continue to be subject to shortages of personnel, particularly among those nurses who are most educated and specialized, throughout the balance of this century [*Nurse Supply* . . ., 1982]. However, these projections are based on a needs-criteria approach; estimates reflect what a panel of experts felt "ought to be" provided in terms of nursing care.

There are no guarantees that perceived needs will in fact be met through health care spending by government, private insurance, industry, and individuals. Demand, as expressed in the marketplace, may be much different from expert perceptions of need. Such possibilities seem particularly realistic in view of extensive efforts at the federal level to restrict funding for health care services of various types. Reduced funding for Medicare, Medicaid, and other health programs will imply reduced employment opportunities for nurses, unless prevailing patterns of practice are changed. Manpower forecasts assume that traditional payment mechanisms will not change, and therefore do not take such possibilities into account. Thus, some possibility exists that the nurse shortage could become a surplus if effective demand for nurse personnel is significantly reduced by the combined effects of the current recession and budget restrictions that reduce access to and utilization of health services.

VIII. Economic Issues in Nursing Education [2]

Nursing education has problems. Total graduations have recently declined, despite relatively favorable employment prospects. Unlike other professions, entry into registered nursing practice continues to be possible through programs of signficantly different character, setting, and length. This is true despite the professional association's long-standing endorsement of baccalaureate-level entry into professional nursing practice. Moreover, in most employment settings, graduates of 2-, 3-, and 4-year programs receive equal or virtually equal wages—a disincentive to choose a baccalaureate program for entry into practice.

Diploma graduations have been declining since the late 1960's; the greatest growth has been in graduations from associate degree programs. One-half of the nation's new nurses now graduate from 2-year programs; approximately two-thirds of nursing students are trained in 2- or 3-year technically oriented programs. Graduates of all types of programs tend to be utilized similarly in practice, undermining implementation of the philosophical base for nursing practice that distinguishes the education for and practice of professional nursing from the education for and practice of technical nursing. Moreover, a number of empirical studies have attempted to explore the effects of nursing education on competency, performance, and quality of care, but the evidence that such differences exist is inconclusive. [3]

---

[2] This section is based upon Richard C. McKibbin, "Nursing Education Trends: An Analysis of the Supply and Preparation of Nursing Personnel," in the National Task Force on Education for Nursing Practice, *Education for Nursing Practice in the Context of the 1980's,* American Nurses' Association, 1983.

[3] This statement is based on the results of 30 previous studies reviewed by Joanne C. McCloskey in "The Effects of Nursing Education on Job Effectiveness: An Overview of the Literature," *Research in Nursing and Health,* 4, 1981, pp. 355-73.

Needed expansion of advanced and specialized nursing education programs is hindered by two factors. First, an inadequate supply of nurses is educated at levels appropriate for staffing these programs, and second, many educational institutions are unable or unwilling to pay salaries sufficient to attract and retain qualified nurse faculty. In addition, nursing continues to be a field dominated almost exclusively by women. While more men are enrolled in nursing programs now than in the past, only some 7 percent of nursing students are male, compared to the more than 25 percent of students in U.S. medical schools who are female. Federal support for nursing education is also eroding.

Moreover, future trends in the potential supply of nursing students, in patterns of career choice, and in federal support for nursing education point toward the continuation of many of these problems.

These are serious problems with far-reaching implications for the economics and the practice of nursing. However, recognition of their existence and development of long-term strategies that take them into account may have important effects.

IX. The Work Setting: Scheduling, Career Ladders, and Alternative Mechanisms for the Provision of Nursing Services

Approximately two-thirds of employed nurses work in hospitals. Hospital nursing involves continuous care, 24 hours a day, 365 days a year. This and other aspects of nursing employment involve work settings and conditions that cannot be considered "ideal" by any stretch of the imagination. Highly stressful situations may alternate with routine activities; non-nursing duties including transportation and housekeeping chores may be expected of registered nurses on a regular basis; rotating hours may take a personal physical toll as well as create problems for personal and family life; jobs may often not be associated with any significant possibilities for career advancement. These are but a few of the problems associated with the work setting for registered nurses.

Scheduling patterns are in a state of flux. Innovative scheduling, including special pay incentives for weekend work, have been implemented in many health facilities and are under active consideration in others. Scheduling includes decisions about the determination of when each nurse will go on or off duty, who will work which shift, and how vacations, special time requests, weekends, and other situations will be handled. Scheduling decisions can also involve choice between alternative workweeks, such as the 4-day/40-hour week, the 7-day/70-hour week, the 12-hour day, and flextime. All of these alternatives can be considered in terms of how well a system meets requirements for coverage of patients' needs, how well nurses like the schedules, how consistent, predictable, and flexible they are, and their costs [Young, 1980].

Substitution, primarily between registered nurses and licensed practical nurses, is another concern. While some hospitals have implemented all registered nurse staffing, these are a small minority. Most facilities utilize both categories of personnel, as well as nursing aides, orderlies, and attendants. Changes in the relative salary levels of each category of worker can be expected to affect, over time, relative employment levels of registered nurses and licensed practical nurses. The desirability of nursing employment in hospitals is related to incomes, but the evidence suggests that incomes of other health care workers have increased more than those of registered nurses. A study by Linda Aiken, Robert J. Blendon, and David E. Rogers found as follows [Aiken, 1981, pp. 1614-615]:

> The relative improvement in income or other health care providers during recent years has, we believe, tended to highlight this problem. A comparison of nurses' incomes with those of other hospital health care personnel indicates that their salaries have been moving upward more swiftly and thus the gap between nurses' incomes and those of allied nursing personnel is narrowing. In 1960, licensed practical nurses' incomes were 70 percent of nurses' incomes; now they arc 76 percent. Nurses' aides' incomes rose from 65 percent of nurses' incomes in 1960 to 71 percent at present.

Thus, changes in relative salary levels create substitution effects in relative employment levels, which also may be a source of dissatisfaction for registered nurses.

Career ladders, structural arrangements to promote meaningful upward mobility among employees at particular institutions, are another relatively new concept in nursing. ANA has recently conducted a survey of institutions known to have or to be developing career ladders for clinical practice. A concommitant development was a study conducted by the American Academy of Nursing to identify "magnet" hospitals—those which, for various reasons, have come to be seen as highly desirable settings within which to practice professional nursing [American Academy of Nursing, 1983]. Both of these studies, only the latter of which has been completed, do appear to provide evidence that concepts such as career ladders for clinical practice hold promise for improving nurses' perception of the settings within which they practice.

In addition, there is renewed interest in alternative mechanisms for the delivery of nursing services. Both solo and group practice possibilities are being explored and developed by nurses, as is the provision of nursing services on a consulting basis. Years ago, many nurses practiced private duty nursing. Most nurses were, in effect, private contractors. Solo and group practice and other possibilities are of interest in terms of the autonomy attached to them, the possibility of direct reimbursement for services rendered in such contexts, and the entrepreneurial character and "ability to be one's own boss" attached to many of them. Legal and practical business impediments exist, however, which often severely restrict the ability of nurses to practice nursing in a manner analogous to the manner in which physicians practice medicine. Still, the drive toward professionalism will certainly include continued interest in alternative models for the provision of nursing services.

A partial substitute for those innovative practice modes, although a very imperfect one from individual nurses' perspectives, has developed rapidly in the form of temporary nurse agencies. The agencies, rather than individual nurses, act as independent contractors for the nurses who are associated with them. While nurses obtain certain benefits from agency employment, such as greater scheduling flexibility, they do not reap other benefits, such as preferential tax treatment and autonomy, which could be associated with solo or group practice of professional nursing.

X. Nurses' Political-Economic Role

Apart from political and economic concerns shared by many Americans, nurses have two specific areas of political-economic interest: health care issues and women's issues. The rationale for these interests is obvious: nursing represents the largest category of health care professionals, and approximately 97 percent of nurses are women.

The role of American Nurses' Association includes representing nurses' interests in government through the political process. The association works to influence national health programs and policy in a manner consistent with the profession's objectives. ANA testifies on behalf of legislation affecting nursing, health care, and women's issues. It also serves as a source of information and of expertise in initiating appropriate legislative actions. ANA has recently been actively supportive of funding for graduate nursing education and nursing research and has been assisting with development of political support for reimbursement mechanisms for proposed community-based nursing centers. These activities are coordinated throught ANA's Washington, D.C. office.

Political objectives are furthered through the association's political action committee, the Nurses' Coalition for Action in Politics (N-CAP). This organization contributes money to political candidates who are supportive of policies and health-related legislation in the interests of nurses and nursing. The importance of nurses as a political force should not be overlooked. There are some 1.8 million registered nurses in the country, a sizable voting "block" for health and women's issues. N-CAP estimates that at least one of every 44 registered women voters is a nurse. Furthermore, employed registered nurses have frequent, ongoing work-related contact with additional millions of health care workers and patients.

Nurses are also a major economic force. Employed registered nurses in this country are estimated by the Policy Analysis Unit in ANA's Center for Research to earn more than $25 billion annually, and to control the expenditure of uncounted additional billions of health care dollars each year [McKibbin, 1982]. Nursing is therefore clearly a major political-economic force for health. Policies and positions of the association over time represent dramatic evidence of this fact.

As a predominantly female occupation, professional nursing has also been closely identified with women's issues. ANA is a staunch supporter of the Equal Rights Amendment; it endorsed the amendment, refused to meet in states that had not ratified it, and most recently, during the association's national convention in Washington, D.C., recessed its House of Delegates on the afternoon of June 30, 1982, so delegates could attend a rally for the amendment. This was a strong gesture of continuing support for the principle of equal rights for women.

Other women's issues with which nursing has been closely identified include pay equity and comparable worth. As long ago as 1975, ANA provided financial and other assistance for the litigation efforts of a Denver-based group known as NURSE, Inc. This group filed a pay equity complaint with the Equal Employment Opportunity Commission (EEOC), arguing that at every level of job classification and salary schedule studied for Denver public sector employees, "starting salaries for male jobs requiring comparable or less qualifications and responsibility were consistently higher than those for nursing" [Jacox, 1979]. More recently, ANA endorsed the concept of comparable worth at its 1982 national convention. Further action can be expected, including support of appropriate legislation, litigation, and research designed to strengthen the attainment of economic equity for all women employees, including nurses.

XI. Reimbursement for Nursing Services

Since 1948, ANA priorities have reflected interest in recognition of third-party payments for nursing services.[4] This interest in reimbursement has centered on several categories of nurses: nurse practitioners, home health nurses, psychiatric and mental health nursing specialists, and nurses providing services to those covered by Medicare. It is recognized that a number of practical problems are associated with the attainment of reimbursement. These include a broad-based, coordinated effort to define the scope of such services, associated costs, appropriate educational levels, and the need to attain approval and acceptance of such changes. Also, concrete data are needed on the

---

[4] The paragraph that follows is adapted from: "A Review of ANA's Stand on Reimbursement of Nursing Services," American Nurses' Association, August 29, 1980, unpublished manuscript.

cost-effectiveness of such proposed changes. The philosophical basis for changing existing reimbursement systems to recognize nursing as a primary health care discipline has been adequately described, but *operational* models, programs, plans, procedures, and studies are lacking.

The interest in reimbursement for nursing services is a part of the effort to upgrade the professional standing and status of nursing. A related effort surrounds separate identification of nursing care costs in hospital budgets. At present, nursing costs are embedded in room rates for hospital stays; nursing costs for hospitals are not separately identified in billing or other presentations of hospital accounts. Rather, daily room rates include nursing costs and a variety of ancillary expenses, including housekeeping, laundry and linen, central supply, and a plethora of other nonnursing services and tasks.[5] Because the cost of nursing care is the single largest component of the room rate, it is frequently confused with it. Increases in hospital room rates thus may be concluded to be the consequence of higher nursing costs. This may or may not be true in any particular case. Cost control efforts, financial accountability and control, and increased recognition of the significance of the role of nursing in the health care delivery process would flow from separation of the costs of nursing care from nonnursing hospital costs. One author has concluded that ". . . the real problem is presenting nursing care costs in their room rate disguise" [Walker, 1982, p. 142]. Further research in the effort to identify and separate the costs of nursing care in hospitals and other institutional settings appears warranted in conjunction with the effort to achieve reimbursement for nursing services.

With rising health costs, there is little chance that federally administered health care financing programs can be amended to cover services such as health promotion and prevention or to provide fee for service for additional providers. In light of these factors, ANA has pursued a legislative strategy that would alter the reimbursement mechanism for currently covered community-based services. This proposal would establish free-standing community nursing centers (CNC's) financed by a pre-determined capitated payment system. The CNC's would provide on-site and in-home services for three major population groups: (1) usual Medicare home health population groups, (2) Medicaid infant and child health service recipients, and (3) previously hospitalized and at-risk rehospitalization, chronically ill Medicare or Medicaid populations. In order to qualify as a CNC, the nursing agency would have to demonstrate that the services are cost-effective at or below the average cost of similar services from other agencies. A bill containing the legislative specifications

[5]See Duane D. Walker, "The Cost of Nursing Care in Hospitals," in Linda H. Aiken (ed.), *Nursing in the 1980's: Crises, Opportunities, Challenges,* Philadelphia: J. B. Lippincott, 1982, p. 134, for a listing of hospital services included in the daily room rate.

for CNC's developed by ANA was introduced during the first session of the 98th Congress.

XII. Other Economic and Employment Issues

A variety of other economic and employment issues affect nurses and nursing. Since it is not possible to describe all such issues in this analysis, the following discussion will be limited to three concerns:

1. Changing ownership and organizations patterns for hospitals
2. The "new federalism"
3. Pro-competitive health care models and nursing.

A. Changing Ownership and Organizational Patterns for Hospitals

The ownership and organization of hospitals is undergoing dramatic and rapid change. The traditional mainstay of the hospital industry—the independent, non-profit, short-term general hospital—is under extreme financial pressure to change by reorganizing its corporate structure, merging with other institutions, diversifying into new business areas out of the traditional acute care hospital arena, or being managed by or sold to a for-profit hospital group. The impetus for such changes comes from reimbursement restrictions imposed by Medicare and Medicaid and, to a lesser extent, by private insurance. Under government programs, hospitals had been reimbursed at a percentage of "reasonable costs," a term not immune to restrictive and redefinition in this era of cost consciousness and intense efforts to reduce federal expenditures for health programs. Limited access to capital funds—the combined results of a reduction in philanthropic contributions and increased interest rates on indebtedness—has exacerbated the problem. A statement from a recent *National Journal* article on this problem is illustrative [Demkovich, 1982, pp. 1131-1132]:

> The one-two punch of federal payment policies and limited access to capital could drive substantial numbers of voluntary hospitals—as many as half, some industry analysts and attorneys say—out of business in the next decade or two.
>
> To help shore up their shaky financial bases, growing numbers of not-for-profit hospitals have begun to restructure. Some are linking into multi-hospital systems or chains as a means of sharing services and management expertise. Others are expanding vertically, opening new lines of business such as nursing and home health services, in some cases as profit-making enterprises.
>
> 'Growth and diversification are going to be the name of the game,' said Sister Irene Kraus, president of Providence Hospital in Washington, which is in the process of implementing a four-phase expansion plan. 'In D.C. or any other large city, it's going to be survival of the fittest.'

How will these developments affect nurses and nursing? Tentative impressions may be formed. These include the probability that employed nurses, at least the two-thirds who work in hospitals, will work in even larger, more bureaucratized, and more complex institutions than at present. Organizational access, the ability to "have a say" or influence the organization in which one works, will become more constrained. Hospital mission statements will be broadened, with less emphasis on the traditional base, care for the acutely ill patient, for which nurses are so essential. Hospital-operated home health services and hospice care, for example, are likely to expand, with accompanying changes in the work nurses do, the skills they need, and the case loads they carry. Increased management expertise, coupled with continued requirements to constrain costs, will lead to more complex and difficult negotiations for contracts covering nurses in organized settings. The same pressures will lead to even more organizing efforts for those nurses who are not organized. Nurses and nursing will experience significant economic and employment effects as a result of these changes.

B. The "New Federalism"

The issues of the appropriate levels of federal involvement in the payment for the delivery for health services, in the financing of health professionals' education and related topics, have been discussed for many years. Most recently, the Reagan Administration has advocated a fundamental realignment of the balance of power and responsibility for a variety of programs among federal, state, and local units of government. Control of numerous programs would be shifted to the states in this plan, which was formally advocated in the president's State of the Union message in January 1982. This proposal is in addition to the nine block grants which were created in the Omnibus Budget Reconciliation Act of 1981.

The administration's proposal has raised many unanswered questions about financing, the continuity of program efforts, the priority-setting process within the states, and the responsibility for regulatory compliance, among others. Lack of political support for the original version of the "new federalism," which would have transferred responsibility for some 50 programs to the states,has led the president to propose a more limited version of the plan. Under that proposal, although details remain unclear, some three dozen programs would be transferred to the states and federal funding for them would be guaranteed for a period of several years ["Reagan . . .," 1982, pp. 1, 6A]. Programs to be transferred include some in the areas of education and training; energy assistance; health, social, and nutritional services, transportation; and community development. In exchange, the Medicaid program would be federalized rather than remaining a jointly financed federal and state arrangement.

It is of course uncertain whether this proposal, or any similar one, will be adopted. But if some form of the proposed "new federalism" is adopted, it will affect nurses and nursing. Those health programs transferred to the states—and many categorical assistance programs, those which provide *specific* health services to defined *special* populations—would be jeopardized. In many states, severe budgetary pressures exist. These could lead to intense competition for federal funds among the various programs, both health and non-health, transferred to the responsibility of the states. Continued support for particular programs would thus become more uncertain in those cases where competition among programs develops, as it would for those programs with no federal "strings" attached.

On the other hand, transfer of responsibility for Medicaid to the federal level of government could lead to reductions in widespread and inequitable differences between states for eligibility requirements, service coverage, and benefit levels. These differences are extreme, but are often inadequately recognized; for example, in Arkansas, only 6 percent of children in the poverty population were eligible Medicaid recipients, compared to the entire child poverty population plus an additional 68 percent of children of non-poor families who were eligible for Medicaid in New York State in 1970 [Davis, 1978, p. 68]. Average benefit payments and service coverage also vary greatly from state to state. Thus, transfer of Medicaid to the federal level could lead to greater consistency and uniformity in the program, although consistency and uniformity might be achieved through a "least common denominator" phenomenon involving decreased benefit levels and/or more stringent eligibility requirements in many states.

C. Pro-Competitive Health Care Models and Nursing

Another concept endorsed by the current administration involves movement toward greater reliance on market forces to allocate health resources, to control utilization rates, and to control costs. The "pro-competitive" approach is viewed as an alternative to the regulatory model for health care delivery that has developed in this country since the passage of Medicare and Medicaid in 1965. In summary, the proposed approach envisions the creation of various incentives through the tax laws and other mechanisms to encourage consumers, employers, providers of health care services, and providers of health insurance and other financing arrangements to be more cost-conscious with respect to health care service delivery.

A number of specific academic and legislative proposals have been made. A recent evaluation of these by the Congressional Budget Office finds that all such proposals rely on one or both of two distinct market-oriented strategies. These involve cost sharing, greater individual "out-of-pocket" financial responsibility for health services utilized, and alternative delivery systems, such as HMO's and other arrangements that avoid fee-for-service incentives to utilize health services more intensively than if revenues were not directly correlated with the volume of services rendered [Congressional Budget Office, 1982, p. ix].

The report identifies three principal ways in which the government could increase the reliance on market forces as a means to control health costs:

- Altering the tax-treatment of employment-based health insurance
- Offering Medicare beneficiaries a voucher to purchase a private health plan
- Other changes in the Medicare reimbursement and benefit structure [Congressional Budget Office, 1982, p. xi].

At the present time, the value of employer contributions to health plans is not treated as taxable income to employees. This creates an incentive, particularly for companies with many employees in high tax brackets, to provide extensive health benefits. In fiscal year 1983, the government indicates that this tax treatment will reduce tax collections from income and payroll taxes by more than $25 billion [Congressional Budget Office, 1982, p. xi]. Limits could be placed on this exclusion, or tax-free rebates could be offered employees who choose less expensive health plans.

Medicare vouchers and other changes in the Medicare program may also be considered. Vouchers would permit people eligible for Medicare to choose a private plan competing with it; other changes might include imposition of tax premiums on insurance plans which supplement Medicare. Changes such as these are believed by some to be viable means for controlling costs by introducing market forces into health care decision making. Certain undesirable side effects of the voucher concept have led ANA to oppose it, however. For example, the voucher concept is associated with larger copayments and deductibles; this could impose a financial burden on the elderly, especially those living on low or fixed incomes.

Interest in pro-competitive health models raises many questions for nursing, such as the following:

- Will reimbursement for nursing services be recognized in these arrangements as a cost-effective alternative means of obtaining certain health services?
- Will physicians and nurses compete for patients if nurses achieve reimbursement for their services in certain contexts?
- Could nurses form independent organizations to contract with employers or the general public for the delivery of primary health care services?
- Will legal barriers to alternative mechanisms for the provision of nursing services be relaxed in conjunction with pro-competitive models?

Although no answers to these or related concerns exist at this time, the

questions illustrate the fundamental changes in the economic and employment environment for registered nurses that could flow from changes, such
as pro-competitive health care strategies, that have been proposed and are
under active consideration.

XIII. Conclusion

Nursing is a major force for the nation's health. The effectiveness with
which nurses and nursing perform in that role is related to the extent to
which individual nurses and the nursing profession identify, explore, understand, and effectively respond to economic and employment issues. This
analysis has discussed the scope, breadth, and impact of many of these
issues; further study is needed to provide fuller information about, analyses of,
policy recommendations for, and discussion of the implications of these
economic and employment issues for registered nurses.

REFERENCES

Linda H. Aiken, Robert J. Blendon, and David E. Rogers, "The Shortage of Hospital
Nurses: A New Perspective," *American Journal of Nursing,* 81:9, September 1981, pp.
1616-618.

American Academy of Nursing, *Magnet Hospitals: Attraction and Retention of Professional Nurses,* Task Force on Nursing Practice in Hospitals, American Nurses' Association, 1983.

American Hospital Association, "1980 Annual Survey of Hospital Personnel," unpublished tabulations—mimeo, 1981.

Edmund Becker, *et al.,* "Union Activity in Hospitals: Past, Present and Future,"
Health Care Financing Review, June 1982, pp. 1-13.

Congressional Budget Office, *Containing Medical Care Costs Through Market Forces,*
Washington, D.C.: U.S. Government Printing Office, May 1982.

Karen Davis and Cathy Schoen, *Health and the War on Poverty,* Washington, D.C.:
The Brookings Institution, 1978.

Linda E. Demkovich, "Urban Voluntary Hospitals, Caught in Price Squeeze, Face
a Bleak Future," *National Journal,* June 26, 1982, pp. 1131-132.

Cynthia Dittmar, "Women and Retirement Income Security," American Nurses'
Association, unpublished draft, 1983.

Roger Feldman and Richard Scheffler, "The Effects of Labor Unions on Hospital
Employees' Wages," *Industrial and Labor Relations Review,* 36:2, January 1982, pp.
186-206.

Paul J. Feldstein, *Health Care Economics,* New York: John Wiley and Sons, 1979.

Audrey Freedman, "Manpower Issues for the 80's," Conference presentation, American Hospital Association Health Manpower Conference, Washington, D.C., October 19,
1981.

Graduate Medical Education National Advisory Committee (GMENAC), *Report,*
U.S. Department of Health and Human Services, DHHS Pub. No. (HRA) 81-652.

"Help-Wanted Ad Index Declined Last Month," *The Wall Street Journal,* August 26,
1982, p. 42

Jesse S. Hixson, *The Recurrent Shortage of Registered Nurses: A New Look at the
Issues,* U.S. Department of Health and Human Services, DHHS Pub. No. (HRA) 81-23.

William C. Hoffman, "The Autonomy Trend: Union Affiliation Among White Collar
Health Care Workers," in *Facing the Hospital Manpower Crisis,* American Hospital Association, 1982.

Ada Jacox, "How Much Is A Nurse Worth?" *The American Nurse,* August 20, 1979.

Charles H. Link and J. H. Landon, "Market Structure, Nonpecuniary Factors, and Professional Salaries: Registered Nurses," *Journal of Economics and Business,* 28:2, Winter 1976, pp. 151-55.

Richard C. McKibbin, "Registered Nurses Wages and Hospital Costs," mimeo, 1982 (portions thereof published as "Nurses' Wages 11 percent of Hospital Costs," *The American Nurse,* January 1983, p. 1).

Edmund J. McTernan and Alan M. Leiken, "A Pyramid Model of Health Manpower in the 1980's," *Journal of Health Politics, Policy and Law,* Winter 1982, pp. 739-51.

Ross Mullner, Calvin S. Byre, and Suzanne F. Whitehead, "Hospital Nursing Vacancies," *American Journal of Nursing,* 83:4, April 1983, p. 547.

Nurse Supply, Distribution and Requirements: 3rd Report to Congress, U.S. Department of Health and Human Services, Bureau of Health Professions, Division of Nursing, DHHS Pub. No. (HRA) 82-87.

Noreen L. Preston, *The Help-Wanted Index: Technical Description and Behaviorial Trends,* The Conference Board, New York, 1977.

"Reagan Offers a New Plan of Federal Powers," *The Kansas City Star,* July 13, 1982.

Frank A. Sloan and Robert Einicki, "Professional Nurse Wage-Setting in Hospitals," in R. Scheffler (ed.), *Research in Health Economics,* Greenwich, Conn.: JAI Press, 1979, pp. 217-64.

Frank A. Sloan and Bruce Steinwald, *Hospital Labor Markets,* Lexington, Massachusetts: D.C. Heath, 1980.

United States Chamber of Commerce, *Employee Benefits 1981,* Chamber Research Center, Washington, D.C., 1982.

"Wealthy Beware: Congress Takes Aim at $100,000-Plus Pension Tax Shelters," *National Journal,* July 3, 1982, pp. 1164-168.

Donald E. Yett, *An Economic Analysis of the Nurse Shortage,* Lexington, Massachusetts: D. C. Heath and Co., 1975.

John P. Young, *et al. Factors Affecting Nurse Staffing in Acute Care Hospitals,* Division of Nursing, (DHHS) Contract No. HRA 232-78-0150, September 1980.

Part Seven

Consumer Preferences and
Health Care Accessibility

Chapter Eighteen

Consumer Preference: The Overlooked Element in Health Planning

KEVIN G. HALPERN, TREVOR A. FISK, and JAMES SOBEL

This paper is divided into three parts. The first part will summarize the evidence from our research and that of others which shows that health consumers possess strong preferences about how they want health care delivered. The second will illustrate one example of a major health planning issue where there appears a significant dichotomy between what consumers want and what planners are proposing. The third will analyze the consequences of overlooking consumer desires in health planning generally.

Consumer Research

We have conducted a series of major public surveys as a basis for our own institutional planning and marketing. We have also compared our findings with those of other authors in this field. From this research we have drawn six broad conclusions about health consumer behavior.

1. Various research findings conclusively show that health consumers do indeed enter the process of seeking care with strong pre-conceived preferences. Several studies show a public with distinct ideas as to the attributes which they are looking for in physicians, in hospitals and other institutional providers [Doyle and Ware, 1977; Market Probe Inc., 1979; IEC Marketing Group, 1981; Halpern and Fisk, 1982]. As one illustration, such studies show that the public most associates a "good hospital" with good doctors, good nurses, up-to-date equipment and accessibility from home and is relatively unconcerned with such factors as modern buildings or private rooms. Failure to meet those expectations produces a relatively high, measurable level of dissatisfaction [Mechanic, 1968; Kelman, 1976]. As they do in other market conditions, consumers respond to such dissatisfaction by actively seeking alternatives. In relation to physicians, our research shows one-quarter of the public at any one time is actively looking for a different physician to the one whom they last used.

Other published findings put this segment of "active searchers" for alternative physicians as high as 50 percent to 55 percent [Klegon, Gregory and Kingstrom, 1982]. Our own surveys show that all but a few members of the adult public have a strong preference as to the hospital which they want to utilize. Also, a majority of interviewees in our surveys volunteered the name of at least one institution to which they would refuse admission under any circumstance. These are the responses of active, not of passive, consumers.

2. Health consumers are not homogeneous however in these preferences, expectations or responses to experience. These perceptions vary by demographic and, more particularly, psychographic segments of the population [Gottlieb, 1959; Ziff, 1971]. Given such distinct psychographic segmentation among health consumers, uniformity of delivery mechanisms is counterproductive.

3. The public desire for more medical information is significant. The active consumer is an information processor [Nicosia, 1966]. Most consumers feel inadequately informed about health care [General Mills, 1979]. Most report that they derive health information substantially from such sources as the news media and informal grapevines because of the failure of official sources to supply either the type of information they want or to supply it in readily understandable methods. Consumers for instance attach a high desire to more information about the meaning of medical symptoms. Health providers hesitate to make such information available because of the complexities surrounding accurate differential diagnosis [General Mills, 1979; Brown, 1980]. They also want information which helps them choose among suppliers to find one that best fits the qualities and benefits that, as individual consumers, they most seek. But health suppliers demonstrate a professional coyness over the self-promotion which provides consumers in other markets with such data [Harris, 1979; Beck, Anders, and Sweeney, 1982].

4. The various official efforts that have been made to provide for "grass roots" consumer input into health planning are no substitute for systematic market research and study of consumer behavior.

Members of local representational bodies focus on advising which actions are "best" for the community. Market research examines how individuals will react to the presentation of choices. The two sets of answers are rarely identical.

5. There is some evidence that satisfied patients have better clinical outcomes [Mechanic, 1976; Hall, Roter and Rand, 1981]. They volunteer more data and follow professional advice more conscientiously. Consequently there is a medical as well as economic imperative to understanding the attitudes and likely behavioral responses which consumers bring to seeking health care.

6. Although health consumers vary in their preferences and priorities, there appears to be one underlying trait in the various responses which our surveys and others have elicited. Health consumers view health care principally as a personal service provided by individual professionals in one-on-one encounters with them as clients. They do not judge the effectiveness

of systems of delivery. They evaluate the individual qualities and actions of each professional provider whom they encounter.

Also, they place the highest value on those individual characteristics which take time to perform well—such as a physician's or nurse's commitment of time to explain what is being done and why. This may constitute a fundamental paradox between consumer preference and the predominant orientation of planners and providers. The latter assess the efficiency of health delivery largely in terms of the speed with which volumes of patients can be processed through any given resource, be it an individual physician office or a hospital department. By contrast, the consumer judges efficiency based on the amount of time and personal attention which was devoted to them as unique individuals. Dissatisfaction with health providers seems closely related to such perceptions of inadequate commitment of time to the individual patient [Anderson, Fleming and Aday, 1981].

Consumer preferences are therefore substantial and dynamic. Failure to evaluate and incorporate these attitudes in health planning may lead both to sub-optimal decisions and to consequences different to those which the planner intended.

Too Many Physicians?

The history of "physician surplus" began in the early 1960's with an assessment of deficit. Analyzed from the viewpoint of consumer preference, the surplus is fictitious. It ignores the consumer demand for more time with and greater access to a clinician. It also miscalculates the impact of the aging of the population.

The process of planning physician supply through the last two decades appears to have consisted of six phases.

Phase 1, a period of assessment, ran from 1959 to 1966. Three commissions, Bane, 1959 ; Millis, 1966; Willard, 1966 — called for more physicians and more primary care physicians.

Phases 2 and 3, periods of decision and action, ran from 1966 to 1976. The federal and state governments and the profession acted to increase physician supply. Legislatively, money was appropriated to aid in training physicians, support increased medical school enrollment, increase the number of medical schools and increase primary care education. Simultaneously, other health professions were augmented by the same process. States, as well, increased the number of medical schools. The profession recognized family practice as the 20th AMA specialty in 1969. This growth represented the decision and action phases in the planning cycle [P.L. 89-129, 89-290, 90-480, 91-623, 92-157, 92-541, 94-484].

Phases 4 and 5 consisted of a period of predictable reaction and feedback. It is interesting however that the reaction and feedback heeded was that of the profession and the health planner on the basis of costs and not of the wishes and concerns of the consumer.

The pressure against increasing the supply of physicians began early. The following are among the most significant instances of this reaction.

- In 1973, the Goals and Priorities Committee of the National Board of Medical Examiners suggested a change in qualifying examinations [NBME, 1973]. Although not strictly part of the numbers planning process, one can read a subtle intent to limit both foreign and American foreign medical graduates.

- P.L. 94-484 in 1976 specifically called for the reduction of foreign medical graduates permitted to enter the United States.

- In 1975, the surgical world issued its *Study on Surgical Services in the U.S.* That report said there were too many surgeons [Moore, 1975; Zuidema, 1975].

- In 1978, the Institute of Medicine of the National Academy of Sciences recommended not increasing medical school enrollment beyond those enrolled in 1978 [NAS, 1978].

All of the instances above created a new consensus demanding reassessment of the earlier growth decisions. Phase 6, the reassessment was finally formalized by 1980 in the report from the Graduate Medical Education National Advisory Committee [DHHS, 1980]. In summary, GMENAC's recommendations included: reducing the number of MD and DO schools and class size, suggesting severe restriction and eventual elimination of both American and foreign medical graduates, and re-evaluating the need for nonphysician providers.

Through this six phase process, health planners went from an initial consensus of inadequate physician supply to a new consensus of an imminent surplus.

Although the calls for restricted physician supply have emanated largely from physicians themselves, it is interesting to note the public has never cried out that there are too many physicians.

Market research typically examines two leading indicators, demographic patterns and psychographic attitudes. Part I has already discussed the psychographic attitudes which consumers bring to health care seeking. This next section will examine future demographic patterns.

The public is beginning to demonstrate anxiety about the consequences of the future growth in the elderly population. The data support this concern. By 2008, the first of the baby boom generation turns 65 years of age. From then until 2035, the over 65 population will grow in both absolute numbers and, given zero population growth projections, will grow as a percent of the population from 11 percent now, to over 18 percent [Statistical

Abstracts, 1980]. The public also seems to perceive of the elderly as high consumers of health services. We know from the considerable data of the National Center for Health Statistics that this perception has some validity.

The rate of office visits/population [NAMCS, 1981] and visits per person [NAMCS, 1982] are significantly greater among the elderly. The accompanying tables show that the older population makes 20 percent to 40 percent more visits than the average visits of all ages. Their visits are for chronic problems and their encounters are longer. Figure I plots percent of visits against age for acute problems in dotted line and chronic problems in solid line [NAMCS, 1982]. Figure II plots duration of visits in minutes against age. As Section I highlighted, people want more information, more time to ask and receive answers to questions [Anderson, Fleming and Aday, 1981]. From clinical experience, 15 to 16 minutes is a rushed encounter with a patient who needs information and/or reassurance.

FIGURE I

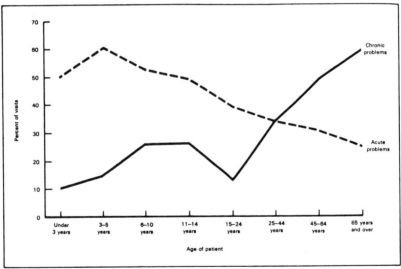

Percent of visits for acute and chronic problems by age of patient: United States, 1979

Cost?

The rebuttal to this argument, however, is typically that increased physicians lead to increased resource consumption. This is not a legitimate assertion. Increased resource consumption depends less on the number of physicians than on the economic incentive to the physician and to the patient. If the third parties, as has been true from 1950 to current, continue to pay big dollars for high cost institutional care and technological studies but not for the less expensive primary care encounter time then increased high technology resources will be used. If however, the third parties will pay for the

FIGURE II

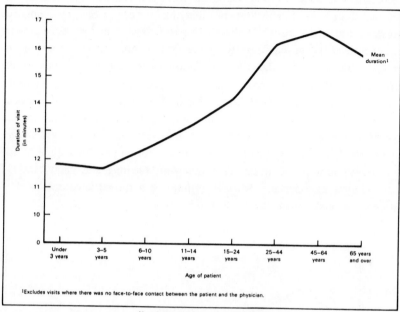

Mean duration of visit by age of patient: United States, 1979

less expensive primary encounter time necessary to treat and reassure patients, then this will not lead to increased total cost, even if primary care provider numbers increase.

The principal current pre-occupation of health economists is to devise methods to limit the total national health bill. This goal is being pursued largely by attempts to restrict utilization of its most expensive components (i.e. hospital-based and high technology services). Containment of the growth of spending in one part of health delivery threatens to result in an imbalanced and nonviable system unless some of the dollars saved are allocated into the acknowledged less expensive modalities of primary care.

Concern about physician supply is shortsighted. There may be some years of abundance but that is not necessarily bad, more costly, nor should it be regulated. Real incentives to primary care have not yet been instituted. People want more information from their clinician and that requires more time. To hold their market share in an era of "surplus" physicians may well extend their availability and accessibility. Finally, because of the aging of the population, no sooner would the reduction in graduates occur than the baby boom generation will attain 65.

Tampering with the supply cycle now for 1990-2000 is premature. To reflect consumer preferences, the cycle needs to run "high" for at least another 10 to 20 years.

The Consequences of Overlooking Consumer Preferences

Overlooking consumer preferences in major health planning decisions can easily produce a dichotomy between the delivery systems offered the public and those it actually wants. In the traditional approach to health planning in our societies, the consumer has been a blind-spot in our field of vision.

This concluding part of our paper examines the major questions which arise from this analysis:

1. How is it that the formalized approaches to health planning which have developed in recent decades succeeded in advancing the health status of our people, without much emphasis on consumer preference but now must do so? What has changed?
2. What will happen if we continue to ignore consumer preference?
3. What should we do differently?

First then, why should health planners change their approaches?

There are two principal reasons why monitoring of consumer attitudes and preferences has been a less well-developed practice in health care than in other areas of major national planning effort.

First, such insights have been regarded as irrelevant. In the era between 1945 and approximately 1970 utilization of health services in the developed economies of the world exploded. This upsurge in the percentage of gross national product devoted to health spending created an environment within which any new service appeared to attract users. This encouraged an assumption among planners and providers that health consumers lacked strong personal preference and that consumers would match any change in the supply of health care with a corresponding demand [Goldsmith, 1981].

Second, insights into consumer preferences have not been actively sought because it has been comfortably assumed that the health consumers are passive in the marketplace. The consumer has been perceived of as willing to surrender the prerogative of personal choice to the planner and health professional.

Both these motivations for ignoring consumer attitudes appear to us now to be invalid.

The rapid transition of modern health care between 1945 and 1970 now appears, in light of more recent trends, atypical of the industry's past and therefore an unreliable indicator of its future. It may well have been a temporary period of transition created by the coincidence of:

1. An explosion in applied bio-medical technology;
2. A corresponding increase in confidence among consumers and doctors that the application of scientific principles had unlimited capacity to improve health status and decrease disease;
3. And an egalitarian insistence on making this scientific knowledge available regardless of the ability to pay.

Such periods of rapid growth have occurred historically in other industries but have seldom been indefinitely sustained.

The fast growth of health care consumption in the 1950's and 1960's, followed by an apparent slowing of growth in the 1970's is beginning to look much more like the traditional shape of a product life cycle curve than the beginning of a perpetual exponential growth in health service consumption. This slowing of growth is being in part stimulated by the doubt among major corporations that they can continue to support such health technology costs on behalf of their employees [Shapiro, 1982].

The doctrine of the passive health consumer is also looking increasingly questionable in the less exuberant and slower growing health market of recent years.

In our high technology societies, consumers are confronted with frequent purchase or usage decisions to which they bring an imperfect understanding. The typical response to such complex market judgements is not one of passive surrender of their right of choice. It is usually a more conscientious effort to evaluate the options offered.

Recognition that health consumers have distinct preferences should not detract from the health planner's or provider's sense of personal responsibility for exercising professional judgement as to health delivery needs. Effective implementation of those professional judgements must however be shaped and conditioned by listening to the expressions of preference being voiced by the consumer.

A Buyer's Market

In the new era that we have entered, health care now possesses the characteristics more of a buyer's market than a seller's market. If our goal remains to deliver health services effectively and efficiently we must find ways of doing so that both meet defined health needs and satisfy consumer wants.

What will happen if we continue to delegate consumer preferences to a back-seat role in health planning?

Because health planners and providers have viewed themselves as exercising professional judgement on behalf of an incompetent consumer public, they have tended to substitute office standards of medical need for observable measures of public demand. They also have attempted to regulate supply to force an artificial equilibrium of need and available service. Such an artificial equilibrium could not exist if consumers act as they do in other marketplaces. Artificial restrictions in demand or supply in such a marketplace leave consumers with unsatisfied demands. Insurance coverage mechanisms may increase that unsatiated demand by lowering its effective price to the consumer.

Consumers who are frustrated will inevitably seek to satisfy their needs in alternatives outside the regulated system. The planner and health professional see themselves as possessing a monopoly control over health care delivery. They do not. There has probably always been a medical counter-system. The current existence and functioning of such a counter-system is beginning to receive some serious attention in both the U.S. and elsewhere [*Lancet,* Ed.; 1982].

A Medical Counter-System

In the United States health spending as currently recorded now exceeds 10 percent of GNP. There is however other health-motivated spending not recorded in this statistic. It is this type of spending which we have termed the "medical counter-system." It includes:

- Wellness spending on health club memberships, diet foods, exercise equipment and fitness literature, all of which are designed to reduce use of the conventional health system by "staying fit."

- Self-diagnostic spending on symptomatic literature and home monitoring devices to enable the consumer to judge more prudently when professional intervention is actually necessary.

- Use of alternative treatment providers such as self-help groups, chiropractors, hypnotists, herbalists and acupuncturists.

The size of this counter-system in the United States has been estimated minimally at 3 percent of GNP [ORC, 1982]. Since that estimate does not include all the items which we mentioned previously, our tentative estimate would put it as high as 5 percent of GNP.

Built-in delays in regulatory and professional response accentuate the disequilibrium of supply and demand. Among the clinical services where consumer dissatisfaction in recent years has generated growing dependence on counter-systems have been alternative birthing modalities, programs for palliation of chronic pain syndromes, support in weight watching, fitness and smoke-ender counseling and growth of self-diagnostic tests for cancer or cardiovascular disease.

In each of these cases the response of the planner and health professional has been slow, somewhat reluctant and often lagging behind the prevalent public demand.

If we continue to ignore consumer preference within the planned and regulated health system, we are likely in a buyer's market to fuel continued growth of a medical counter-system. We make no value judgements about that counter-system. Many aspects of it seem highly desirable. We assert, however, that it makes a mockery of the whole idea of health planning if it results in the parallel existence of two industries—the one highly planned and regulated but unresponsive—the other unplanned and unregulated but highly responsive to the consumer.

Finally, what should health planners do differently?

All planning processes must contend with time and with the associated phenomenon of unavoidable delay. Obtaining and analyzing data, deciding upon and implementing actions and then monitoring feedback consume time. We have been impressed with how similar to a sine-wave the planning cycle appears.

As with any process containing time delays, planning tends to follow a cyclical progression of assessment-decision-action-reaction-feedback-reassessment. The case example of the physician supply debate followed precisely this pattern.

The more protracted these delays, the greater the risk that when planned actions take effect the circumstances which appeared to necessitate them have changed to such a degree that the new action exacerbates a new problem rather than ameliorates the former problem. National and regional health care planning is such a complex process.

In other major planning arenas, regulatory agencies have come to rely on "leading indicators" of incipient change in market behavior.

We believe that health planning must rely not only on data that count utilization of services but also on systematic investigation of consumer attitudes, preferences and satisfaction levels. Economists and marketing scientists have much to offer in the further understanding of these attitudes and behavior patterns and of their significance to the planning of health delivery.

Our own efforts to utilize these concepts in planning the future of our hospital appear to demonstrate their relevance.

TABLE 1
Growth of Physicians

	# Med.Schools	# Med.School Grads.	# Physicians
1955	81	6977	
1960	85	7081	250,000
1965	88	7409	292,000
1970	101	8367	334,000
1975	114	12714	394,000
1978	122	14393	437,000
1980	126	15135	468,000
1990	127	18151	536,000

TABLE 2
Average Annual Office Visit Rate
Per/1000 Pop (1977-78)(NAMCS, 1981)

	All Ages	45–64	65+
Women	3167	3729	4299
Men	2251	2800	3913

TABLE 3
Annual # of Office Visits/Per Person/Yr. (NAMCS, 1982)

		1975	1980
All Patients		2.7	2.7
Women	45–64	4.0	3.4
	65+	4.4	4.3
Men	45–64	2.8	2.6
	65+	4.0	4.0

REFERENCES

American Medical Association, Citizens Commission, *The Graduate Education of Physicians,* John Millis, CHRM, Chicago, Illinois 1966.

American Medical Association, *Meeting the Challenge of Family Practice, The Report of the Ad Hoc Committee on Education for Family Practice,* William Willard, CHRM, Council of Medical Education, Chicago, Illinois, 1966.

American Medical Association, *Physician Characteristics and Distribution in the U.S. 1981 Edition,* Survey and Data Resources, Chicago, Illinois, 1982.

JAMA 1968:106(9):2017, *Undergraduate Medical Education."*

R. M. Anderson, G. V. Fleming and L. Aday, "Study Points Out Medical Manpower Needs," *American Medical News,* November 20-27, 1981.

L. Beck, G. Anders and D. Sweeney, "Effective Marketing," *Pennsylvania Medicine,* January 1982.

S. Brown, "Comparing Attitudes and Opinions of Arizona Physicians and Consumers," *Arizona Medicine,* April 1980.

Department of Health and Human Services, *Report of the Graduate Medical Education National Advisory Committee,* Vol. H. Modeling, Research and Data Technical Panel, No. HRA 81-652, pp. 282-84, pp. 273, 262.

B. Doyle and J. Ware, "Physician Conduct and Other Factors that Affect Consumer Satisfaction with Medical Care," *Journal of Medical Education,* 52, October 1977.

General Mills, Inc., *Family Health in an Era of Stress,* 1979.

J. Goldsmith, "Can Hospitals Survive?" *Dow Jones,* 1981.

M. Gottlieb, "Segmentation by Personality," *Advanced Marketing Efficiency*, L Stockman, ed., American Marketing Association, 1959.

J. Hall, D. Roter and C. Rand, "Communication of Affect between Patient and Physician," *Journal of Health and Social Behavior*, March 22, 1981.

K. G. Halpern and T. A. Fisk, "The Pure Competitive Model: Hospitals Don't Fit, But What Does?" *Hospitals*, July 1, 1982, p. 69.

Lou Harris Organization, Poll Reported in *Snowmass Advisory*, September 1979.

IEC Marketing Group reported in *Snowmass Advisory*, March 1980.

H. Kelman, "Evaluation of Health Care Quality by Consumers," *International Journal of Health Services*, 6:3, 1976.

D. Klegon, D. Gregory and P. Kingstrom, "Planning for Ambulatory Care Delivery Systems: A Market Segmentation Approach," *Health Care Management Review*, Winter 1982, pp. 35-45.

Lancet, Ed., *Disparities in European Medicine*, July 3, 1982, pp. 26-7.

Market Probe Inc.: quoted in *Health Care Planning and Marketing*, October 1981.

D. Mechanic, *Medical Sociology*, The Free Press, 1968.

D. Mechanic, *The Growth of Bureaucratic Medicine*, Wiley, 1976.

Francis Moore, "Report on the (SOSSUS) Manpower Subcommittee," *Annals of Surgery*, 1975; 182(4):526-30.

National Academy Sciences, *A Manpower Policy for Primary Health Care*, Institute of Medicine, Washington, D.C., 1978, pp. 41-2.

National Board of Medical Examiners, *Evaluation in the Continuum of Medical Education*, Report of the Committee on Goals and Priorities of the National Board of Medical Examiners (GAP), pp. 11-12, 78, Philadelphia, 1973.

National Center for Health Statistics, *Vital & Health Statistics–The National Ambulatory Medical Care Survey*, U.S. 1979, Department of Health and Human Services Public No. (PHS) 82-1727, Hyattsville, Maryland, September 1982.

National Center for Health Statistics, *Vital and Health Statistics–Patients Reasons for Visiting Physicians*, The National Ambulatory Medical Survey, U.S. 1977-78, Department of Health and Human Services Publication No. (PHS) 82-1717, Hyattsville, Maryland, December 1981.

F. Nicosia, *Consumer Decision Processes*, Prentice Hall, 1966.

ORC (Princeton, New Jersey) study reported *Advertising Age*, July 26, 1982, p. 52.

I.S. Shapiro, *Health Care, The Price of Success*, DuPont Company, 1982.

U.S. Congress, *Health Professions Educational Assistance Act*, P.L. 88-129, 1963.

U.S. Congress, *Health Professions Educational Assistance Amendments*, P.L. 89-290, 1965.

U.S. Congress, *Health Manpower Act*, P.L. 90-490, 1968.

U.S. Congress, *Emergency Health Personnel Act*, P.L. 91-623, 1970.

U.S. Congress, *Comprehensive Health Manpower Training Act*, P.L. 92-157, 1971.

U.S. Congress, *V.A. Medical School Assistance and Health Manpower Training Act*, P.L. 92-541, 1972.

U.S. Congress, *Health Professions Educational Assistance Act*, P.L. 94-484, 1976.

U.S. Department of Commerce, Bureau of Census, Statistical Abstracts of the U.S., 1980, 101st Edition, pp. 30-1.

Kerr White, "General Practice in the United States," *Journal of Medical Education*, 1964, 39(4):333-343.

R. Ziff, "Psychographics for Market Segmentation," *Journal of Advertising Research*, Vol. 11, April 1971.

George Zudema, "SOSSUS and the Outlook for American Surgery," *Annals of Surgery*, 1975; 182(4):531-37.

Chapter Nineteen

Marketing Strategy in the Changing Environment

ALGIN B. KING

I. Introduction

Management of health care facilities must be aware of the changing needs of the markets that they serve. Marketing might be defined as the professional management of activities which seek to accomplish the objectives of an organization by anticipating and meeting the needs of the customer or client and directing appropriate goods and services from producer to customer or client. In health care this concept has been largely ignored with management perceiving the mission to be to provide the services that the organization believes the patient needs or desires. Where marketing has existed in hospitals, it has generally been a middle-management staff function and few resources have been channeled into it. At best, some hospitals have seen marketing as simply "communication focused" or "sales promotion" oriented.

Hospitals have been involved in marketing but many do not know it. The average hospital must have about 70 percent of its beds full in order to cover costs from the business office, the emergency room, the operating room, the laboratory, the OB/GYN unit, the maintenance department, the psychiatric unit, and the administration, and break even. Many costs are involved in the operation of the average hospital—whether for profit or for non-profit—and it must be run like a modern business to survive. The non-profit hospital must not only reclaim costs involved with a physical facilitiy but the costs involved with replacing equipment as technology improves and the modernization of the physical facility is required. This requires occupancy above break even.

All health care facilities have one thing in common: they must make enough to cover costs and (1) pay the owners and provide for the continuation of the services or (2) provide for the continuation of the services. No health care unit can provide for services, which is the main concern in most cases, if it can no longer pay for salaries, hard goods, and the like. In order to cover costs, any health care facility must operate on a financially sound basis as concerned with break-even occupancy, and this involves meeting the needs of the patients and the admitting physicians; and this means modern marketing concepts *must* be used.

279

We have been concerned to this point with the relationship between the health care facility and the consumer or patient. In the health care environment today, is the patient or potential patient the main concern of health care marketing in hospitals? In all respects, over the long run, yes. However, who admits a patient to a hospital and why? Should emphasis be given first to the attending physician and second to the patient as far as policies, public relations, and the like are concerned? If patients are brought to a hospital by the physician and the financial viability of the hospital depends on this, shouldn't the management of the hospital be concerned about its relationship with the physician as well as with the patient? Many hospitals are on the brink of financial disaster and, therefore, their ability to provide health care is declining due to a lack of consideration of marketing to identify and meet the needs of the patient *and* the physician.

This study will be concerned with an aspect of health care marketing dealing with a hospital in a new environment. Despite being a new facility in an area needing health care facilities of that type, this hospital (called Hospital A) was on the brink of failure due to a lack of consideration of modern marketing techniques. Simple changes to a market-orientation dealing with the needs of patients and with physicians quickly brought this hospital to financial stability and brought better care to the population served by the hospital.

II. Background of the Study

Less than 50 percent occupancy of the new physical facilities of Hospital A in the fastest growing suburb of a city of 400,000 prompted the need to gather certain data for decision making purposes and to better identify how certain problems could best be solved. On the assumption that the types of health care services and facilities offered by Hospital A were "in high demand" by the general public in the Standard Metropolitan Statistical Area (SMSA) and the location of the hospital was in the fastest growing census tracts (sections) of the city, the logical question arose as to why the health care services and facilities of Hospital A were underutilized.

III. Objectives of Research Study

The major purposes of the research study were as follows:

A. Identify some of the major policies and strategies of Hospital A.

B. Identify the various types of health care facilities and services currently provided by Hospital A.

C. Determine the general public's awareness of Hospital A as a health care facility. In addition, determine what type of general image Hospital A had among the general public in the SMSA as a health care facility.

D. Determine the medical profession's perception of Hospital A as a health care facility; and determine what type of general image Hospital A had among the medical profession in the SMSA as a health care facility. Specifically, the image of the hospital would be examined in terms of the variety of services offered as perceived by the medical profession, versus its image as primarily an obstetrical facility.

E. Determine if there were any operating policies and procedures presently employed by the hospital that were identifiable deterrents to the utilization of Hospital A as a health care facility by the medical community.

IV. Methodology of Research Study

A. Personal interviews were conducted during May and June, 1981, with key members of the administrative staff of Hospital A to determine policies and procedures employed by the hospital in providing health care services and to identify problem areas as perceived by the various professional personnel in the hospital.

B. During the period June 12-23, 1981, structured personal interviews were conducted by professional interviewers with a stratified random sample of 50 physicians in the city of 400,000 population. A cross section of different types of medical specialists which might use the hospital facilities was used to stratify the sample and insure representation. Types of data discussed in the objectives of the study were sought in an in-depth interview with each physician. Interviews with each physician ranged in length between 45 minutes to 60 minutes. The personal interview with the selected sample of physicians was designed to determine a variety of opinions among the local medical profession; for example, the reasons why the physician did or did not utilize Hospital A for his/her patients; how much knowledge the physician had of the current facilities and/or services offered by Hospital A for the physician to care for his/her patients.

It was deemed desirable to determine what kind of image Hospital A had among the general public in its primary service area. The primary service area was defined by the hospital officials as being the suburb of the city (SMSA of 400,000) and most of the nearby country (excluding possibly one district). To secure the requisite data on the type of image Hospital A had in its primary service area, structured personel interviews were conducted between June 10-21 with a random sample of 210 consumers in this defined primary service area of the city and the county (a population area of about 100,000). Each interview with each consumer was an in-depth survey of the consumers' perceptions of Hospital A, their knowledge of the hospital's existence, its current physical location, and the types of health care services offered. Interviews with each consumer took approximately 30 minutes. The sample size of 210 consumers was sufficient to enable the data results to be accurate, plus or minus three points.

V. Data Findings—Physicians Survey

1. Table 1 indicated that physicians practicing affiliations were about equally dispersed among the three hospitals in the area: Hospital A, Hospital H, and Hospital R.

2. Physicians respondents reported that they practiced at Hospital R and Hospital H slightly more than Hospital A but utilization for their pateints was not fairly evenly spread among the three major hospitals in the area, as may be noted in Table 2. Data on the proportion of the patients referred by physicians to a hospital indicated that a substantially higher percentage (proportion) of patients were referred to Hospital R and Hospital H than to Hospital A.

3. Over two-thirds of respondent physicians reported that their offices were within 10 miles or less of Hospital R and Hospital H. Only one in three doctors (36 percent) indicated their office was located within 10 miles of the location of Hospital A.

4. The most commonly cited and important perceived strengths of hospitals utilized by respondent physicians were: in the case of Hospital R—facilities, equipment, diagnostic services, staff and general services; in the case of Hospital H—location, facilities and equipment, staff and general services; in the case of Hospital A—staff, facilities and equipment. (See Table 3.)

5. Hospital A's most commonly perceived weaknesses were lack of speciality equipment, special services and specialization consultants, and location. (See Table 4.)

6. Analysis of data in Table 5, "General Image" of Hospital A among the medical profession, indicated the following perceptions were held by a substantial portion of respondent physicians:

Hospital A was:
    a. A good hospital 54%
    b. Not well known as a general hospital 40%
    c. Perceived as having limited services and equipment 68%
    d. Not particularly convenient geographically 16%

7. The degree of familiarity of the respondent physicians with service and facilities of Hospital A is a problem since one-third of the respondents indicated they were not familiar with at least 25 percent of Hospital A's services and 16 percent were not familiar with 50 percent or more of the hospital's services and facilities. (See Table 6.)

8. Analysis of data in Table 6 showed that the three most common rationale for non-affiliation on the staff at Hospital A by respondent physicians were:

    a. Time factors limited physicians' practice to one hospital;
    b. Geographical location of Hospital A was inconvenient to the physician

in his/her practice;

c. The hospital lacked requisite diagnostic services and equipment and/or requisite equipment for patient treatment and surgery.

9. The data findings in Table 7 showed that the doctor was the dominant influence in the determination of hospital facility for the patient. Analysis of these data showed that in over half of the cases the choice of hospital was solely the physician's and in three-fourths of cases the physician chose or influenced the choice of hospital.

10. The three most important rationale cited by respondent physicians for using the hospital for patients (where they are currently practicing) in rank order were:

a. Facilities and services "good";
b. Convenience of location to physician;
c. Excellence of staff.

V. Data Findings—Consumers Survey

1. The existence of Hospital A appeared to be well known throughout its primary service area with 94 percent of respondents having heard of the hospital and 89 percent being aware of its physical location. There were no significant differences in consumer awareness of the existence of Hospital A based on age, sex, or income.

2. Hospital A had an image as a good, to very good, health care facility in the eyes of the public in its primary service area. Table 8 shows two out of every three respondents (67 percent) rated Hospital A as an excellent health care facility. Another 14 percent of respondents rated it reasonably good, with only 3 percent of respondents perceiving Hospital A negatively. There were no significant differences in the respondents' perceptions of the image of Hospital A based on sex, age, or income, with two exceptions. A higher proportion of respondents over 65 and in the over $40,000 income category rated Hospital A as an excellent health care facility.

3. Analysis of data in Table 9 showed that a large proportion of respondents in the hospital's primary service area were not aware of a significant number of the medical facilities of Hospital A. A little more than one-third (35 percent) were familiar with many or most of the medical facilities of the hospital. There were no significant differences in the respondents' degree of familiarity with the variety of health care services/facilities offered by Hospital A, with one exception. Respondents in the over $40,000 income category indicated a higher degree of familiarity with a variety of services and facilities than did total respondents.

4. Based on their own personal experiences, respondents indicated that the most likely decision factor in the selection of a hospital was the physician.

Analysis of data in Table 7 revealed that in over half (54 percent) of the cases, a physician was the decision-maker in the selection of a given hospital. In about one-third of the cases (30 percent), the patient or the patient's family chose the hospital. Geographical convenience and location was also an important decision variable.

5. Analysis of data revealed that the most important factors to the individuals in selecting a hospital in order of importance are: type of services or facilities offered (56 percent), convenience and location (44 percent), their physicians practice there (25 percent), and the general image or reputation (23 percent). As might be expected, most respondents cited more than one factor as being important to their decision.

6. Analysis of data reinforced prior findings that the physician was the key element in the choice of a hospital for the patient. Only 31 percent of respondents indicated that the physician offered them a choice in the selection of a hospital. Conversely, 60 percent of respondents indicated that they were offered no choice in the selection of the hospital.

7. From the data in Table 10, it appeared that Hospital R and Hospital A enjoyed the best image and reputation as the best hospitals in the SMSA. Thirty-seven percent of respondents believed that Hospital R enjoyed the best reputation as a hospital, while 36 percent of respondents believed that Hospital A had the reputation as the best hospital in the SMSA. Hospital H was not perceived by many individuals as enjoying a best reputation image. Some respondents (14 percent) believed that all three hospitals had about the same reputation as a health care facility.

VI. Conclusions

A. Survey of Physicians

1. While a substantial number of physicians had practicing staff affiliation with Hospital A, the physicians were not utilizing it to the same degree that they were utilizing either Hospital R or Hospital H.

2. The breadth and depth of the various services and facilities offered by Hospital A were not well known to a significant proportion of the medical community in the SMSA. Therefore, the scope of services and facilities available at Hospital A needed to be communicated to the medical community. Hospital A should educate those segments of the medical community that were simply not aware of the variety of services and facilities offered by Hospital A, and they should then persuade the medical community to use the hospital by promoting the advantages of utilizing the services and facilities.

3. A substantial portion of the medical profession perceived the physical locations of Hospitals H and R to be more convenient and in greater proximity to their office than the location of Hospital A. The construction of

a physicians' office building near the hospital, with attractive rent, could attract physicians to practice at Hospital A.

4. From the data findings, it can be concluded that Hospital A had an image problem among a substantial portion of the medical community as a health care facility lacking the requisite diagnostic services and equipment for their medical practice, and requisite equipment for patient treatment and surgery. Whether or not this was a fact or not, so long as a substantial portion of the medical profession held this opinion, it would be a serious limitation to the utilization of Hospital A.

5. One of the most seriously perceived weaknesses of Hospital A among a portion of the medical community was the inadequate availability of specialized medical consultation. Whether this was a fact or not, so long as this perception was held by a sizeable portion of the medical profession, it presented a serious limitation to the utilization of the hospital by the medical community.

6. Hospital A enjoyed the image as "a good hospital," and its nursing care was particularly accorded high marks by a substantial portion of the medical community. It was concluded that Hospital A enjoyed a "good" image in its primary service area as a health care facility, i.e., good in terms of the quality of health care services and particularly in terms of the quality of its nursing care.

7. Many physicians preferred to limit their practice to one hospital, or at least concentrate the majority of their patient workload in one hospital because of the time factor. Given this significant constraint, many physicians chose what they considered to be the "best" hospital, either from the standpoint of the services and facilities capability of the hospital that best satisfied the demands of their practice or for their own convenience.

8. Physicians did have distinct decision rationale in choosing the hospital where they did the majority of their practicing. Many physicians even rank ordered the variables that influenced their choice of hospital for utilization. The three most important rationale in rank order influencing the physicians' choice of a hospital were:

   a. The various medical services and facilities available and the perceived quality of such services and facilities;
   b. Convenience of location of the hospital to the physician;
   c. The hospital staff in terms of its quality and excellence.

Some of the same factors that influenced physicians in their choice of a hospital for their practice were also important to consumers and influenced their choice of a hospital. From the data findings of both the physicians' survey and consumers' survey, the same three factors were the most important to *both* groups in the *same* rank order, i.e., (1) types of services and facilities offered by the hospital; (2) convenience and location of the hospital; (3) general image or reputation of the hospital as a health care facility (nursing care and staff).

9. From the data findings, it was concluded that the physician was the dominant factor in the selection of a hospital for a patient. This was a strong conclusion from the survey of physicians and from the survey of consumers.

B. Survey of Consumers

1. The existence of Hospital A as a health care facility was well known by the public in its primary service area (94 percent awareness level). Further, they were also aware of the hospital's location (89 percent awareness level). It was concluded that the existence of Hospital A as a hospital (i.e., a health care facility) was well known and not a problem.

2. A substantial proportion of the public in Hospital A's primary service area believed that Hospital A's image was one of a hospital offering a limited number of health care services and facilities (i.e., primarily an OB/GYN hospital). Hospital A appeared to have a substantial problem in its primary service area in terms of public awareness of the wide range of medical services and facilities offered by Hospital A. Increasing public awareness of the breadth and depth of the different types of health care services and facilities the hospital had to offer the public is very important.

3. A substantial proportion of consumers believed that Hospital A's image as a hospital or health care facility was excellent and ranked among the "better" hospitals in the SMSA.

VII. Recommendations

There is little doubt but that most health care organizations (profit or non-profit), such as hospitals, are competing in many areas of health care services with similar organizations in the same service area. Thus, in many ways, the hospital is much like a business in the private enterprise sector in that it is in direct competition with other hospitals in the area when it comes to utilization of health care facilities *by physicians* for their patients or by the public in the choice of a hospital either for themselves or members of their families. Any decision-makers (e.g., Board of Directors, top hospital administrators) who do not recognize and understand this fact and do not develop policies and strategies to implement the offering of health care facilities on a competitive basis are not assessing the situation realistically.

The following are the general recommendations resulting from the study:

1. Hospitals should develop a communications program designed to educate and familiarize the medical community in their service area regarding the breadth and depth of health care services and facilities offered.

2. A separate communications program needs to be developed and di-

rected toward the medical community in the service area, stressing the convenience of the hospital's location, both in terms of convenience to a large number of the medical profession in the area and to the general population. Specifically, attention should be focused on such issues as the convenience of the hospital in terms of arterial roads, distances expressed in number of minutes from the downtown city, distances from population centers in the service area, parking, and distances from physicians' offices. It might also be advantageous to cite the trend of population movements in the SMSA to highlight the fact that the present location of the hospital is strategically located to accommodate population trends.

3. A third phase of the communications program to the medical community should stress the advantages of the particular hospital, i.e., more personalized patient care, less red tape and bureaucracy for the physician and the patient, faster turn around time for diagnostic services and traditions of high quality nursing services.

4. Hospitals should explore the possibilities and opportunities of soliciting "a first affiliation" from new physicians coming into the SMSA.

5. The hospital should explore the possibilities and opportunities to encourage the development of a large doctors' office complex in physicial proximity to the hospital. Physical convenience of the hospital is a major decision determinant to the physicians in their selection and utilization of a hospital for their practice. Of course, physicians should be consulted concerning their interest and later concerning the design of offices. Rent (or lease) arrangements should be favorable to the physician.

6. Top administration of the hospital should carefully and objectively assess the present range of equipment and facilities against those of competing hospitals. If such an assessment reveals that there is a major equipment deficiency area, then serious consideration should be given to remedying this equipment deficiency. For example, lack of neuro-surgical equipment at Hospital A was very evident from this survey. The lack of requisite equipment can be a serious competitive disadvantage.

7. Top administration of the hospital should insure an appropriate range of consulting expertise availability on the staff as a service to encourage greater utilization of the hospital by the medical community.

8. Hospitals should initiate a tasteful communications program directed to the general public, particularly in the primary service area, to educate the public as to the range of health care services and facilities offered. Among some of the items that deserve particular stress in the communications effort would be the high quality of nursing care, individual patient attention and care, advantages of convenient location, and the like. The key strategy suggested in this communications program would be to highlight the advantages of the hospital in a tasteful and low-keyed way.

9. Top administration should carefully and objectively assess the hospital's advantages and weaknesses with the objective of determining a strategy of how it can provide health care services to the general public and for the use of physicians better than its competitors do.

VIII. General

Marketing in health care is becoming established but is viewed by most hospital administrators as being a discipline concerned with communications. This was one of the findings of a national study by the task force of the American Society for Hospital Public Relations (ASHPR) that was completed last July. Many hospitals, such as Hospital A, and other health care facilities have engaged in public relations efforts for many years. These have included employee newsletters, letters (or newsletters) to donors and patients, and letters to physicians. These activities are orientated to sales, promotion, and education, which are only a part of modern marketing.

Many health care marketing programs, if they exist, are viewed as being little more than communications work positioned as a middle management, staff function. To many, it is P.R. work with a fancy name and with little definition, low authority, and few resources. Those doing marketing work in health care often have little, if any, formal education, training, and experience in marketing. Public relations practitioners often view marketing as a threat since they lack the necessary qualifications—although an increasing number are obtaining training and education in marketing and now view this as an area of opportunity. There is an increasing demand in health care for individuals well-educated and trained in marketing, and they are being positioned in top management.

Marketing in health care might also be defined as the professional management of activities (analysis, planning, implementation, and control) to anticipate patient or client needs and direct a flow of need-satisfying services from the health care facility to the patient or client in order to achieve the objectives of the organization. This concept is much, much more than P.R. work, although communications is a part of the modern marketing concept. Public relations deals with image management to influence opinions and attitudes about the health care organization. On the other hand, marketing deals with the patient or client to identify wants or needs so that the organization can offer appropriate services. The objectives of the organization may be many, such as "x" percent profit, better patient care, and provision of a needed service at a place, price, and time convenient to the consumer. Public relations could be used to educate and inform the potential consumer about the service or this could be done within marketing.

Since hospital P.R. is a well-established function (and a very useful one) in many health care facilities, it should be continued. Marketing should encompass the P.R. function as it is brought into the health care facility as depicted in Figure I.

FIGURE I

Relationship of Marketing and Public Relations

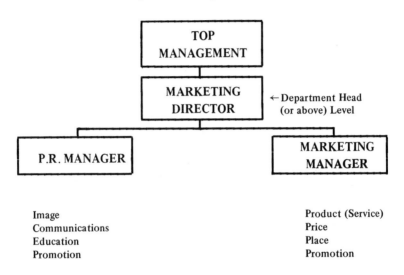

This concept shows a separation of the two functions but under one manager. The concept of ASHPR showed the functions to be separate but with overlap in the area of communications. Public relations personnel would require additional training and education to function in such a set-up.

As in the "Hospital A" example, marketing research could be aimed at the physicians and the patients. An understanding of consumer attitudes about the hospital could then be developed to assist in meeting the needs of the physicians and patients on a continuous basis. Public relations could then be used to inform and educate the physicians, patients and the public. This effort would require close coordination between the two functions. This would benefit the consumer, the physician and, ultimately, the hospital in its goal of providing better patient care.

Who forgot the M.D. as well as the patient?

TABLE 1
Practicing Patterns of the Medical Profession in
the City SMSA as to Hospitals

Name of Hospital	Practicing Status	
	No.*	%*
Hospital H	23	46.0
Hospital R	23	46.0
Hospital A	20	40.0
Other Hospitals	5	10.0
TOTAL SAMPLE	50	100.0

*Total Sample of physicians is 50 and many doctors practice at more than one hospital.
 Percentages were figured using total sample number of 50.

TABLE 2
Hospitals In the City (SMSA) Currently Utilized
by Physicians for Their Own Patients

Name of Hospital	Patient Utilization	
	No.*	%*
Hospital H	23	46.0
Hospital R	24	48.0
Hospital A	15	30.0
Other Hospitals	10	20.0
TOTAL SAMPLE	50	100.0

*Total Sample of physicians is 50 and many doctors practice at more than one hospital.
 Percentages were figured using total sample number of 50.

TABLE 3

Strengths of Hospitals Utilized as
Perceived by Respondent Physicians

Hospital and Strengths	Responses	
	No.*	%*
Hospital H		
Location	11	22.0
Facilities/Equipment	15	30.0
Staff (Administrative & Nursing)	14	28.0
Services	7	14.0
Consulting Staff	3	6.0
Other	3	6.0
Hospital R		
Location	3	6.0
Facilities/Equipment/Diagnostic Services	21	42.0
Staff (Administrative & Nursing)	8	16.0
Services	9	18.0
Other	2	4.0
Hospital A		
Location	1	2.0
Facilities/Equipment	12	24.0
Staff (Administrative & Nursing)	22	44.0
Services	3	6.0
Other	6	12.0

*Total sample of physicians is 50 and percentages were figured using total sample number of 50.

TABLE 4

Weaknesses of Hospitals Utilized as
Perceived by Respondent Physicians

Hospital and Weaknesses	Responses	
	No.*	%*
Hospital H		
Facilities	1	2.0
Staff	3	6.0
Services	3	6.0
Other	4	8.0
None	14	28.0
Hospital R		
Facilities	6	12.0
Staff	11	22.0
Administration	3	6.0
Other	7	14.0
None	6	12.0
Hospital A		
Location	7	14.0
Facilities/Equipment	1	2.0
Staff	6	12.0
Lack of Speciality Equipment, Special Services & Specialization Consultants	12	24.0
Other	5	10.0
None	4	8.0

*Total sample of physicians is 50 and percentages were figured using total sample number of 50.

TABLE 5
Perceived General Image of Hospital A Among the Medical Profession in the City SMSA

Image Picture Options	Physicians' Perceptions									
	Agree or Strongly Agree		Neutral		Disagree or Strongly Disagree		No. Response		Total	
	No.	%	No.	%	No.	%	No.	%	No.	%
Favorably Perceived as a Good General Hospital	27	54.0	9	18.0	13	26.0	1	2.0	50	100.0
Not Well Known as a General Hospital	20	40.0	1	2.0	27	54.0	2	4.0	50	100.0
Perceived as a "Poor" Hospital	3	6.0	3	6.0	39	78.0	5	10.0	50	100.0
Perceived as a Hospital Having Limited Services/Equipment	34	68.0	4	8.0	9	18.0	3	6.0	50	100.0
Perceived Primarily as a Hospital Specializing in Obstetrics	14	28.0	8	16.0	26	52.0	2	4.0	50	100.0
Thought of as an Unneeded Third Hospital	11	22.0	6	12.0	31	62.0	2	4.0	50	100.0
Thought of as Being Geographically Inconvenient	8	16.0	13	26.0	27	54.0	2	4.0	50	100.0

TABLE 6

Reasons Cited By Physicians for not Currently
Being on the Staff at Hospital A

Reasons Cited For Non Affiliation at Hospital A	Physicians Reporting Reason	
	No.*	%*
Time Dictates Limit Practice to One Hospital	19	38%
Not Aware That Hospital A Offered Wide Range of Facilities	2	4%
Geographical Location of Hospital A Inconvenient To Me	12	24%
Major Policies of Hospital Are Not Conducive to My Practicing There	2	4%
The Hospital Does Not Have Diagnostic Services/Equipment Needed	5	10%
The Hospital Does Not Have Equipment Needed For Patient Treatment/Surgery	5	10%
Other Reasons	1	2%
No Response**	24	48%
TOTAL SAMPLE	50	100%

*Total Sample of Physicians is 50 and many Doctors listed more than one reason.
**All these respondents were on the staff at Hospital A.

TABLE 7
Decision Maker/Decision Factor in Selection of Hospital*

Types of Decision Makers / Decision Factors	TOTAL SAMPLE		SEX				AGE						INCOME									
			Male		Female		< 40		40 – 65		65 >		<$15,000		$15-24,999		$25-39,000		$40,000>		No	
	No.	%	No.	%	No.	%	No.	%	No.	%	No.	%	No.	%	No.	%	No.	%	No.	%	No.	%
Patient	42	20.0	15	7.0	27	12.5	26	13.0	13	6.0	3	1.5	20	9.0	17	8.0	10	5.0	0	0.0	0	0.0
Patient's Family	21	10.0	5	2.5	16	7.0	13	6.0	7	3.0	2	1.0	10	5.0	4	2.0	3	1.5	1	0.5	2	1.0
Attdg. Doctor Generally	104	50.0	35	16.5	69	33.0	60	28.5	35	17.0	4	1.5	25	11.5	37	17.5	32	16.0	5	2.5	4	2.0
Attdg. Doctor Always	7	3.0	3	1.5	4	2.0	5	2.5	6	3.0	1	0.5	4	1.5	1	0.5	1	0.5	1	0.5	0	0.0
Surgeon Inv.	2	1.0	0	0.0	2	1.0	0	0.0	0	0.0	0	0.0	0	0.0	0	0.0	0	0.0	0	0.0	0	0.0
Geog. Convenience to Family & Patient	29	14.0	12	6.0	17	8.0	19	9.0	8	4.0	1	0.5	7	3.0	10	5.0	5	2.5	3	1.5	1	0.5
Emergency Factor	5	2.0	3	1.5	2	1.0	6	3.0	0	0.0	0	0.0	0	0.0	2	1.0	5	2.5	0	0.0	0	0.0
TOTAL	210	100.0	73	35.0	137	65.0	129	62.0	70	33.0	11	5.0	66	30.0	71	34.0	56	28.0	10	5.0	7	3.0

*Total sample of consumers is 210 and percentages were figured using total sample number of 210.

TABLE 8

Hospital A's Rating By Respondents as a Health Care Facility*

DEMOGRAPHICS	Excellent Health Care Facility No.	%	Reasonably Good Health Care Facility No.	%	Poor Health Care Facility No.	%	No Opinion No.	%	Total No.	%
Total Sample	140	67.0	30	14.0	6	3.0	34	16.0	210	100.0
Sex Male	44	21.0	12	6.0	2	1.0	15	7.0	73	35.0
Female	98	47.0	15	7.0	4	2.0	20	9.0	137	65.0
Age < 40	83	39.0	15	7.0	5	2.5	26	12.0	129	62.0
40 – 65	50	24.0	12	6.0	0	0.0	8	4.0	70	33.0
65 >	10	5.0	0	0.0	1	0.5	0	0.0	11	5.0
Income < 15,000	39	18.0	9	4.5	4	2.0	14	6.5	66	30.0
$15-$24,999	50	23.5	8	4.0	4	2.0	9	4.5	71	34.0
$25-$39,999	39	18.0	9	4.5	0	0.0	8	4.0	56	28.0
$40,000 >	9	4.5	0	0.0	0	0.0	1	0.5	10	5.0
No Response	2	1.0	3	1.5	0	0.0	2	1.0	7	3.0

*Total sample of consumers is 210 and percentages were figured using total sample number of 210.

TABLE 9
Degree of Respondents' Familiarity with Variety of Health Care Services/Facilities Offered by Hospital A*

DEMOGRAPHICS		Yes		Familiar with Many Facilities		Only Partially Aware Of Facil.		Not Aware Of Facil.		Total	
		No.	%	No.	%	No.	%	No.	%	No.	%
Total Sample		61	29.0	13	6.0	35	17.0	101	48.0	210	100.0
Sex	Male	20	10.0	2	1.0	13	6.0	38	18.0	73	35.0
	Female	41	19.0	10	5.0	22	10.5	64	30.5	137	65.0
Age	< 40	34	16.0	6	3.0	18	9.0	71	34.0	129	62.0
	40 – 65	23	11.0	5	2.5	11	5.0	31	14.5	70	33.0
	65 >	2	1.0	0	0.0	5	2.0	4	2.0	11	5.0
Income	< $15,000	18	8.5	5	2.5	10	4.5	33	14.5	66	30.0
	$15-$24,999	19	9.0	2	1.0	13	6.0	37	17.5	71	34.0
	$25-$39,999	16	8.0	5	2.5	9	4.5	26	13.0	56	28.0
	$40,000 >	5	2.5	0	0.0	1	0.5	4	2.0	10	5.0
	No Response	0	0.0	3	1.25	1	0.5	3	1.25	7	3.0

*Total sample of consumers is 210 and percentages were figured using total sample number of 210.

TABLE 10

Ranking of Three General Hospitals in Newport News—Hampton
SMSA as to Overall Image—"Best Reputation"*

HOSPITALS	TOTAL SAMPLE		SEX				AGE						INCOME									
			Male		Female		< 40		40 – 65		65 >		<$15,000		$15-24,999		$25-39,000		$40,000>		No Opin.	
	No.	%	No.	%	No.	%	No.	%	No.	%	No.	%	No.	%	No.	%	No.	%	No.	%	No.	%
Hospital H	5	2.0	0	0.0	5	2.5	5	2.5	0	0.0	0	0.0	3	1.5	0	0.0	1	0.5	0	0.0	0	0.0
Hospital R	76	36.0	23	11.0	53	25.0	48	23.0	26	12.5	4	2.0	17	8.0	24	11.0	29	14.0	3	1.5	2	1.5
Hospital A	77	37.0	26	12.0	51	24.0	51	25.0	20	10.5	5	2.5	25	11.5	26	12.0	23	11.0	3	1.5	3	1.5
All About the Same	29	14.0	14	7.0	15	7.5	12	5.5	12	5.5	2	1.0	12	6.0	11	5.0	1	0.5	3	1.5	1	0.5
Hospital H & Hospital A above Hospital R	0	0.0	0	0.0	0	0.0	0	0.0	0	0.0	0	0.0	0	0.0	0	0.0	0	0.0	0	0.0	0	0.0
No Opinion	23	11.0	10	5.0	13	6.0	13	6.0	12	5.5	0	0.0	9	4.0	10	5.0	2	1.0	1	0.5	1	0.5
TOTAL	210	100.0	73	35.0	137	65.0	129	62.0	70	33.0	11	5.0	66	31.0	71	33.0	56	27.0	10	5.0	7	4.0

*Total sample of consumers is 210 and percentages were figured using total sample number of 210.

Chapter Twenty

Who Should Receive Health Care?

MARTHA S. ALBERT

The subject of this presentation, "Who Should Receive Health Care?" is customarily dealt with either in terms of philosophy or from an economic framework. Rather than bipolar and fundamentally irreconcilable perspectives, I have chosen to attempt an integrated approach which examines the political milieu in which such decisions are made; politics is the interface between philosophy and economics for the health care industry.

Usual treatments of this subject are very global and general and do not start with an analysis of populations which do or don't receive health care, yet we can deduce a society's economic and philosophic premises from the outcome: Whose health care is funded? It is these latent social realities which must be attended to because extensive changes in provision of services or the structure of the health care system reflect the premises of the majority of citizens in a democratic society.

The author's bias should be displayed for the reader because no treatment of this topic can really be unbiased. My belief is that health care is a right not a privilege and that the individual's primary covenant is with the government in a free society rather than with health practitioners, who must, in the final analysis, be guided in their professional relationships by self-interest, however enlightened that self-interest may be. I think that there must be constraints on what society will provide to individuals of different ages and health conditions and this must be related to the total resources available for health care. In brief, the day of rationing and prioritizing of services has been reached in many countries. In the past, health care needs have been simply met as they have been identified. This is no longer possible, largely due to technological advances. These advances will be limited in their application by the recent international movement to control increases in health care expenditures. For example, Britain's increase in health care expenditures will be under 2 percent in the next fiscal year. In the United States, application of incentives for conservation of health care system usage and behavior modification on a societal scale are being attempted.

My basic contention is that health care policy follows economic and social trends and that economics, philosophy and politics are inextricably linked. To this point, technology, physician preference and patient ability to pay have been forceful determinants of who receives care. As the tolerable level of discomfort for individuals has been reduced, human needs for health care in the affluent nations have escalated beyond institutions' ability to pay.

Health care can be envisioned as a lifeboat and we can ask "Who is in the lifeboat and why?" There are problems in the regulated sector affecting health care availability. Considerations such as efficiency, cost benefits and the effects of available care on the health status of the nation are regularly debated. The potential exists to deny health care overtly. For example, institutions can and do turn away patients by referring them to public facilities if the patients lack a third party payment source and also lack the means to pay their own health care bills. More subtle and covert denial occurs when patients receive "the runaround," going from one facility to another, being turned away repeatedly because their care does not fall within institutional guidelines. Some give up without ever reaching the "right" facility. For others, there is no facility at all. For example, patients with terminal illnesses who do not fit research protocols for experimental treatments may be either expelled from the system entirely or forced to use treatments which have no hope of curing them.

One recent innovation to improve this referral system and to avoid denial of care entirely is called triage. Triage or "sifting and sorting out" may be defined as [Zwick and Bobzien, 1982] "the provision of immediate brief medical evaluation of all incoming patients and the determination of the general nature of the problem, the type of service needed, and the appropriate referral." Nurses or physicians assess multiple available health care resources in relation to the patient's physical condition and resources, and a decision concerning referral is usually made soon after the patient is admitted to the emergency room of the facility. The severity of the patient's problem is evaluated and classified as emergency, urgent or non-urgent, with each designation requiring different disposition. Full and complete records are kept, indicating the seriousness of the triage process as part of an institutional commitment toward quality health care for the public. Triage, in brief, substitutes a series of activities designed to find help for the patient for refusal of care or admission with a write-off of the patient's bill. Triage is especially significant in the United States because hospitals might otherwise simply refuse admission; 25 percent of acute care hospitals have operational deficits and the threat of bankruptcy may force hospitals to refuse care regardless of legality, or the ethics involved, and in the absence of provider participation in the decision-making process [Robbins, 1982].

A recent and especially intriguing effort to "add people to the lifeboat" or increase the quality of their lives has been the creation of incentives to encourage development of new remedies for rare diseases by private pharma-

ceutical companies. This legislative change is a consequence of national attention in the media, and hearings since 1980 before the U.S. House Subcommittee on Health and the Environment, which raised public awareness
of the need to develop orphan drugs. Persuasive individuals testifying included Marjorie Guthrie, the singer's widow, actor Jack Klugman, star of the
television show Quincy (which featured an episode on Tourette's Syndrome),
and researchers, including Dr. Melvin Van Woert of New York's Mount Sinai
Hospital; he investigates myoclonus, a nervous disorder affecting 2,000
Americans. Lack of availability and exhorbitant cost of medication for the
chronically ill with exotic diseases was amply demonstrated by testimony
related to cystic fibrosis (40,000 afflicted), Tourette's Syndrome (10,000
Americans), Prader Willi Syndrome (2,000), Wilson's Disease (1,000) and
Huntington's Chorea (14,000) as well as rare cancers. Drug companies receive a $9 million appropriation for orphan drug development, a seven year
period of exclusive marketing rights for unpatentable orphan products and
in the absence of alternative treatments, orphan drugs are available to patients
by drug firms during the testing period [*Time*, 1982]. This effort does indicate proportionately high spending for a few people, but the encouraging
note is the built-in incentives for drug development.

The issue raised implicitly by both triage and orphan drugs is basic to the
American perspective: "Is health care a right?" The American people have
traditionally believed that health care is a right, although the patchwork of
private and public decisionmaking has not comprehensively operationalized
this belief. If health care is a right, then one can ask "For whom and under
what circumstances?" This question has been consistently answered by the
courts in the United States reflecting the lack of societal consensus, sheer
cost of total provision, and frequent conflict among and between health care
providers, patients and their families and third party payment sources. The
debate concerning the boundaries of life is by no means resolved.

Generous third party payment sources and thriving economies delayed
societal questioning on a large scale concerning the uses of medical discovery.
Insurance coverage has frequently been generous, and consumers have not
consistently scrutinized uses of technology. Statistics indicate that Americans
maintaining health insurance seek health services at double the rate of the unin-
sured, suggesting overutilization. Tax subsidies have been incentives for obtaining coverage. Employer contributions are not part of gross taxable income
for employees. Half of out-of-pocket private health insurance expenses (up to
$150) are deductible from personal income tax. Expenses above 5 percent of
adjusted gross income are also deductible from personal income taxes. Medicare and Medicaid overlap private plans, and the former account for almost
10 percent of all federal expenditures and 2 percent of the gross national
product [Unger, 1982].

Under some circumstances, regardless of coverage, individuals are temporarily welcomed into the lifeboat, usually via diligent triage efforts when national disasters shock people throughout the country. The Hyatt Hotel disaster is one exemplar. In 1981 during a tea dance at this luxury hotel, two giant skywalks collapsed killing 100 people and injuring many more. This was the worst disaster in the history of Kansas City, affecting almost everyone living there. Physicians, nurses, policemen and citizens volunteered to help in arranging care for the victims. Organizations assisted, including the American Red Cross and the Salvation Army. Participants were briefly and totally involved in rescue, and they describe the experience as enormous in its personal impact [Campbell and Pribyl, 1982]. The need for local emergency health disaster plans by American cities was raised immediately afterward [Orr and Robertson, 1982]. Similar responses were elicited by the Martinez bus accident in 1975, when a chartered bus with 51 members of a student choir rolled off a freeway ramp, with 29 passengers dying and 22 casualties [Lewis, et. al., 1980].

It appears that the right to health care has been historically well accepted in the United States. It has been presumed that the federal government would subsidize the elderly and the poor, that national disaster assistance was available for everyone, and that the middle and upper income groups would enroll in private health insurance plans. Yet there has never been an absolute safety net. Who slips through this "safety net?" About five million Americans without health insurance do. So do children whose parents, usually for financial reasons or reason of disability, do not seek health care for them. Sometimes the elderly in nursing homes do not obtain care. A few recent examples of groups slipping through the safety net are instructive because they describe the dislocations in health care coverage which have appeared or increased due to recession, a lesser emphasis on community public health and the inability of current institutional arrangements to fill the needs of a higher proportion of people without employment (and thus without health insurance).

The Miami Herald noted that Dade County, Florida public schools temporarily excluded 10,000 students from the public due to failure to show evidence of measles vaccination. That was one quarter of the students in the public schools. There was an outbreak of measles in the county, stimulating the desire to enforce the regulation. Temporary immunization clinics were opened to deal with the measles emergency [Silva and Macari, 1982]. Parents' lack of initiative was one cause of the absence of immunization. Another was probably poverty, as the Dade County public schools primarily enroll poor Blacks and Spanish-Americans.

A few months later, The New York Times quoted a panel of health experts who warned that cutbacks in the federal government's childhood immunization program could result in new epidemics of polio, measles, rubella and other childhood diseases which have almost been eradicated. Dr. Frederick C. Robbins, president of the Institute of Medicine at the National Academy of Sciences was quoted as stating that [Reinhold, 1982] "Most of the disease agents are still present in the population, just waiting for the number of susceptible children to be large enough that a wave of disease can sweep through them."

The Miami Herald, in the same week described infant mortality statistics in Michigan townships with a high rate of adult unemployment as about equal to the infant mortality rates in poor Central American countries. Detroit, with unemployment at 18.3%, had an infant mortality rate of 21.4 per 1,000 in 1981. City officials claimed that the city had unused maternity facilities for pre-natal care ["Heartland," 1982]. Presumably, the mothers involved did not know about these facilities or did not qualify for their usage.

While state laws define child abuse, parental autonomy is protected, up to a point. In most cases there is sufficient clarity concerning the state's right to intervene; for example if a child is repeatedly battered or if lifesaving care is refused by parents or religious groups. When a child is defective and the parents refuse care, the "best interest" of the child may be abjudicated, especially if a persistent advocate of the particular child requests legal determination. The most recent case to receive national attention was that of Phillip Becker, an institutionalized boy with Down's Syndrome, a form of severe retardation. His "psychological parents," who cared for him in their home, succeeded in obtaining a court order for Phillip to have a cardiac catheterization procedure, which would be in the child's best interest. The natural parents, who had never lived with the child, refused to give their consent [Cushing, 1982].

The Des Moines Register included a recent article which described physicians' unwillingness to visit patients in nursing homes because "it's too much hassle, pays too little and is too depressing." Doctors described nursing home patients as "human rejects" and nursing homes as "human dumps." The economic reasons were primary, according to the study on which the article was based, which was commissioned by the federal Health Care Financing Administration and done by the Center for Health Economies Research in Chestnut Hill, Massachusetts [Ager, 1982].

The Albuquerque Journal described the efforts of the nation's 5,000 family planning clinics to stay in business, some without federal funds from now on. New Title X regulations issued by Reagan's Secretary of Health and Human Services require that clinics with federal funding tell parents within ten days when a minor receives a birth control medication or device. This rule, ostensibly to "promote family communication," will discourage teenagers from using birth control. The rule will affect over half a million patients, divert $2.7 million per year to administrative expenses and the means test will result in withdrawing services from over 71,000 low income women and teenagers ["Family Planning," 1983].

When we discuss slippage in the "safety net," we reach into a more subtle area, that of where health care needs should be identified. There is some slight shift toward the schools. Communities are fragmented by geographically mobile one parent nonnuclear families. The majority of families' health problems are attended to informally, especially because more women are part of the work force. The care of ill children has become a national issue, both in terms of home nursing care and also the escorting of children to sources of medical care. The cost of getting children to health care services they need has thus increased, without formal social mechanisms to deal with an economically induced difficulty. Few health services are directly available in the public school, nursery school or day care center. Low income families presumably use individuals in their informal social networks to "take up the slack" or lose income to escort their children to medical care facilities or do not obtain needed care for their children at all. With over 50 percent of adult American women employed, and many of them heading one parent households, there is a gap between real and apparent availability of health care for children at a reasonable cost, i.e., without loss of wages [Carpenter, 1980].

The model for care in the public health model could be public school nursing programs, if incentives existed for school administrators to deal adequately with children's and adolescents' needs. The case of adolescents who are pregnant indicates clear bureaucratic reluctance to extend care beyond the minimum. Many of these teenagers now keep their children. There is sufficient reason to believe that [Zellman, 1982] "The schools neither seek nor want an active role in dealing with student pregnancy or parenthood. As a result, schools treat the problem passively, foregoing opportunities for early detection, counseling and medical referral. By not acknowledging a pregnancy at an early date, school staff members may succeed in avoiding involvement with a student's decisions to have an abortion, but schools also lose the opportunity to discuss the implications of pregnancy with the student." The quality of such programs is unstable; they are created due to the persistence of some one individual in each situation and administrators usually view the programs as very expensive. This issue of programs for pregnant teenagers which include health care information and referral is important because medical complications and infant mortality rates are quite high for adolescent mothers and their babies.

Loopholes in legislation and insurance coverage also allow people to "slip through the safety net," including the very poor who don't readily fit into established Medicaid categories and those too poor to have private health insurance but just above Medicaid income limits. Disabled persons must wait until two years after an injury or accident causing disability before receiving Medicaid. Middle class individuals can be bankrupted by catastrophic illnesses not adequately covered by their private insurance plans and by limitations on reimbursement for medications and nursing home care [Schramm, 1980]. State-sponsored health plans for the public differ incredibly among the states, often limiting the geographic mobility of wage earners with ill family members whose care is affordable and available in one state but is unavailable or available at insurmountable cost in another state.

The context for the issue of disparity in care among the states is the historical American ambivalence about a central government which could tyrannize the people and curtail their liberty. The result of national pressure on Congress, though, has been a 20 year effort toward "the Great Society" including many more federal benefits, benefits which are being curtailed now due to federal deficits and a shifting political climate. Prior to 1965, states and localities spent more on health care than did the federal government, but by 1978, 68.2 percent of all government spending for health care was federal expenditures [Clarke, 1981]. States are financially pressed and the traditional relationship of states to residents has been irrevocably altered by "the Great Society" era of dependence on the federal government.

Some current cutbacks are not in programmatic areas where the states are likely to pick up expenses, in part because they are extensions of national health care experiments. For example, the federal government is eliminating the $35 million yearly appropriation for fledgling HMO's which offered enrollees full medical coverage for a prepaid fee. While HMO enrollments have soared 60 percent in five years, they require startup assistance, especially so that they can serve the elderly and marginally poor who are not covered by expensive private plans and are not eligible for sufficient public assistance ["Costly Cuts," 1982].

A direct or indirect conclusion can be drawn, and that is that denial of care does occur as a consequence of a changing societal consensus fueled by recession. However, it is not yet apparent how quickly dislocations will be addressed or in what form. The Reagan administration in the United States is now supporting legislation providing health care insurance for the unemployed, suggesting a "floor" for federal coverage of the calamity of unemployment.

Federal discretionary social program funds are being cut, and many programs will be administered through the states, which will receive block grants from the federal government. With deregulation and a more competitive marketplace for health services, the emphasis is likely to be upon provision of cost-effective and profitable services. There will now be federal limitations upon Medicaid expenditures and a 25 percent reduction in funding for the categorical programs which will be replaced by block grants. State and local tax revolts are further lowering the availability of health services. Reduced aid under Title XX of the Social Security Act (a 25 percent cut) affects homemaker, home health and adult day health services. Medicaid regulations in the Omnibus Budget Reconciliation Act of 1981 raise deductibles significantly. Some states have already restricted Medicaid eligibility [Estes, 1981].

Block grants will transfer not only money but power over funds and their usage to the states in areas such as alcohol, drug abuse and mental health, maternal and child health services, primary care, and preventive health. President Reagan stated that "Our task is to restore the constitutional symmetry between the Central Government and the States and to reestablish the freedom and variety of federalism" [Brandt, 1981]. The "variety of federalism" translates, positively, into the ability to respond easily to local problems but negatively into the temptation for financially pressed states to deny local funding, thus reducing the volume of actual health services delivered. Further, "variety in federalism" can mean unequal health service provision between rich and poor states. The needs of small groups of people with unusual diseases may also be all too easily forgotten.

A further problem in state assumption of responsibility for health services is the effect in poorer states on viability of public hospitals. The entire public hospital system in the United States is on the verge of collapse and large urban public hospitals have been described as "dinosaur(s) on the edge of extinction" [Harrigan, 1981]. Without public hospitals, there would not be service to the indigent in many urban centers.

Moral and ethical dilemmas also affect the availability of health care. The abortion debate, a potent national issue, involves the use of federal funds when the request comes from an indigent woman. Administrative guidelines now limit federal government payment stringently. Supreme Court decisions, however, have liberalized women's right to abortion. State and local laws often seek to discourage the procedure, constraining medical autonomy and patients rights [Kapp, 1982]. Providers may also limit availability by refusing to perform the procedure or assist in caring for the patient having an abortion. The issue is one of belief, rights and consensus and is not susceptible to simple resolution [Fromer, 1982].

State authority and responsibility may be insufficient in terms of resources or legal accountability in areas like environmental health where the needs may be enormous and almost impossible to fully identify or fund. Politically, this is an inflammatory subject which has in the past required national popular press dramatization for public health care to be offered. The Love Canal disaster and other environmental health hazards amply demonstrate this point. The environmental health issue in the United States has produced another class of people who do not receive health care or receive limited care. The potential for political and economic upheaval if their illnesses were publicly recognized and acknowledged has constrained provision of services [Brown, 1981]. Environmental health issues affect Americans exposed to Agent Orange in Viet Nam and the victims of many diseases resulting from hazardous work situations. Some groups have sufficiently dramatized their situations so that care has been funded by the federal government and by private corporations, such as asbestos workers and coal miners. Others have not yet been as fortunate.

There is a further class of patients whose needs are expensive but have traditionally been met to some extent by the federal government. Patients receiving organ transplants are part of a surgical renaissance, the crossover of research and health care. They may receive hearts, lungs, kidneys, livers, bone marrow and pancreas. Success rates are higher than ever before, but the availability of donor organs is low and the cost is high. For example, a heart or liver transplant costs $55,000 and a kidney or pancreas transplant costs $25,000 ["A Renaissance," 1982]. The shortage of transplant organs raises ethical problems concerning the choice of recipient. A physician recently stated that "the liver should go to the child whose parents made the effort to get the organ" while a professor of religious studies stated that "The moral decision should hinge on who had been waiting the longest, or even decided by lottery." The AMA recommends that decisions be made strictly on a medical basis rather than "social worth." The case which brought the debate forward was that of Jamie Fiske, whose father, a hospital administrator, launched a remarkably skillful national campaign which located a suitable donor who specified that the liver should go to Jamie, who also fit the AMA guidelines. Scholars are very concerned, however, at the media's role in determining which patients will live or die ["Which Life," 1982]

The American experience with kidney dialysis is the cutting edge of a crucial question: "Should people be denied lifesaving care due *entirely* to its long-term cost to the taxpayer?" Kidney dialysis has been described as "a taxpayer's nightmare," costing about $25,000 annually for each of the 68,000 people with chronic kidney disease. The issue has been complicated by fraud on the part of physicians, hospitals and treatment centers [Robinson, 1982]. In 1980 the program cost 1.4 billion and it is estimated by the Senate Finance Committee that it will cost $2.4 billion by 1984. The program has been described as a medical success and a financial disaster ["The Kidney Experiment," 1982]. The Reagan administration has suggested Medicare cuts in the kidney dialysis program, based on the potential switch from hospital to home dialysis and to curb the high profits derived by private treatment centers [Schorr, 1982].

It should be evident from the material presented thus far that there is a lack of full and current resolution within the United States about health care as a right or a privilege. A patchwork of fragmented public and private programs is the rule rather than the exception. Whether people are "on the lifeboat" is a consequence of a large number of variables, including: (1) Socio-economic status; (2) Personal characteristics, i.e., age, employment, assertiveness and knowledge of how to "work the system;" (3) Health status, i.e., disease type, intensity and popularity; (4) Quality of triage provided by accessible hospitals; (5) Geographic location, which often determines cost and availability of services; (6) Attractiveness to providers, affecting care of the elderly and the disabled; (7) Morality, whether the health condition is regarded as a consequence of defective patient character, as in the case of birth control and abortion; (8) Legality, which is clear in issues such as parental consent for childrens' health care and the use of life support systems; (9) Cost, as in the current debates concerning kidney dialysis and organ transplants; (10) Necessity, especially where the benefits have not yet been fully demonstrated in relation to costs, as in preventive health maintenance; (11) Recognition, as in the case of some environmental pollutants such as Agent Orange; (12) Bureaucratic regulations, including the effect of loopholes and waiting periods; (13) Glamour and dramatization, the extent to which the media can be utilized to build national support for programs, patients seeking lifesaving care or national disaster assistance.

Americans appear to be willing to debate the issue of "Who Should Receive Health Care?" in the media, with occasional physicians' opinions expressed. The debate has generally been undertaken by economists, philosophers, sociologists, and members of special interest groups. What is most noticeable after a review of the literature is the scarcity of health care providers' commentary or serious study of their attitudes and behaviors concerning the selective distribution of health care in practice in this country. One can conclude that there is a profound uneasiness about the issue and that health care professionals can and do hide behind vague codes of ethics which are not explicit enough to encourage challenges of institutional practices facilitating a maldistribution of care. This maldistribution could be interpreted as denial of care.

A second reason for the lack of providers at the center of the debate on who should receive health care is what I call "telescoping." Health care providers have a compressed and narrowed field of vision limited by presenting patients who *do* receive care. Most health care providers do not participate in inpatient admission and rarely are fully aware of a patient's economic constraints. Those issues are dealt with by office staff personnel. Thus it is quite possible for health care providers to be unaware of those individuals who "slip through the safety net as a consequence of institutional guidelines." The "null data" or missing information about denial of care is largely buried and does not affect the daily work lives of providers.

A third reason for the lack of providers in the mainstream of the debate concerning health care criteria and availability is provider socialization. Broad ethical knowledge is included in the educational process without wrestling with the complexities and ambiguities of the law, economics, patient preference or institutional policy. In such a milieu, educational impacts on students' awareness are comfortably removed from decisionmaking or social responsibility. Thus professional education in health care is usually lacking in depth and the issues of practitioner risks and preferences are carefully avoided. Triage represents an effort to extend care to everyone to the satisfaction of providers, but does not address the problems of patients who do not appear at all. Triage fits crises rather than chronic dilemmas.

Any plan for total health care for all Americans is politically vulnerable and, conceptually vulnerable, since there has been no determination of the individuals, groups or institutions fully legitimated for delivery of full spectrum care. One assumption of a Democratic society is that imbalances and inequities will surface and be equitably handled. There is certainly lag time between the appearance of a health problem, creation of a special interest group to dramatize its needs and obtaining sufficient political influence to fund research and treatment.

One wonders about the needs which do exist, are reported on, but may never be dramatized because they would not be exciting to read about, such as the chronic problems which nursing home care has produced in the past few decades. Some issues aren't ever systematically and comprehensively studied because they have no powerful constituency. For example, there are no studies of potential incentives for health care maintenance by the poor (vitamins, exercise plans, dietary change, smoking withdrawal) and health care maintenance is clearly the province of the upper middle class at this time. The debate concerning health care availability has accumulated greater momentum recently. This momentum results from an increase in provider awareness. Providers are now turning away patients with whom they already have professional relationships. Denial is no longer primarily a bureaucratic maneuver without provider complicity. *The New York Times* described this sort of situation, quoting an administrator, a physician and a nurse associated with the Comprehensive Family Care Center in the Bronx (New York). At the end of February 1982 the Center would have to turn away 1,500 of the 2,500 low income elderly and working adults served if they could not afford the higher fees necessitated by the Center's loss of a $350,000 federal grant. Patients would have to use other facilities, primarily the emergency rooms of city hospitals. The Center's director indicated that the clientele might be expanded with an appeal to middle class patients [Rule, 1982].

The effort to change provider perspectives, namely those of physicians concerning their obligations in an ethical context has begun. It exists in the context of a redefinition of provider relations with patients and provider significance *vis-à-vis* the government of a democratic society. Norman Daniel, a social scientist, in a recent article entitled "What is the Obligation of the Medical Profession in the Distribution of Health Care?" asserts as his thesis that [1982, p. 129] "the primary obligations in the distribution of health care are social rather than individual or professional obligations of physicians (and other health care providers)." Professor Daniel states that [1982, p. 130] ". . . we can account for the special importance ascribed to health care needs by noting the connection between meeting those needs and the opportunity range open to individuals in a given society. This suggests that the principles of justice governing the distribution of health care should derive from our general principles of justice guaranteeing fair equality of opportunity . . . we have the foundation for important social obligations in the distribution of health care." Professor Daniel suggests that physicians desiring reimbursement for their services be licensed by the government in a given health care planning region in accord with physician-patient ratios applicable to their specialty areas. Professor Daniel believes that [1982, p. 133] ". . . health care providers acquire obligations in the distribution of health care through specific contractual arrangements when they enter into roles within the social system of health care institutions."

A physician's counter-argument focuses on the freedom and liberty of individuals to contract with other individuals where personal accountability is significant. Dr. Mark Siegler states that [1980, p. 1595] "If a right to health care is granted, irreversible modifications in the original physician-patient relationship may result, such that both physician and patient become responsible to and dependent on societally imposed definitions of health and disease and on a societally imposed notion of what health services are appropriate." Dr. Siegler rejects the notion of a right to health care on these grounds [1980, p. 1596] "(1) The language of rights provides an improverished moral vision of what a properly constituted society ought to provide its citizens in the way of health care. (2) A right to health care is unworkably ambiguous in the absence of a restricted normative definition of health and of health care. (3) Such a right would have a detrimental and destructive effect on the practice of medicine, particularly in limiting the freedom of both patients and physicians and in changing the physician-patient relationship from a covenantal to a contractual one. (4) The right to health care would reduce substantially the liberty and freedom of all citizens, patients and prospective patients alike."

The issue of liberty was considered by Professor Daniel, who indicated that physicians could still choose specialties and work settings and locations, but with awareness of the limitations on income related to those choices since health care is a precondition of "life, liberty and the pursuit of happiness." Certainly the Great Society legislation suggested a consensus (which may be fading) that health care is a basic human right. The more basic issue is one of justice in a society where some children do not receive innoculations and where some areas have third world infant death rates but there is a surging (and well served) demand for face-lifts and similar procedures for self-enhancement.

Under the current system, [Summers, 1981] "the intense provision of health care services (and their high cost) has not resulted in a healthier population." One problem may be the oversupply of surgeons leading to enormous incidences of certain surgical procedures, including the hysterectomy, tonsillectomy, appendectomy, cholecystectomy, cardiac revascularization, gastrectomy and radical mastectomy. One article stated that [Huston, 1983] "at the present rate, more than half of all United States females would have hysterectomies by age 65." Educated patients and second medical opinions may reduce the frequency of these procedures in the future, unless redistribution of services takes care of this problem.

Physicians are asked to make, on behalf of society, decisions concerning life sustaining care, especially with high technology available to maintain bodily functions. The welfare of the patient and the saving of his or her life may be opposing considerations. A new version of the Hippocratic oath is emerging. Life support systems, genetic engineering and access to medical care are being studied by the Institute of Society, Ethics and the Life Sciences, the Kennedy Institute of Ethics at Georgetown University and the President's Commission for the Study of Ethical Problems in Medicine and Biomedical Behavior Research ["Doctors' Dilemma," 1982]. The legal definition of death will have to be redrawn because it is too narrow. Up to 5,000 permanently unconscious patients are kept "alive," including Karen Ann Quinlan, who has been fed but not regained consciousness since 1975 suffering from partial brain death with no possibility of recovery.

Still more difficult issues are those of the crossover between abortion and premature birth and surgical or other lifesaving treatments for infants with Down's Syndrome, especially if the child must live with continual pain and the parents with uncertainty about the child's care after they die or the cost of care while they are alive. Physicians, the government and parents make life and death decisions idiosyncratically. Patients in general are refusing medical care when they are seriously ill, sometimes invoking the courts to counter physician's orders. When the patient is incapable, it is unclear who has authority: physicians, nurses, the family, the government or the courts.

Rationing seems inevitable, but the conflict between traditional notions of the sanctity of life and quality of life are debated. The issue of sheer cost must be approached, even in a wealthy society. Arthur Caplan of the Hastings Center says that ["Doctors' Dilemma," 1982, p. 56] "We are faced with a tough moral question. There will not be enough heart transplants for everyone who needs one. By the year 2050, there will not be enough artificial hearts for everyone who could benefit. What will be the standards for giving out scarce medical technologies—particularly to old people?" Some hospitals are implicitly rationing. For example, Massachusetts General Hospital no longer performs heart transplants because too few people benefit at too high a cost.

Technology increases the ability to prolong lives, while insurance covers the cost of doing so. For hospitals, cost containment may mean lowered quality of care, [Fifer, 1981] unless criterion are generated which prioritize health care expenditures. Some countries have already begun rationing. For example, Britain's National Health Service does not provide hemodialysis for patients over age 65. Sweden denies organ transplants to those over age 65 ["The Staggering Cost," 1981].

In the United States the issue is not simply one of rationing the use of technology, but that of physicians' services to keep costs within a controllable range, compatible with reduced optimism about the American economy. Professor Mechanic recommends prepaid group practices, a form of implicit rationing consistent with both administrative needs and professional autonomy. Clearly some patient demands would remain unmet and services might be denied as unnecessary or as a low priority according to physician-developed institutional norms. This could be a serious problem, especially for minority groups and women who are unlike the majority of their providers with respect to important defining characteristics. According to Professor David Mechanic, a medical sociologist with a world-wide reputation, "It is inevitable that efforts to contain medical care costs will increase. Approaches to cost containment vary substantially and have different effects on access, equity, and professional performance . . . Physicians should contribute to the development of regulatory approaches consistent with the responsible exercise of clinical judgment and professional autonomy" [Mechanic, 1980].

The British system may have greater ease in rationing because it is governmentally operated, while third party payments in the United States are in the hands of private organizations which have not found any incentives to restrict utilization to that which is truly necessary. The tasks of both systems are similar: (1) To establish resource expenditure limits; (2) To determine what care will be provided and to whom under what circumstances; and (3) To establish a means of efficiently using the available resources. The major defect of the health care system in Britain is also the means of rationing. It is called queuing, or people's willingness to wait for health care [Spicer, 1981].

Four interpretations of justice have been proposed by Professor Ruth B. Purtilo, a specialist in health care ethics at Massachusetts General Hospital. Each addresses health policy goals, rights and justifications for availability of health care for everyone. The *utilitarian approach* measures a high level of health in society by low mortality and morbidity and high rates of return on investments in health resources. The *needs-based approach* focuses upon at least a minimal standard of health regardless of the expected return on resource investments in health; priorities are established in different health areas for provision of services above the minimum. The *social contract approach* emphasizes the contractual ways in which the policy is developed rather than its goals. The *skeptical approach* examines what is practically possible without making any moral judgments or hoping for more [Purtilo, 1981].

The philosophy of the Great Society was needs-based while the current social environment appears to be a mixture of utilitarian and social contract approaches without an emphasis on health care availability for everyone. It is time for large-scale interdisciplinary research to predict alternative future scenarios for American health care, with an honest assessment of the trade-offs involved in each—economic, political, sociological and medical. I would agree with Dr. Andrew W. Nichols, an Associate Professor of Family and Community Medicine at the University of Arizona that [1981, p. 38] ". . . government has the responsibility for guaranteeing access to a level of health care which is compatible with a basic quality of life. Increased access can best be achieved through implementation of a "fairness" doctrine in the distribution of limited or scarce resources. Given the many opportunities for action currently available, it is quite likely that a multiple program approach will emerge containing everything from catastrophic health insurance for all citizens of the state to some form of prepaid health care for the medically indigent as well as the non-indigent. Such a complex package is always the result of compromise and this requires the participation of all concerned parties in its development.

Cost-benefit analysis is most popular today as an interpretation of utilitarianism during this country's "Age of Social Timidity" [Jain, 1981]. In cost-benefit analysis, according to Dr. Benjamin A. Barnes, an Associate Professor at Harvard Medical School [1982, p. 745] "aggregated data provide a basis for decisions that will maximize the benefits to society in the sense of the greatest good for the greatest number or a maximum-net-benefits approach. Other goals have been advocated by ethicists, including special provision for the most disadvantaged in society or a distribution of goods and services that minimize the variance and maximizes equality regardless of what happens to the average welfare. Others expound on the absurdity of presuming to determine the value of a life. Cost-benefit analysis/cost-effective analysis operationally says if a policy change increases net health benefits in the aggregate, do not worry about the distribution."

Cost-benefit analysis may not work well as a means of affecting the health status of the very poor, because they are sick about twice as frequently as the general population and have a much greater incidence of chronic illness, such as heart disease, arthritis and hypertension. This may explain in part the statistics indicating that the gap in health between the rich and poor hasn't been bridged over the past 15 years. Some researchers believe that the gap can be closed only with (1) More emphasis on the social and psychological components of health care in social programs; (2) Improvements in the treatment of chronic illness through social programs; (3) A federal payment system which facilitates coordination among the various programs for the impoverished chronically ill. "The problem is not one of fine-tuning but rather of having the band play a different tune altogether" ["Income, Illness," 1981].

In a modern industrial nation the question "Who Should Receive Health Care?" is answered by the government, presumably acting upon the wishes of the majority of its citizens. Ultimately, obtaining greater equity is a consequence not only of correct timing, but of the proposal of programs that can be controlled in terms of cost and where outcomes have a high degree of predictability. A whole variety of changes in the American health care system would have to occur to satisfy the predictability criteria, including a separation between medical needs and medical wants, development of mechanisms for physicians to share in the costs they generate, a redefinition of public and private hospitals and their responsibilities and use of business methods to determine real costs of medical procedures and technologies individually.

Why is there such a patchwork in American health care? This is the result of tradition, market forces, shifting political alliances in a heterogeneous country, and the fact that most people are satisfied. Healthier people are also more influential in the political process. What would it take to radically change the American health care system? Aside from timing and changes in the factors described above, a media campaign would have to be successfully launched by a charismatic leader forming a whole new coalition. Unfortunately, the prospects for this in the near future are unlikely. What can we expect? Pessimistically, piecemeal rationing and increased inequity without a net increase in "people in the lifeboat." In fact, with block grants to states we can expect even greater divergence in capabilities for health care among the states and further fragmentation of health care system benefits.

The most frustrating questions are probably these: (1) When should health care be terminated? (2) How can health care dollars be increased for some purposes and decreased for others? and (3) How should providers' roles in generating health care costs be managed, especially when providers oppose patients and their families?

Concerning the first issue, medical care should surely be terminated when there is no possibility of the patient ever recovering, i.e., regaining consciousness. The Karen Ann Quinlan case remains as a reminder that terminating care would mean, in some instances, withdrawing intravenous feeding. Ms. Quinlan may have been a symbol of hope in the early stages of the medical technological revolution as well as a reminder of the lack of a fully adequate definition of death. Where the patient has signed a right to die instrument, surely this should be respected by the courts. When there has been repeated failure of treatments, these should be discontinued, whether organ transplants or alcohol detoxification. Certain procedures might be limited to individuals in an age range which suggests that their entire physical systems are not in a stage of breakdown, as in the British system, where organ transplants are not financed for individuals over 65 years old.

How can health care dollars be increased for a more ethical distribution of care? The Internal Revenue Service could be utilized. Sizable charitable deductions could be legislated for donations to national disasters. A limited and specific list could be generated annually by Congress and a general health fund could be available for contributions by taxpayers. This would help the country in dealing with specific environmental disasters (such as the Love Canal) as well as infant mortality in economically hard pressed states. Corporate as well as private sources could receive tax credits on some sliding scale based on federal revenue requirements as well as urgency of national need.

How can practitioner role in generation of health care costs be handled? Physicians and other providers could be required to participate in payments for costs they generate which fall outside the norms for the classifications of type of patients served. Using a system similar to DRG's, physicians and other providers could be taxed or receive tax credits based upon their economic performance. One consequence would be provider awareness of costs generated, something that is currently absent from the health care economic matrix.

Clarification of the legal responsibilities of health care providers, patients, families and the courts concerning cessation of care would greatly affect costs. An inability of physicians to agree to cessation of care has been linked to traditional medical ethics, and this could be dealt with through changes in physician's education as well as in the legal system governing physicians' freedom to make treatment choices in the absence of rewards or penalties.

The basic question is primarily: "How do we integrate ethical dilemmas into the health care mainstream?" and secondarily: "How do we change the behavior of the American citizen to enlarge the value of money spent on health care to provide essential care to as many people as possible?"

These questions are likely to be answered in the context of increased corporate dominance of the health care system. Many projections support the belief that 90 percent of hospital beds will be owned or controlled by private enterprise in less than a decade. Unless the public and the government develop ethical standards and practical guidelines rapidly, decisions concerning refusal or cessation of care or termination of life may be made strictly on financial bases. In the United States, the report of the President's Commission for the Study of Ethical Problems in Medicine and Biomedical and Behavioral Research has been encouraging. In general, the Commission favors allowing informed, competent patients to make their own decisions. When the patient is not competent to do so, the Commission believes such decisions should be made by a surrogate, usually a family member. Weaning some patients from physician dominance may be painful while it will be rewarding for others.

Regardless of the locus of decisionmaking—physician, patient or family, the American dream of equality must be satisfied. The ethical context for choosing who should receive health care must pass the scrutiny of the people in a democracy. If it appears to be arbitrary or based on social, economic or ethnic group preferences, then the very basis of democracy will be challenged. The societal bonds, already weakened by recession, lack of cohesive values or life style consensus, and by ethnic discord, could be further weakened. With a larger proportion of the elderly and technological advances in health care, resolution of ethnical dilemmas affecting health care decisionmaking is both more difficult and more crucial.

REFERENCES

Susan Ager, "Sixty Percent of Doctors Avoid Nursing Homes," *Des Moines Register,* December 5, 1982, p. 8E.

Benjamin A. Barnes, "Cost-Benefit and Cost-Effective Analysis in Surgery," *Surgical Clinics of North America,* Vol. 62, No. 4, August 1982, p. 745.

Edward N. Brandt, Jr., "Block Grants and the Resurgence of Federalism," *Public Health Reports,* Vol. 96, No. 6, November/December 1981, pp. 495-97.

Michael Brown, *Laying Waste,* New York: Washington Square Press, 1981.

Patricia M. Campbell and Catherine A. Pribyl, "The Hyatt Disaster Two Nurses' Perspectives," *Journal of Emergency Nursing,* Vol. 8, No. 1, January/February 1982, pp. 12-6.

Eugenia S. Carpenter, "Children's Health Care the Changing Role of Women," *Medical Care,* Vol. XVIII, No. 12, December 1980, pp. 1208-218.

Gary J. Clarke, "The Role of the States in the Delivery of Health Services," *American Journal of Public Health,* Vol. 71, Supplement, January 1981, pp. 59-69.

"Costly Cuts for Health Care," *The New York Times,* May 29, 1982, p. 22.

Maureen Cushing, "Whose Best Interest? Parents Vs. Child Rights," *American Journal of Nursing,* February 1982, pp. 313-14.

Norman Daniel, "What is the Obligation of the Medical Profession in the Distribution of Health Care?" *Social Science and Medicine,* Vol. 15F, 129, 1982.

"Doctor's Dilemma: Treat or Let Die?" *U.S. News and World Report,* December 6, 1982, pp. 53-56.

Carroll L. Estes, "Policy Shifts and Their Impact on Health Care For Elderly Persons," *The Western Journal of Medicine,* Vol. 135, No. 6, December 1981, pp. 511-18.

"Family Planning Clinics Will Fight Federal 'Squeal' Rule," *Albuquerque Tribune,* Wednesday, January 26, 1983, p. 1.

William R. Fifer, "Cost/Quality Tradeoffs Will be the Next Medical Care 'Crisis,'" *Hospitals,* June 1, 1981, pp. 56-9.

Margot Joan Fromer, "Abortion Ethics," *Nursing Outlook,* April 1982, pp. 234-40.

Susan Harrigan, "Grady Hospital, Haven for the Poor in Atlanta, Calls Itself Critically Ill," *The New York Times,* March 2, 1981, pp. 1, 17.

"Heartland Has Death Role Like That of Third World," *The Miami Herald,* Thursday, November 25, 1982, pp. 16D-17D.

Phillips Huston, "Seven Common Operations We May No Longer Need," *NEXT Magazine,* Regency Hotels, January 1983, p. 40.

"Income, Illness and the Health Gap," *Science News,* January 24, 1981, p. 59.

Sagar C. Jain, "Introduction and Summary" National Symposium, January 1980, 608, sponsored by the American Public Health Association, the North Carolina Department of Human Resources and the Robert Wood Johnson Foundation, *American Journal of Public Health (AJPH),* Vol. 71, Supplement, January 1981, pp. 5-8.

Marshall B. Kapp, "Abortion and Informed Consent Requirements," *American Journal of Obstetrics and Gynecology,* Vol. 144, No. 1, September 1, 1982, pp. 1-4.

"The Kidney Experiment," *The New Republic,* August 30, 1982, pp. 12, 14.

Frank R. Lewis, Donald D. Trunkey and Muriel R. Steele, "Autopsy of a Disaster: The Martinez Bus Accident," *The Journal of Trauma,* Vol. 20, No. 10, October 1980, pp. 861-66.

David Mechanic, "Rationing of Medical Care and the Preservation of Clinical Judgment," *The Journal of Family Practice,* Vol. 11, No. 3, 1980, p. 431.

Andrew W. Nichols, "Beyond Medicaid," *Arizona Medicine,* Vol. 38, No. 1, January 1981, p. 38.

Steven M. Orr and William A. Robertson, "The Hyatt Disaster: Two Physicians' Perspectives," *Journal of Emergency Nursing,* Vol. 8, No. 1, January/February 1982, pp. 6-11.

Ruth B. Purtilo, "Justice in the Distribution of Health Care Resources: The Position of Physical Therapists, Psychiatrists and Rehabilitation Nurses," *Physical Therapy,* Vol. 61, 1981, pp. 1594-1600.

Robert Reinhold, "Experts Warn Cutbacks May Revive Serious Childhood Epidemics," *The New York Times,* February 5, 1982, p. 19A.

"A Renaissance in Transplant Surgery," *U.S. News and World Report,* October 4, 1982, pp- 68-9.

Dennis Robbins, "Reduced Federal Monies: Conflicts in Ethics and Policy," *Journal of Emergency Nursing,* Vol. 8, No. 4, July/August 1982, p. 208.

Donald Robinson, "Kidney Dialysis: A Taxpayer's Nightmare," *Readers Digest,* October 1982, pp. 149-52.

Sheila Rule, "Aid Loss to Force Clinic to Turn Away Some Poor," *The New York Times,* February 14, 1982, p. 41.

Burt Schorr, "U.S. Plan to Cut Payments by Medicare for Kidney Dialysis Nears a Showdown," *The Wall Street Journal,* October 18, 1982, p. 5.

Patricia C. Schramm, "Cooperating in the Health Care System," *Delaware Medical Journal,* Vol. 52, No. 10, October 1980, pp. 539-41.

Mark Siegler, "A Physician's Perspective on a Right to Health Care," *Journal of the American Medical Association (JAMA),* Vol. 244, No. 14, October 3, 1980, p. 1595.

Mark Silva and Ann Macari, "Dade Schools Bar 10,000 Pupiles Over Measles Shots," *Miami Herald,* Tuesday, November 23, 1982, pp. 14A-15A.

Michael W. Spicer, "British and American Health Care Systems: A Comparative Economic Perspective," *British Medical Journal,* Vol. 282, April 18, 1981, pp. 1334-36.

James W. Summers, "Money, Health, and the Health Care Industry," *Hospital and Health Services Administration,* Winter 1981, p. 23.

"The Staggering Cost of Prolonging Life," *Business Week,* February 23, 1981, pp. 19-20.

Walter J. Unger, "Challenges in the New Era of Competition," *Southern Hospitals,* January-February 1982, pp. 14-24.

"Which Life Should Be Saved?" *Time,* November 22, 1982, pp. 100-01.

Gail L. Zellman, "Public School Programs for Adolescent Pregnancy and Parenthood: An Assessment," *Family Planning Perspectives,* Vol. 14, No. 1, January/February 1982, p. 20.

Dianne L. Zwicke and William F. Bobzien, "Triage Nurse Decisions: A Prospective Study," *Journal of Emergency Nursing,* Vol. 8, No. 3, May/June 1982, pp. 132-38.

Contributors

Contributors

John M. Virgo, editor of this book, is a specialist in manpower, labor, and economic theory, as well as personnel, business law, and social responsibility. He is author of five books and over 30 articles and has served as consultant to the U.S. Department of Labor, State of California, State of Virginia, and numerous regional private and public groups. Dr. Virgo founded the Atlantic Economic Society and the *Atlantic Economic Journal* in 1973, where he serves as Executive Vice-President and Managing Editor, respectively. In addition, he recently founded the International Health Economics and Management Institute. He currently teaches at Southern Illinois University at Edwardsville.

Martha S. Albert is a health systems consultant specializing in strategic management of health care, business and educational structure. Dr. Albert is an adjunct Associate Professor at the Robert O. Anderson Schools of Management at the University of New Mexico and the author of numerous published articles and chapters of books in the health field.

Claude E. Ameline graduated from Ecole Nationale d'Administration in 1972. He was responsible for Child Welfare Services at the Department of Social Affairs and National Solidarity in Paris. From 1977 to 1980, he worked at the French Embassy in London as Counsellor for Social Affairs. In 1980-1982, he was in charge of personnel recruitment and training at the DSANS. He is now Under Secretary for Health Services Planning, French Ministry of Health.

John E. Baird, Jr. is Managing Partner of Baird, DeGroot and Associates, an employee relations and organizational development consulting firm located in Mountain View, California. Dr. Baird also is active in the publishing field, having written and published seven books and over 30 articles dealing with effective communications and management in organizations. He also serves as advisory editor for several major publishing houses.

Carolyne K. Davis is the Administrator of the Health Care Financing Administration (HCFA), Department of Health and Human Services. Dr. Davis oversees the functions of the Medicare and Medicaid programs, which help to finance health care services for nearly 50 million poor, elderly and disabled Americans.

Alfonso D. Esposito is Director of the Division of Hospital Experimentation, Office of Research and Demonstrations, Health Care Financing Administration (HCFA). Mr. Esposito directs HCFA's demonstration programs to test alternative hospital payment methods for the Medicare and Medicaid programs.

Robert B. Fetter is a professor of management at Yale University, School of Organization and Management. His current research and consulting activities include development of DRG's; management information and control systems in the HMO environment; applications of computer simulation for the analysis of operating problems of management; and development of database structures and computer languages for decision support systems. He is the author of *The Quality Control System,* which has been translated into Japanese, Italian, Spanish, and Yugoslavian.

Frederick S. Fink is Vice President of Booz, Allen & Hamilton and Managing Officer of the Health and Medical Division. In this capacity he is responsible for all of the firm's activities in the Health Care Industry. His studies have included strategic planning, marketing strategy, health manpower planning, corporate reorganization, health program planning, and financial consulting assignments.

Trevor A. Fisk is Executive Vice President/Marketing & Planning for Cooper Hospital/University Medical Center. His responsibilities include market research to establish future viability of existing and proposed programs, direction of strategic planning, design and management of promotional activities, governmental relations, and public relations. His previous positions include marketing in industry and education and being a Sloan Fellow in Management, M.I.T.

Dorothy H. Fox is currently a Nursing Management Consultant. Her previous positions include Vice President for Nursing, St. John's Mercy Medical Center; Director of Nursing, Bethesda General Hospital; and Director of Special Admissions Program, St. Louis University School of Nursing. She has published in major nursing and health care journals and has presented numerous papers at professional conferences on the subject of nursing management.

Richard T. Fox, a health care economist, is now Director of Planning–Service Programs, Peoples Community Hospital Authority, Wayne, Michigan. Formerly he was Professor of Hospital and Health Care Administration, St. Louis University; and Research Consultant to the Catholic Health Association, Inc. He is Economic Editor of *Hospital Progress.*

Jean L. Freeman is an assistant in research at Yale University. Her research activities include development of DRG's; analysis of hospital utilization patterns; development of statistical methods for multivariate analysis; and product definition in ambulatory care.

Kevin G. Halpern is President and Chief Executive Officer of Cooper Hospital/ University Medical Center. He has full responsibility and accountability for operations of a 530 bed tertiary/university medical center. He is also an Adjunct Assistant Professor of the University of Medicine and Dentistry of New Jersey–Rutgers Medical School at Camden.

Gloria S. Hope, until 1982, was Deputy Director, VA Nursing Service where she helped in setting national policies, programs, standards, and legislation affecting nursing services in 172 VA medical centers. Before becoming Deputy Director, Dr. Hope served as Chief, Education and Training Division, VA Central Nursing Service. She has been recognized in *Outstanding American and Community Leaders, Who's Who in Government,* and is in demand around the world as a speaker and leading authority on nursing.

Algin B. King is the Dean of the School of Business and Economics, Christopher Newport College. He is also President, Algin B. King & Associates, Ltd, Management Consultants-Market/Economic Analysts; former partner and manager, Fine Virginia Foods, Williamsburg, Virginia; and Chief, Economic Analysis Branch, District Office, Office of Price Stabilization, Columbia, South Carolina. Dr. King has published 13 books and monographs and over 40 articles dealing with health care, marketing, and economics.

Robert J. Maxwell is Secretary for King Edward's Hospital Fund for London. He has written extensively on health policy and management, particularly on international comparisons, health service expenditures, and value for money. He is a Justice of the Peace for Inner London, currently chairing the Juvenile Court in Tower Hamlets; a member of the Council of the Royal Institute of Public Administration; and a Governor of the National Institute for Social Work.

Richard C. McKibbin is the Director of Policy Analysis for the American Nurses' Association where he is responsible for economic and manpower policy analysis, projects, reports, and programs, analysis of federal legislation and policies which affect health care and nursing, and economic consultation services to association executives, staff and officials. He has published and appeared extensively on programs dealing with the economics of health, and is on the editorial board of a major health journal. He has been listed in *Who's Who in Health Care, Who's Who in Wichita,* and *American Men and Women of Science.*

Gilberto Muraro is currently Professor of Public Finance and Director of the Institute of Public Finance, University of Venice. He has written many contributions in the field of public economics, with special reference to taxation, collective choice, environmental and urban economics, and health economics. He also serves as a member of the ministerial commission for the reform of local finance and as a member of the editorial board of *Resources Policy* and *Ricerche Economiche.*

Harry M. Neer has a total of 19 years experience in hospital administration and consulting. He is currently the Chief Executive Officer, President, and member of the Board of Trustees of Presbyterian Hospital, Inc. His former positions include: Hospital and Medical Consultant with Booz, Allen and Hamilton; Assistant Director of Institutional Services at Mt. Sinai Hospital of Cleveland; and neurobiologist at Barrows Neurological Institute in Phoenix, Arizona.

324

Arthur M. Randall is currently the Director of National Sales of the Health Services Division of McDonnell Douglas Automation Company. He has previously held positions as Marketing Manager of IBM, Branch Manager, Service Bureau Corporation, Vice President of Marketing for Kidde Computer Services, and General Manager, System Development Corporation in New Jersey. Mr. Randall is also the contributing editor and columnist for major national publications in the computer and health care fields such as *Computers In Health Care* and *National Report Computers and Health.*

James Sobel is Associate Professor of Clinical Family Medicine, Rutgers Medical School, and Chief/Department of Family Medicine, Cooper Hospital/ University Medical Center. He had formerly been Assistant Professor and Associate Director for the Division of Family Medicine, Hahnemann Medical College & Hospital, Philadelphia.

Lyndsey Stone is Vice President of Operations and Nursing Administration at Presbyterian Hospital and adjunct Professor of Nursing at the University of Oklahoma College of Nursing. He has a total of 40 years experience working in clinical nursing and nursing administration, including 22 years of duty with the U.S. Army Nurse Corp attaining the rank of colonel. His former positions include Chief, Department of Nursing, Hawlew Army Hospital, Indianapolis; Assistant Chief Nurse, U.S. Army Hospital, Fort Carson, Colorado Springs; Chief Nurse, 24th Evacuation Hospital, Republic of Viet Nam; and Chief Nurse, 7th Army and 7th Medical Brigade, Europe.

Charles T. Wood is currently the General Director for the Massachusetts Eye and Ear Infirmary where he has been since 1963. Previously he was with the Roanoke Memorial Hospital in Virginia, Jefferson Hospital in Virginia, and was a Chemical Engineer at Virginia Electric & Power Company. He serves on the board of directors of several health care groups and is the immediate past chairman of the American College of Hospital Administrators.